ELECTROMAGNETIC MAN

This book is dedicated to all those pioneers in bioelectromagnetics, past, present and future, and especially to Professor Herbert Fröhlich, FRS, as well as to our respective wives, Eileen and Penny, without whose patience and support it would never have been completed.

ELECTROMAGNETIC MAN

Health and Hazard in the Electrical Environment

Cyril W. Smith and Simon Best

J. M. Dent & Sons Ltd.
London

First published in Great Britain 1989

© Cyril W. Smith and Simon Best
© Hilary Bacon, chapter 8, first section

All rights reserved. No part of this publication may be reproduced, stored in a retrieval system, or transmitted, in any form or by any means, electronic, mechanical, photocopying, recording or otherwise, without the prior permission of J. M. Dent and Sons Ltd

Printed in Great Britain at The Bath Press, Avon
for J. M. Dent and Sons Ltd,
91 Clapham High Street, London SW4 7TA

British Library Cataloguing in Publication Data
Smith, Cyril W.
 Electromagnetic man
 1. Man. Health. Effects of radiation
 I. Title   II. Best, Simon
 613

ISBN 0–460–04698–5

Contents

	Foreword	vii
	Introduction	1
1	History of a phenomenon	8
2	Basic concepts: scientific fundamentals	18
3	The cosmic connection	35
4	Human biology and electromagnetic fields	53
5	Electromagnetic fields in medicine	67
6	Electrical sensitivity and allergy	85
7	Alternative medicine – the potential breakthrough	104
8	Electromagnetic environmental pollution	126
9	Chronic electromagnetic field exposure, health risks and safety regulations	165
10	Beware: military at work	209
11	Old wisdom, new understanding	238
12	The last frontiers	258
	Conclusion	270
	Postscript	279
	Glossary	290
	References	298
	Name index	331
	Subject index	339

Foreword

by Professor Herbert Fröhlich, FRS

The sensitivity of biosystems to electromagnetic fields has been known for a long time. Only recently, however, has it been shown that the laws of physics permit extraordinarily high sensitivities when biosystems are activated through energy supply. Unlike machines and instruments, however, the non-activated state does not exhibit a particular construction. It is the supply of random energy (food) above a critical magnitude, rather, which causes a highly organised mode of behaviour, usually in the form of coherent electric oscillations. The transformation into this activated state has features of a phase transition in that it is very sharp in terms of the magnitude of the supplied energy − in contrast to the case of ordinary systems where energy supply leads to heating.

In principle, such sharp transitions can, of course, lead to great sensitivity to outside stimuli.

The structure of biosystems is, of course, very complex so that treatment of a specific case requires far-reaching investigation. The recent developments, mentioned above, do, however, indicate the possibility of sensitivities which, before the discovery of coherent states, seemed impossible.

Such sensitivities do, of course, give rise to difficulties in the reproduction of experiments and, in fact, a new subject, 'Deterministic Chaos', has arisen to deal with this.

The present book does provide examples which in earlier years might have been rejected as unphysical but which now give rise to the hope of an understanding in terms of the recent developments which show through examples how some systems starting from minutely different situations can develop in vastly different ways.

Introduction

> Negative Capability, that is, when a man is capable of being in uncertainties, mysteries, doubts, without any irritable reaching after fact and reason.
>
> John Keats (1795–1821), Letter to G. and T. Keats, 21 December 1817

The ability to tolerate uncertainty is a characteristic of being adult; this book – for adults of all ages! – was conceived in the mind of the editor, Malcolm Gerratt, through reading an account of a demonstration of electromagnetic hypersensitivity that was laid on for the Press by Dr Jean Monro and myself on a fine August Bank Holiday in 1984. The account was written by my co-author, Simon Best, in the *Guardian* (24 October 1984) and a copy is included in the BBC's mammoth video disc *Domesday Project*, produced in 1986, the 900th anniversary of the original, to portray all aspects of life in Britain in the 1980s. When Malcolm Gerratt telephoned me to ask whether I would write a book for him, I said that he would get a book rather than a thesis if he could persuade Simon Best to write it with me. Even then, with the amount of material for, and against, the existence of electromagnetic phenomena in man, it was a daunting prospect and has taken years longer than expected. That this book is at last published is testimony to Malcolm Gerratt's patience with us.

This is not the beginning of my involvement with electromagnetic phenomena in living systems. I had already done my doctorate at Imperial College, London, on the application of television to the viewing of clinical X-ray images. At Salford University in the 1970s, I was concerned with initiating and running a course, the first in the UK, on Biomedical Electronics. This was chopped, like most interdisciplinary activities in our universities, following the government resource cuts of 1981. This was a *déja vu* experience for me; I am old enough to have witnessed various governments' inability to lead this country's radar research from a wartime success story to peacetime success in harnessing the same scientific energies to post-war economic recovery. When one looks back at the Old Country from the New World, one realises that attitudes have not really altered since the Pilgrim Fathers set sail. But, as I write this in 1988, I am delighted to place on record that the Vice-Chancellor has instructed me to re-establish Biomedical Electronics at Salford University. It is through understanding how living systems use electronics and quantum fields at the molecular level that the jump from micrometre to nanometre scale electronic devices will be made, and with it will come a revolution as great as that engendered by the silicon chip; this is what 'Molecular Electronics' is all about.

It was in 1938 that Professor Herbert Fröhlich first realised that biological membranes were extremely good electrical insulators and, in co-operation with Lord Rothschild, began to consider the theoretical implications of this in biology. But then came the war and it was not until 1965, when he was invited to give the introductory lecture at a meeting on Theoretical Physics and Biology at the Institut de la Vie, in Paris, that he returned to the topic. He had then moved from Bristol University to Liverpool University and it was in 1973 that he began to come to Salford University through the encouragement of its Head of Electrical Engineering, Professor J. H. Calderwood. I was then working on electrical insulating materials and gladly added biological materials to my list of interesting substances to measure.

We published several papers on these measurements, but they only showed what was already known, namely that 'wet' biological materials show a lot of electric charge effects. A breakthrough came when we found that the measurements were affected by magnetic fields in an unexpected way. The results were sufficiently like room-temperature superconductivity that we interpreted them according to this model. Professor Fröhlich had of course already, in 1950, made a fundamental contribution to the theory of superconductivity. Such advances in science (Hyland, 1987) are only possible with a broad outlook and a constant awareness of the possible relevance of concepts and techniques to branches of physics in which they did not first arise. This success stands as a '...strong indictment against fragmentation and overspecialization in theoretical physics' (Fröhlich, 1950) – a situation so common today in organised science, which is largely the self-fulfillment of prophecies made in funding applications and only gratifies the administrators.

We did not clear up all the difficulties with these electrical and magnetic measurements for many years. They eventually proved to be due to contamination with living organisms. What was an interesting dielectric material was also dinner to any stray organism that chose to come into the laboratory, and we had to combine our facilities for electric, magnetic and electromagnetic measurements with the sterile conditions of a biological laboratory.

The medical and social implications of this work also began to appear. Since the end of the Second World War, people had been concerned that there might be harmful effects due to the electromagnetic fields which had suddenly become so widespread throughout the environment. In North America, it took 20 years of pressure against those vested interests, who wanted to retain unrestricted use of any part of the electromagnetic spectrum, to get the New York State Power Lines Project set up. In 1973, the New York State Power Authority announced plans to build a 765 kV transmission line from Canada. Environmental groups cited studies that pointed to health risks; the state's Public Service Commission approved the line but acknowledged that the record of the hearing contained 'unrefuted inference of possible risks that we cannot possibly ignore' and ordered the utilities to fund a $5 million research programme on the health effects of electromagnetic fields. In 1981, the New York State Department of Health began soliciting research proposals. In all, it funded 16 projects and reported in July 1987, to considerable world-wide press coverage, that overall the studies indicated a 'variety of effects' not 'previously appreciated' and that, 'Several areas of potential concern for public health have been identified.'

I did try to get a project of my own funded, but without success. Not wishing to leave a good idea lying about after its disclosure, I published it (Aarholt and Smith, 1982). What I said was that currents induced in a person near a power line can be greater than those known to stimulate pain-relieving natural opiates, therefore one must not be surprised to see withdrawal symptoms among persons chronically so exposed. Dr Jean Monro, a nutritionist and clinical allergist in London, read this and wrote to me saying that she had many such electrically sensitive patients and could I help? Since then, I have been privileged to be the fly on the wall of her clinic and have seen what I would describe in scientific terms as sensitivities at the theoretical limits of physics, and, in engineering terms, as the failure of human regulatory or control systems.

Cyril Smith

My interest in bioelectromagnetics has a more modest beginning than Cyril Smith's although no less significant for me. After declining a clinical psychology course place at the University of Surrey in 1979, I entered medical journalism. Among my first assignments was a feature on the claims of illness caused by overhead powerlines by the inhabitants of the hamlet of Fishpond in Dorset, led by Hilary Bacon, whose account of her struggles appears in Chapter 8. Impressed by the evidence she had gathered both locally and from the literature, I realised that the 'story' was much bigger than it appeared.

Pursuing it led to contact with other researchers such as, in Britain, Dr Stephen Perry, Dr Leslie Hawkins, Dr David Melville and Dr David Dowson, in the Republic of Ireland, Mr John Royds, and in the USA, Dr Robert Becker, Dr Andrew Marino, Dr Milton Zaret and Dr Louis Slesin, all of whose assistance I gratefully acknowledge. I met Cyril Smith in 1981 while writing other articles and, through him, became acquainted with the work of Dr Jean Monro and the Environmental Medicine Foundation. This, in turn, led to the *Guardian* article mentioned above and, in due course, to helping to research a *Panorama* programme on powerlines and cancer in 1988.

The four years of writing and researching *Electromagnetic Man* have involved help from many unnamed people, all of whom I thank. It has also stimulated many exciting mental and intellectual journeys, some of which are unfinished but for most of which I owe a considerable debt to my co-author.

Simon Best

This is the starting point in real time for this book, but the signpost also has an arm pointing back to the earliest recorded history of man's realisation that he was able to perceive these extremes of electromagnetic sensitivity even if he could not understand them.

We acknowledge the pioneering work of octogenarian Professor Herbert Fröhlich in this field, thank him for many years of co-operation and guidance to the senior author and for writing our Foreword.

The history of the phenomenon of man's electromagnetic sensitivity is traced from the folklore of antiquity to the dawning of experimental science. Once convictions and opinions became established, controversies arose; these were a reflection of the contemporary society, its philosophies and religions. This happened in Europe over many centuries and is now happening in other parts of the world.

The whole terminology of this area is coloured by the name of Antoine Mesmer – Mesmerism. His great error was to be successful in making money; if he had not, his work would have been ignored as irrelevant.

We have tried to emphasise how the spirit of the times – the 'zeitgeist' – is reflected in contemporary sciences. Today we are preoccupied with 'zapping' the enemy en masse, whether real or imagined: bacteria with bacteriocides, weeds with herbicides, pests with pesticides, humanity with genocides. We shall stop and pose the question, has man also shot himself in his own foot with his electrical thunderbolts? The father of electrical engineering, Nikola Tesla, became what was probably the first well documented but non-diagnosed case of electromagnetic hypersensitivity.

Some basic science that will assist the reader to follow our arguments is presented, non-mathematically, in Chapter 2. The fundamental concept for understanding how living systems use electromagnetic fields for communication and control is that of coherence, or precision, in time and in space. The human body is restricted in time to the present and, in space to the immediate few metres of its environ. The mind of man can contemplate the whole world and beyond; the present day, and past ages through the records that our forebears have passed down to us.

To function in real time, the body and its cells must be able to use communication frequencies at least up to those of light. Beyond light, we soon enter the spectral region of ionising radiation where the very success in making measurements causes difficulties in regulating the use of ionising radiation for peaceful purposes. The disintegration of a single atomic nucleus can be detected; yet even millions of atoms of other environmental pollutants cannot be detected or controlled, although both can produce free radicals which may be hazardous (see Glossary).

Man's coherence in time extends only to his three score years and ten. We have used the products of the minds of men from all ages, cogent and coherent even today as we write this and which will reach beyond to the day you, the reader, peruse this book. There is an essential randomness about Nature, but a purposeful randomness. It is not the randomness of a shuffled pack of cards, but the randomness with which a player sorts out the cards to solve a game of Patience. 'Ordered chaos' is becoming increasingly important in the theory of living systems.

At present there is no theory of health and disease, nor any money to be made in preventative medicine, unless, like the ancient Chinese, the doctor is only paid while the patients remain well. One cannot quantify precisely how many times lightning will not strike during a storm; neither can one quantify how many times in life a person will not be struck with illness. We here examine the concept of disease as the failure of body and mind control processes or regulation.

Man has long considered the influences of energies from outside himself and beyond his purview. In Chapter 3 we consider the effects of the Earth's geomagnetic field on human psychological and physical functioning, emphasising the extreme sensitivity of the pineal gland to electromagnetic changes and its important role in maintaining and regulating the body's biological cycles.

Widespread use of electromagnetic fields is already to be found in medical therapy (Chapter 4). This serves to emphasise a considerable and widespread scientific mental blockage to effects of very weak electromagnetic fields. A doctor once said how horrified he had been to learn that it was known in the 1920s that cancer tissue had a different electrical capacitance from healthy tissue and yet, a quarter of a century later when he was in medical school, no one had told him about it. This mental blockage is to the advantage of those who want unrestricted use in the environment of all the electromagnetic frequencies available, and to those who feel able to solve all medical problems with chemicals. We propose that even here they may unwittingly be synthesising chemicals which are in fact sophisticated electromagnetic resonators.

Man is not unique in the living world in having a vital dependence on things electromagnetic. In Chapter 5 we emphasise the importance of electromagnetic forces throughout all the orders of living systems and their role in communication and control. Only in recent years with the development of modern control theory is it becoming possible to see how this can happen. Things can go wrong with the ability of a living system to communicate and regulate effectively. This was made clear to us when we met with Dr Jean Monro and later with American pioneer Dr Bill Rea. They deal with the unfortunate victims of our twentieth-century environment – the environmentally sick. Their work (Chapter 6) has led to an extension of the concept of allergy that includes illnesses, often non-specific but none the less real, triggered electromagnetically and affecting regulatory systems in the broadest sense.

In 1810, Samuel Hahnemann wrote his classic *Organon of Medicine*. The father of homoeopathy was in revolt against the medical establishment of his time. Modern 'orthodox' and 'high-tech' medicine have since spent more than was spent developing the atom bomb and still cannot deliver the promised cures for man's illnesses. A consequence of taking account of electromagnetic man is to be able to see a rationale and scientific basis to many of the 'alternative medicines' which the orthodox medical establishment can neither assimilate nor refute and to which more consumers are turning (Chapter 7).

Specific example of illnesses which appear to have been triggered by the highly coherent fields from overhead power transmission lines are provided in Chapter 8, partly written by Hilary Bacon, herself a former sufferer in the Dorset village in which she used to live. An attempt is made towards interpreting the many effects in terms of man's electrical sensitivities and regulatory system failures. Because of a duality between coherent frequencies and chemical structures, or molecules, which is as fundamental as the chemical bond itself, we consider synergistic effects involving both electromagnetic and chemical factors in the environment and nutrition. This leads to concerns of safety and public health (Chapter 9) and to the uses made of electromagnetic fields in matters offensive and defensive (Chapter 10). These merit a separate chapter which has been written solely by Simon Best from material available in the public domain; this was so as not to compromise any indiscretions which may have been imparted to the senior author at any time.

The awakening of man's realisation of his electromagnetic sensitivities is like entering a New Year, and is a time to look backward as well as forward. In Chapter 11 we look back to man's unexplained sensitivities recognised from antiquity. The technique of dowsing is a particular example, so also are the prescriptions in the Bible and Talmud on water, that most uncommon common substance so vital for life and health.

A peep through the scientific fence, beyond the last frontiers, takes us into the realms of mind and matter, extra-sensory perception and psychic phenomena, life and death, the necrotic radiation at the transition. Reputable laboratories are now producing evidence that man has an ability, by conscious mental exercise, to affect the operation of a wide range of mechanical and electrical systems, albeit with a low probability, but with a probability that would not be tolerated as a fault incidence in space technology. Is this an opening in the frontier fence of science through which it will be possible to 'peek' and 'poke' the psychic?

Because bioelectromagnetics research is moving so fast, we have included a final 'Postscript', written at the last minute, which updates certain subject areas in which significant developments have occurred since the time of first discussion in the book.

We have written this book for a number of different audiences, perhaps an unwise objective. The average reader should not be put off by the scientific detail (making full use of the Glossary), but should try to grasp the main concepts involved in order to gain a broad understanding.

Dr Cyril Smith
Simon Best
January 1989

CHAPTER 1
History of a phenomenon

Chaque âge a ses plaisirs, son esprit et ses moeurs.
Nicolas Boileau (1636–1711)

The spirit of an age

At certain times in the history of mankind successful developments in science and technology have taken place simultaneously in widely separated parts of the world by independent workers who had no obvious direct contact or collaboration, but who were fortunate to live and work in a period when the spirit of the times – so well expressed by the German word *Zeitgeist* – was favourable to their endeavours. There is no force so great as an idea whose time has come. Others have had all the right ideas but at the wrong time and in the wrong place so, in spite of many struggles, they were never able to bring them to fruition. Now is the time to look afresh and in depth at the implications of electromagnetic fields in living systems.

Electric fields are a property of electric charge at rest, magnetic fields a property of electric charge in motion, and radiation a property of electric charge being accelerated or decelerated. Close to their source, the fields may appear as electric or magnetic according to the way in which they are generated, but from a distance they appear as combined electromagnetic fields. As Brillouin (1934) states: 'Les electrons indépendants sont une fiction. Il va fallour maintenant tenir compte de leurs couplages magnétiques.' (Free electrons are a fiction. It is always necessary to take their magnetic interactions into account).

Many writers have used the term electromagnetic as a synonym for magnetic. This is because the use of the word magnetism in a biomedical context results in its instant dismissal as Mesmerism (see below). We prefer to use electromagnetic to indicate the more general idea.

There are long-standing differences between two fundamental concepts of man-made law. For the Anglo-Saxon, law is an instrument of justice, while the Justinian concept of law sees it as an instrument of public order; these concepts persist into the contemporary *Zeitgeist*. In the EEC, we find the Anglo-Saxons disadvantaged by trying to observe, to the letter, regulations for which there should be 'accomodazione'. Conversely, those countries with the Justinian tradition for 'bending the law' are liable to suffer the environmental consequences of trying 'accomodazione' with the laws of science.

The laws of science are laws of Nature and unlike the laws of kings, emperors and governments, they cannot be changed by whim or public opinion. The only option is the use which is made of the different laws and techniques available.

When a prominent rebel in Britain's American Colonies, Benjamin Franklin of Philadelphia, was engaged in diplomacy against the British in Paris, controversy raged over whether lightning conductors on buildings should be pointed or rounded. Sir John Pringle, the then President of the Royal Society, made the classic reply to King George III of England who had allowed himself to be drawn into the controversy on the side of rounded conductors: 'Sire, I cannot reverse the laws and operations of nature.'

Benjamin Franklin retorted that he hoped that the King would bring the thunder of heaven upon himself by dispensing with lightning conductors altogether.

Electromagnetism and medicine in history
The ancients

Throughout the history of science, needs have dictated which scientific instruments were developed at any particular period. The skills of the craftsmen, and particularly the instrument makers, had reached the limits of the unaided human hand and eye by 1500 BC. Because the precision with which things could be weighed was then adequate for dealing in precious metals and detecting adulteration, there was no incentive to improve the accuracy of the balance until three millennia had elapsed, that is from 1500 BC to 1500 AD.

New instruments can open up whole new worlds awaiting man's discovery and interpretation. A very important example in the history of medical science is the development of the microscope into a scientific instrument by that very controversial character, Galileo. In fact, it was probably based on prior Dutch inventions. The microscope showed that there was much to be discovered on a scale of dimensions far smaller than the anatomical drawings of Vesalius could envisage, just as in its turn the electron microscope has now shown so much detail existing beyond the capabilities of the optical microscope. It seems that the computer-aided human brain is now all set to make discoveries in personal and collective thought processes perhaps even greater in importance than those made by the microscope-aided eyes of scientists over past centuries.

What society permits to be observed dictates in some measure what will be observed. Until the seventeenth century the teachings of the second-century Greek physician Galen were accepted without critical examination. The *Zeitgeist* within which he lived did not permit him to dissect the human body, so the sciences of anatomy and physiology which he did so much to found remained based upon animal anatomy and his observations of injured gladiators. This state of affairs persisted until the middle of the sixteenth century when Vesalius began to investigate how Nature actually goes about things; he soon discovered inaccuracies in Galen's work.

William Gilbert

William Gilbert, physician to the Court of Queen Elizabeth I of England, published a treatise *De Magnete* (Gilbert, 1600/1958), in which his proposal for 'trustworthy experiments' heralded the arrival of a new scientific spirit. The origins of the discovery of loadstone, probably by iron-smelters or miners in veins of iron ore, and the phenomena of magnetism are lost in antiquity; Plato, Aristotle and others recorded that the loadstone attracts iron. Gilbert, the earliest classical writer on terrestrial magnetism, considered the mariner's compass to have been brought to Venice by Marco Polo from China about the year 1260. However, by then, it was already in use in Europe by the Catalans and Basques.

In his chapter, 'Of other properties of the loadstone and of its medicinal virtue', William Gilbert wrote:

> Not a few physicians have thought that loadstone has power to extract an iron arrow-head from a human body: but a loadstone attracts when it is whole, not when reduced to a powder, deformed, buried in a plaster; for it does not with its matter attract in such case, but serves rather to heal the ruptured tissues by exsiccation, so causing the wound to close and dry up, whereby the arrow-head becomes fixed in the wound. ... Nicolaus puts into his 'divine plaster' a good deal of loadstone, as do the Augsburg doctors in their 'black plaster' for fresh wounds and stabs; because of the exsiccating effect of the loadstone without corrosion it becomes an efficacious and useful remedy. Paracelsus in like manner and for the same end makes loadstone an ingredient of his plaster for stab-wounds.

The *Zeitgeist* of the sixteenth century was not ready for the scientific investigation of the claims of magnetic field enhanced wound and bone fracture healing techniques. Then, it was still the job of the physician to philosophise about illness. 'I am dying with the help of too many physicians', said Alexander the Great, who lived from 356 to 323 BC. His words were still applicable in the sixteenth century and, dare we suggest it, may still be applicable in the latter part of the twentieth century. The practicalities of healing became the task of the barber, the apothecary, the midwife and the herbalist when the men of medicine became philosophers.

Luigi Galvani and Alessandro Volta

It is the person with the clinical experience who has the feel for how living systems will react, however subjective and unscientific this feeling might be. Galvani, an obstetrician and an anatomist, concluded from his many years of experiments on the relation between biology and electricity, that 'animal electricity' was the long sought after 'vital force' and announced this to the Bologna Academy of Science in 1791. The injury potentials (about 50 mV) he eventually found were also similarly interpreted.

However, within a couple of years, Volta, a physicist of the University of Padua, had disagreed and concluded that the electricity was not animal but, in effect, electrochemical in origin. He went on to develop the battery, which enabled the science and technology of electrochemistry to start its development. Volta presented his discoveries to Napoleon, who then controlled the city of Bologna, and was duly honoured. Galvani had no stomach for controversy; he ceased to communicate and died quietly. However, his nephew Aldini, a physicist, carried on a prolonged and acrimonious debate with Volta.

Sanity was eventually injected by Humboldt, who showed that both Galvani and Volta were partly correct and partly incorrect. Subsequently, Matteucci did an experiment which confirmed Galvani's experiment: he made contact with a nerve, so as to stimulate muscle contraction, and showed that the electrical action potential preceded the muscle contract (Geddes and Hoff, 1971; Becker and Marino, 1982; Becker and Selden, 1985). Even without modern electronic apparatus able to record and measure the millivolt nerve and muscle potentials, it was still possible to demonstrate the basic phenomena of bioelectricity in the eighteenth century by doing the right experiments.

Antoine Mesmer

Antoine, or Anton, Mesmer is described as the author of the doctrine of animal magnetism (Didot, 1861). He was born on 23 May 1733 at Mersbourg, near Lake Constance, which forms the Swiss–German border, and he died there on 5 March 1815. He studied and qualified in medicine in Vienna. In 1766 he published a dissertation with the title *De Planetarium Influxu*; this was his point of departure into animal magnetism. In it, he proposed that the sun and moon exerted a direct action on the component parts of living systems, particularly the nervous system. Back in 1609, Kepler, in an attempt to give astrology a scientific basis, had deduced the laws of planetary motion from the careful observations of Tycho Brahe (1546–1601). These ideas have been around for a long while.

During the years 1773–4, Mesmer treated a lady, Frauline Oesterline, who had suffered for many years from a convulsive illness with many unfortunate symptoms, including delirium, vomiting and fainting. Attempting to reproduce artificially the natural geophysical tidal variations, he placed magnets on the patient's stomach and legs. These resulted in extraordinary internal sensations of painful currents flowing towards the lower part of the body and which during six hours cleared up all the symptoms. This is the sort of reaction frequently encountered in the treatment of hypersensitive allergic patients (see Chapter 6).

About the same period, a Jesuit by the name of Hell also tried using a magnet to cure nervous complaints. Both claimed priority of invention and a violent polemic ensued. It was resolved when Mesmer announced that his discovery consisted not only in the use of the magnet, but that 'animal magnetism' was essentially distinct from the magnet. Mesmer pursued with ardour the applications of his method amid further controversy. Following what he called 'persecutions', he left Vienna for Paris. He published his propositions on animal magnetism and his methods in 1779; these became doctrines and fed the flames of the political and religious scepticism of the philosophical *Zeitgeist* of that century. In Mesmerism was seen a strong analogy with that other importation from across the Rhine, homoeopathy. The controversy and partisanship developed until Mesmer was offered, in the name of Louis XVI, a sum of money and a stipend on the only condition that he should initiate into the secrets of his discovery ... three persons to be named by the government. This Mesmer refused; subsequently his disciples subscribed for him nearly twenty times the amount offered by the King. The growing enthusiasm eventually led the government to appoint a commission consisting of four doctors and five members of the Academy of Sciences, including Lavoisier and Franklin, to examine the 'doctrines'.

The main conclusion of the report, described as a masterpiece of clarity, was that there was nothing in animal magnetism which could explain the observed healing influences that individuals exerted on one another by their presence. The report, intended for the eyes of the King, was leaked to the press even before the Academies had considered it and was given great publicity by the government. Mesmer, realising that nothing could be recovered, left France with his 'subscriptions' and returned, via England, to retirement in his birthplace where he died, forgotten.

One is left wondering whether there were some environmental factors present in the lives of eighteenth-century Parisians which, like pesticide exposure, could have predisposed Mesmer's obviously large supply of wealthy patients to allergic responses. The expected incidence of some degree of allergic reaction in any modern population is about 15 per cent. The events in Paris took place about the time that chlorine was discovered by Scheel in 1774. There is a report that the over-enthusiastic use of chlorine for bleaching candles once led to the production of so much hydrochloric acid gas that a room had to be evacuated. This suggests that, under normal conditions at this time, persons wealthy enough to be able to enjoy 'night-life' could have been chronically exposing themselves to a variety of chlorinated hydrocarbons in the fumes from the candle-lighting.

Nikola Tesla

Nikola Tesla, a prolific inventor and visionary in many fields of electrical engineering and electronics, was born in 1856 in a hamlet on the borders of the Austro-Hungarian Empire, in what is now Yugoslavia. He was weak in health, but strong in his determination to succeed in electrical engineering. In his youth he had suffered both malaria and cholera. John J. O'Neill (1968), whom Tesla himself said understood him better than anyone else in the world, wrote in his Pulitzer prize winning biography of Tesla:

> Always an indefatigable worker, always using up his available energy with the greatest number of activities he could crowd into a day, always rebelling because the days had too few hours in them and the hours too few minutes, and the seconds that composed them were of too short duration, and always holding himself down to a five-hour period of rest with only two hours of that devoted to sleep, he continually used up his vital reserves and eventually had to balance his accounts with Nature. He was forced to discontinue work.

O'Neill then describes in detail Tesla's illness, which has many of the features of environmental hypersensitivity disorders:

> The peculiar malady that now affected him was never diagnosed by the doctors who attended him. It was, however, an experience that nearly cost him his life. To doctors he appeared to be at death's door. The strange manifestations he exhibited attracted the attention of a renowned physician, who declared that medical science could do nothing to aid him. One of the symptoms of the illness was an acute sensitivity of all the sense-organs. His senses had always been extremely keen, but this sensitivity was now so tremendously exaggerated that the effects were a form

of torture. The ticking of a watch three rooms away sounded like the beat of hammers on an anvil. The vibration of ordinary city traffic, when transmitted through a chair or bench, pounded through his body. It was necessary to place the legs of his bed on rubber pads to eliminate the vibrations. Ordinary speech sounded like thunderous pandemonium. The slightest touch had the mental effect of a tremendous blow. A beam of sunlight shining on him produced the effect of an internal explosion. In the dark he could sense an object at a distance of a dozen feet by a peculiar creepy sensation in his forehead. His whole body was constantly wracked by twitches and tremors. His pulse, he said, would vary from a few feeble throbs per minute to more than one hundred and fifty. Throughout this mysterious illness he was fighting with a powerful desire to recover his normal condition. He had before him a task he must accomplish – he must attain the solution of the alternating-current motor problem.

Tesla did eventually recover and later moved to America where, although his inventive and visionary powers flourished, they exceeded his financial prowess; he died in 1943, a poor man. Among his more spectacular research activities, he succeeded in setting his neighbourhood buildings in mechanical resonance, producing a near-earthquake phenomenon to the alarm of the residents. Following his artificial lightning experiments he tried to set the Earth into electrical resonance as a means of communicating with the antipodes but this was thwarted by his overloading the power supply system. He considered that in the process of thinking, the brain probably produced waves, and that there was no reason why the waves sent out by one mind should not be received by another, with the resulting transfer of thought, an idea also put forward by Lakhovsky (1939) (see below) and Professor J.D.Bernal (1939).

Like others who become electromagnetically hypersensitive, Tesla experienced phenomena bordering on the psychical. In his case, these included premonitions and the visualisation of his life events. Tesla's hypersensitive experiences must have helped his intuitive appreciation of the invisible electrical forces which he did so much to harness, and with such success. It is fascinating to realise that the person who can justly be called the 'Father of Electrical Engineering' must have received enough long-term exposure to electromagnetic fields and frequencies through his pattern of obsessional working that he himself became what is probably the first well-documented case of allergic responses leading to hypersensitivity triggered by electromagnetic fields.

Georges Lakhovsky

Georges Lakhovsky was an engineer who was born in Russia and who settled in France where he became a naturalised citizen. He wrote a book called *The Secret of Life* in the 1920s under the sponsorship of

Professor d'Arsonval; its English translation (Lakhovsky, 1939) contains additional new material as an appendix. Lakhovsky was the first to use high-frequency electromagnetic fields in biological experiments. These were at a frequency of 150 MHz, for which the corresponding wavelength is 2 metres. His original experiments on cancerous plants published in 1924 are supported by remarkable photographs. In a book entitled *La Cabale*, Lakhovsky wrote, 'I have been attacked by physicists ignorant of biology and by biologists ignorant of physics who can consequently neither understand my theories nor judge my experiments.'

Lakhovsky's fundamental principle was that, 'Every living being emits radiations; the great majority of living beings are capable of receiving and of detecting waves.' Health is equivalent to the oscillatory equilibrium of living cells, disease is characterised by oscillatory disequilibrium. The fight between the living organism and invading microbes is fundamentally a war of radiations. A number of workers subsequently found and photographed mitogenic radiation in the ultra-violet part of the spectrum. Gurwitsch and Frank worked with growing plants and vegetables; Reiter and Gabor worked with embryonic tissues and malignant tumours; in 1930 Cremonese made direct photographic records of radiations emitted by human subjects as well as from their saliva or blood specimens.

The theme of cancer is the *Leitmotiv* of Lakhovsky's work and he approached it from the biophysical point of view. Needless to say, his views brought him into conflict with the medical establishment in Paris, just as Pasteur's did in his day. Lakhovsky, too, went further than theory – he evolved a piece of 'radio-electrical apparatus' which he called his 'Multiple Wave Oscillator'. This generated an electric field containing all frequencies from 750 kHz to the infra-red (see Fig. 2.1). These gave him practical results, with many types of cancer and in various hospitals, that confirmed his theoretical views. The apparatus and therapy achieved sufficient reputation and respectability that they were used to treat Pope Pius XI in January 1937, giving success only to the extent of a possible two-year remission.

Lakhovsky also took into consideration the geographical distributions of cancer and the geological nature of the soil and possible causative connections. In this respect, it should be realised that geological conditions and ground water retention affect the propagation, penetration, absorption or reflection of electromagnetic waves incident upon the Earth's surface. He considered the possibility of phenomena ranging from physiological effects and illnesses to the quality of Bordeaux wine vintages being correlated with solar activity over the eleven-year sunspot cycle and the concomitant electromagnetic and meteorological effects.

Lakhovsky treated his plants by placing them within 'an open metallic circuit of 30 cm in diameter kept in position with an ebonite rod'. In effect this was a Hertzian resonator for about 2 metres wavelength (150 MHz) which would enhance any natural oscillations emitted by the encircled plant or present in its environment. Two months after inoculation with a plant tumour the treated plant remained healthy, while the untreated 'control' plants had all died.

Lakhovsky specifically considers the role of water in relation to cancer, citing examples, 'to show that water does not play a part in the incidence of cancer except when its electric constants and the form of its...water-beds... are of such a nature as to affect the field of cosmic radiation which may break up the equilibrium of cellular oscillation.... We are in a position to realise why many reputable writers have drawn attention to the existence of "cancer streets," "cancer villages," and "cancer districts."' Lakhovsky's ideas continue to be supported by the current work of Dr Deiter Aschoff (1986) who has measured a number of different physical parameters at geopathic zones, and by the findings of dowsers (see Chapter 11).

Lakhovsky concludes by summarising his theory in the form of a threefold principle:

> Life is created by radiation;
> Life is maintained by radiation;
> Life is destroyed by oscillatory disequilibrium.

What he had not begun to appreciate is the extreme degree of sensitivity, precision and coherence involved in Nature's applications of electromagnetic oscillations, nor the wide spectral range of frequencies which need to be considered under his term 'cosmic radiation'.

Historical perspective

To A. J. P. Taylor (1967), the originator of the 'cock-up' theory of history, the 'scientist who believes that he has discharged his duty by working devotedly in his laboratory evades his responsibility as Ranke did; and will end in the same service of blind power. It is tempting to believe that government is a special calling and that the calling will always be of God. If history has any lesson it is that men should resist this temptation and should recognise that no member of the community can escape responsibility for its actions. The historian or scientist does well to lead a dedicated life; yet, however dedicated, he remains primarily a citizen. To turn from political responsibility to dedication is to open the door to tyranny and measureless barbarism....'

In the present book we are dealing with the electromagnetic attributes of men and women who have travelled to the present day through the generations of their ancestors in what we call history, but which to each in their own time was their present. The presence today of each individual is also an historical statement. Written into his or her genetic material is a unique program which can be implemented according to laws of Nature which have remained unchanged for so long as can be known. Kingdoms have been won, lost and fought over, on the basis of the genetic inheritance of certain persons throughout the course of history.

A.J.P. Taylor does not see men and women at the end of the twentieth century sitting back in helpless contemplation like their predecessors waiting for the end of the world. Yet, if we are to dismiss with him all the charges of decadence levelled at modern man, what are we to make of the assertion by Dukes (1965) that,

> It is a part of the doctor's function to make it possible for his patients to go on doing pleasant things that are bad for them – smoking too much, eating too much, drinking too much – without killing themselves any sooner than is necessary.

It may now be necessary to add to this list of things pleasant but potentially harmful in excess – the television and all the other electromagnetic devices of twentieth-century convenience and delight, which contribute to the so-called 'electromagnetic smog' of today's environment. It may be cynical to point out that there are considerable economic advantages for governments in having people smoking. A loss in life expectancy of twelve years at the expensive, pension and health care demanding, non-productive end of the life-span gives governments financial rewards which far exceed the tobacco duty they collect. The same may also be found to apply to other environmental pollutants.

Personalities, both the mutally compatible and the mutually antagonistic, and even the straight confidence tricksters, have greatly influenced the course of scientific events throughout history. 'Electroquackery' (Stillings and Roth, 1978) has thrived along with legitimate research and the practice of electromedicine, just as the 'Patent Medicine' man thrived during the development of modern pharmaceuticals. The basic requirement for any confidence trick is that the recipient shall have no opportunity of checking impressions against reality and since no one then understood electrical phenomena, this was not difficult. This is, of course, also the basis of the 'double blind' trial.

The above examples show that over many centuries there have been people prepared to carry out research into phenomena which required both a strong belief and the suspension of disbelief. When the Pandora's Box containing man's electromagnetic secrets is finally unlocked, the responsibility for their proper use will still remain. And that may open up an even bigger 'can of worms' – scientific, medical, legal, military, commercial and social.

CHAPTER 2

Basic concepts: scientific fundamentals

> To see a World in a Grain of Sand
> And a Heaven in a Wild Flower
> Hold Infinity in the palm of your hand
> And Eternity in an hour.
> William Blake (1757–1827), *Auguries of Innocence*

The speed of light

The three major 'forces' of the physical world are gravitational, nuclear and electrical. Gravitational forces are too weak to be responsible for the structure and organisation of living systems, while nuclear forces are too short in their range of action — less than the dimensions of atoms. Electromagnetic forces are just right since they can operate over the distances of the atoms and molecules which make up living systems. To a physicist, therefore, man is an electromagnetic organism. Not only are electromagnetic signals important to the working of the body, but man the tool-maker has found out how to make and use electromagnetic oscillations and fields as a medium of communication around the world and far beyond. All that is required for this are suitable transmitters, antennae and receivers together with enough time in which to await the reply. It is generally recognised that the energy of electromagnetic fields does not travel faster than the speed of light, 186,000 miles per second (3×10^8 m/s). So saying, there have been measurements around since 1977 reporting faster-than-light events in electrical measurements based on the Obolensky circuit (Pappas and Obolensky, 1988). The most recent measurements indicate a definite anisotropy of the normal velocity of light depending on the orientation, the time of day and the polarity of the current. Certain signals travel up to twice the above speed of light.

To give some idea of a scale of distances in the universe so far discovered, even if one could move through space at the 3×10^8 m/s velocity of light it would still take tens to hundreds of years to reach the stars, millions of years to cross to other galaxies, but only eight minutes to reach the sun, just over a second to reach the moon, and a fraction of a second to orbit the earth. The relative scales of the universe in space and time and the physical quantities used to make measurements are shown in Figure 2.1.

Around the year 1900, the physics of time and light began to discover anomalies. To the accuracy obtainable in physical experiments, Michaelson and Morley found that the velocity of light did not depend upon its direction of travel in space; this was not in accord with what Newton's Laws had led scientists to expect.

Considering man-sized distances, light travels a foot in a nanosecond (1 nanosecond = 1ns = 10^{-9} second). It is now even possible to photograph by the nanosecond the progress of a light wave as it crosses a room, using a high-speed electronic camera. Biological cells are micrometres to hundreds of micrometres in size (1 µm = 10^{-6} metres), so light only takes femtoseconds (1 femtosecond = 1 fs = 10^{-15} second) to cross them. But, the frequency of visible light is of the order of 10^{+15} Hz (1 Hz = 1 Hertz = 1 cycle per second), so there is still time, at the speed of light, for one or more complete wavelengths of light to span the dimensions of a biological cell.

The quantum of energy

Just as the tissues of living matter cannot be subdivided indefinitely (eventually the biological cell would be reached), and as a drop of water, if successively subdivided, would eventually have to be separated into one atom of oxygen and two atoms of hydrogen, so within the continuity of the oscillations of an electromagnetic wave the energy it carries cannot be subdivided indefinitely into smaller and smaller packets of energy by going to lower and lower intensities. (The intensity is the power of a light beam, the frequency is its colour.)

The ultimate subdivision of energy is that which gives the single quantum of energy. The quantum theory (Mott, 1972) originated in the year 1900 with the work of the physicist Max Planck. He was trying to find an explanation for the properties of radiation which is in equilibrium with a hot surface, like the heat radiation inside an oven. Until Planck's work there was no reason to suppose that there were any restrictions on the minimum values of energy transfer which could take place. He

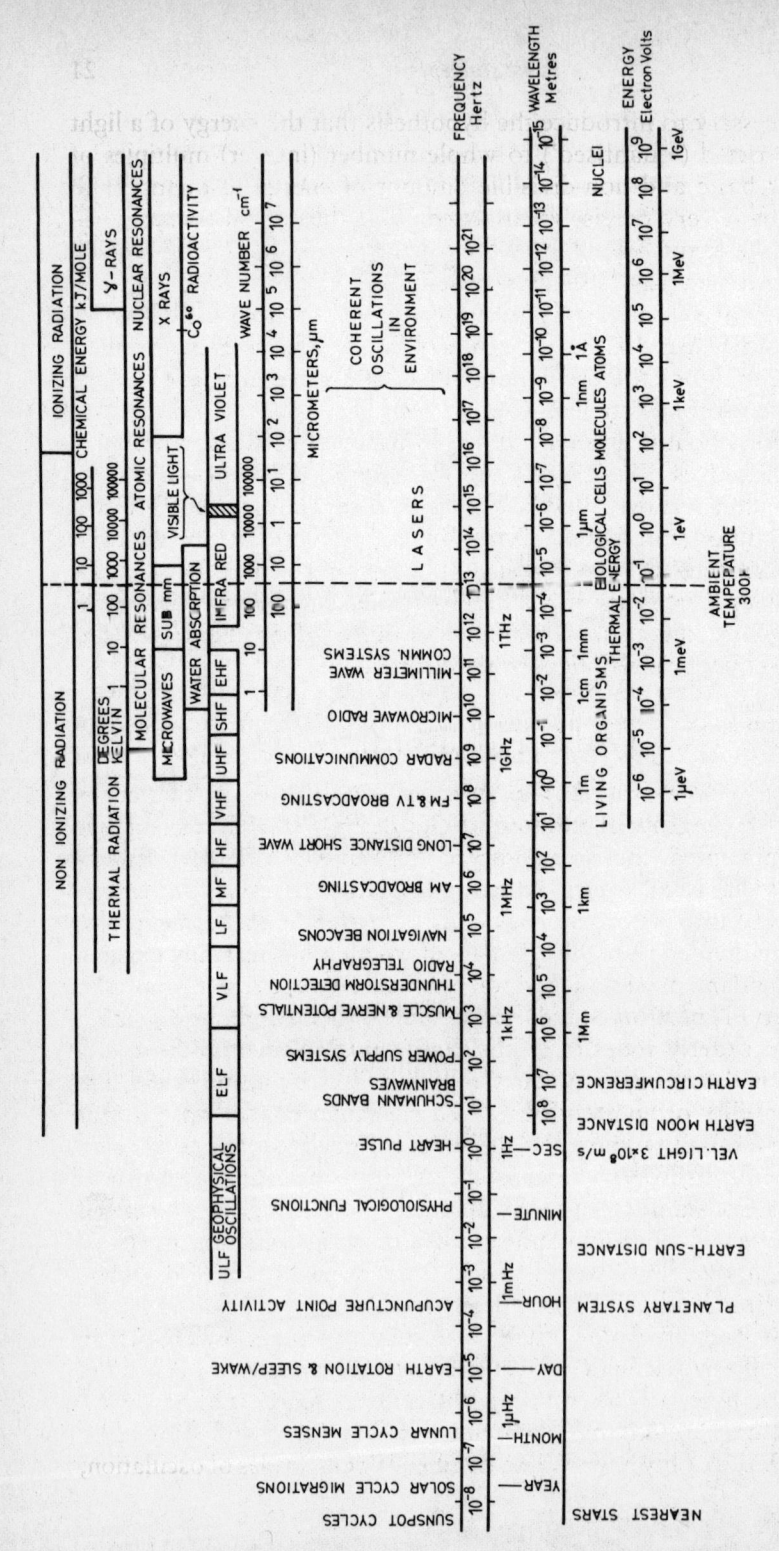

Fig. 2.1 *The Scales of the Universe* This shows the most general relations between the time and distance scales of the Universe, decreasing from right to left. The year correlates with the seasons and animal and bird migrations; the day with sleeping and waking cycles; the second with the heart beat and so on, through the other coherent oscillations in the environment. In the vertical direction, the descriptive scales are for the non-scientific reader, the various numbered scales are to enable the scientific specialist to correlate the scales to a particular scientific discipline. Few speak all the 'energy-languages' of science!

found it necessary to introduce the hypothesis that the energy of a light wave is restricted ('quantised') to whole number (integer) multiples of a particular basic and non-divisible amount of energy (a quantum of energy). This is very precisely expressed in mathematical terms as the product of the frequency of the wave (usually given the Greek symbol v, pronounced 'new') and Planck's constant (h).

The motion of a child's swing or the pendulum of a clock are examples of oscillations. Their frequency is measured by counting the number of complete cycles of the oscillation which take place in a unit of time (second, microsecond, etc.). If you are near the sea, you can see that the motion of a boat is given a certain frequency of oscillation (up-and-down) as the waves pass it by. If you look from the top of a cliff, you can see all the successive waves rolling in from the horizon. From a calibrated photograph taken then, you could measure the distance between the successive crests or troughs – this would be their wavelength. The speed with which they travel in towards the shore is the wave velocity. These three quantities are mathematically inter-related; velocity is equal to frequency multiplied by wavelength.

Order and disorder

The world around us is a paradox of order and disorder. In the forests of Germany trees grow at random; along Berlin's streets not only are the trees regimented, they are numbered in sequence. In 1850, Rudolf Clausius distinguished energy which is available for use, from energy which is locked into the order or structure of matter. Scientists and philosophers were divided over the question of whether atoms really existed. Ludwig Boltzmann passionately stood out for their existence (Bronowski, 1973) and to his memory stands the formula which defines the number of ways that orderly states of atoms can be assembled from disorderly states. This is the Boltzmann equation, which states that the logarithm of the probability of an atom being in a particular energy state is proportional to a quantity known as the 'entropy' of the system, a measure of its degree of disorder. The constant of proportionality is known as Boltzmann's Constant. It is usually denoted by the symbol k and is one of the fundamental constants of physics. The more 'information' it is possible to have about any system, the less must be its degree of disorder. (Ideas about information and energy are elaborated on in Chapter 12.)

This applies equally to a system of electrical oscillations. Frequency can only be measured with perfect precision if the oscillation persists for an infinite time, as shown in Figure 2.2. In practice, it must always be switched on, and off; the clock must be wound up and allowed to run down, thus we only have a finite number of ticks, cycles of oscillation,

Basic concepts

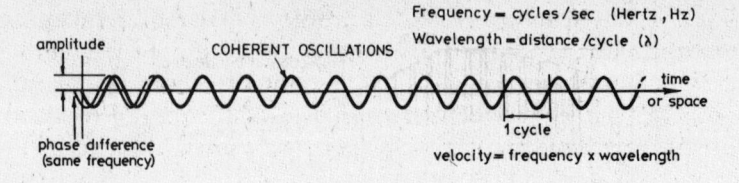

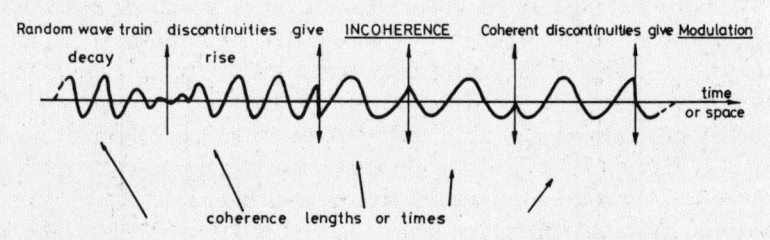

Fig. 2.2 Coherence and Incoherence Oscillations must start and stop. The shorter a burst of oscillation, the less coherent it is. Even if the frequency of two oscillations is the same, they may not be in phase. For any wave, its frequency multiplied by its wavelength gives the constant velocity with which it travels. The velocity only depends on the medium through which the wave is travelling. An exception is within highly coherent systems where the wavelength is constant and the velocity is proportional to the frequency.

heart-beats in a life-time, upon which to base our estimate of the frequency. This limits the precision of 'coherence' attainable within the confines of space and time. In the interactions of oscillations with living systems, the incoherent are not recognised; coherent, in-phase oscillations can write information into a memory or store; coherent out-of-phase oscillations can erase stored information (Popp, 1979). There is an inverse relation between coherence and the life-time of an oscillation, as shown in Figure 2.3. This allows the possible interpretation that in the course of evolution a living system has survived by having a coherence or life-time exceeding that of its competitors. If a living system has evolved so as to give its communication systems an optimum signal-to-noise ratio (see below), then purely from the fundamental physical constants, the size of the basic biological cell should be about 10 μm (Popp, 1979), which is what is found in Nature. This result is also obtained by Del Giudice and co-workers from quantum field theory (Del Giudice et al., 1986).

We live in a chaotic world in many senses of the word but, in one special sense the atoms, molecules and photons around and within us are chaotic. However, they have a random statistical distribution of chaotic energies superimposed upon their energy states. This is because the world is warm, at least warmer than outer space. The physical model for this concept of temperature is the so-called 'perfect gas'. The energies

Basic concepts

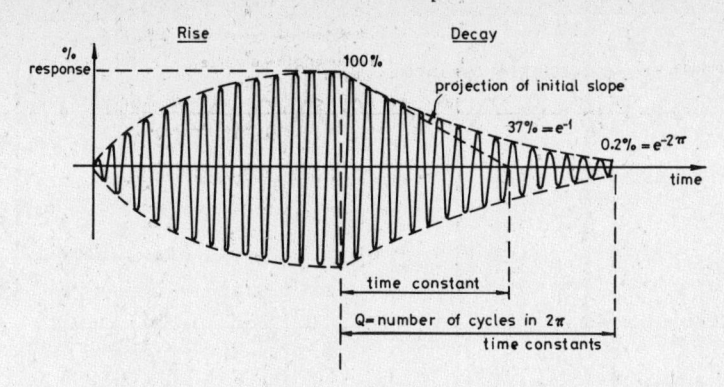

Figure: Rise and Decay waveform diagram with labels: %response, 100%, projection of initial slope, 37% = e^{-1}, 0.2% = $e^{-2\pi}$, time, time constant, Q = number of cycles in 2π time constants

The quality (Q) of a resonant system is the ratio of the energy stored/energy lost per cycle. It expresses the sharpness of resonance and response rate.

Fig. 2.3 Resonance Response Rate The more precise an oscillator is in frequency (the 'sharper' its resonance) the longer it takes the oscillation to build up and decay. The sharpness of a resonance is called its 'Quality' or 'Q', and is the reciprocal of the fractional 'bandwidth' or 'selectivity' obtained.

of all the colliding molecules give rise to a pressure. When they reach the walls of their container they push against them. The relation between the pressure, the volume of the container, the number of molecules it contains and the temperature, which must be measured from the absolute zero of temperature (−273 degrees Celsius, formerly centigrade), is Boltzmann's constant (k), making another appearance. It has the value of 1.3805×10^{-23} Joules per degree of temperature on the Absolute or Kelvin scale (K) of temperature. Ice melts at 273 K, water boils at 373 K, and room temperature is usually taken to be about 300 K. The latter corresponds to an energy of 4.142×10^{-21} Joules, or the equivalents in other units of measuring energy, namely: a quantum of $\frac{1}{40}$ electron-volt (eV), a frequency of about 6×10^{12} Hz, a wavelength of 50 microns (μm), a wave number of 200 cm^{-1}, or a chemical energy of about 2 kilojoules per mole (0.5 kcal/mole). Table 2.1 compares the various measures of energy.

Signal-to-noise ratio

Frequencies greater than 6×10^{12} Hz have quanta (photons) which are more energetic than those corresponding to the chaotic thermal background, so such single quanta should be detectable. This includes visible light – green light has a frequency of 6×10^{14} Hz. At frequencies below 6×10^{12} Hz, the wave properties will predominate over the quantum

Table 2.1 Electromagnetic radiation and energy systems

Type of radiation	Frequency (Hz)	Wave-length	Wave number (cm^{-1})	Quantum (eV)	Chemical (kcal/mole) (kJ/mole)	Thermal (K)	Energy*
Ionizing	3×10^{15}	100 nm	100,000	12.4 eV	260 (1088)	130,000	2×10^{-18}
UV	10^{15}	300 nm	30,000	3.7 eV	86 (360)	43,000	6×10^{-19}
Visible light							
IR[†]	10^{14}	3 μm	3,000	0.37 eV	8.6 (36)	4,300	6×10^{-20}
	10^{13}	30 μm	300	37 meV	0.86 (3.6)	430	6×10^{-21}
Ambient[†] thermal	6×10^{12}	50 μm	200	25 meV		300	4×10^{-21}
Sub-mm[†]	10^{12}	300 μm	30	3.7 meV		43	6×10^{-22}
Mm[†]	10^{11}	3 mm	3			4.3	
Radar frequencies							
(cm)	10^{10}	3 cm					
(dm)	10^{9}	30 cm					
Radio frequencies	10^{8}	3 m					
	10^{6}	300 m					
Audio	10^{4}	30 km					
Power supply	10^{1}	30,000 km (Earth's circumf.)					
Geophysical	10^{-3}						

* Joules or spectral power density (Watts/Hz of bandwidth).

properties and large numbers of quanta will be needed to have enough energy to exceed the thermal background, or 'noise' level or, in the language of communications, to give a signal-to-noise ratio (coherence-to-incoherence ratio) greater than unity.

Communications engineers are usually concerned with the signal power in a communications channel of specific bandwidth rather than the energies involved, although this spectral power density, expressed in watts per cycle of bandwidth, is numerically the same as the energy if a bandwidth of 1 Hz is taken. However, it is necessary to consider the number of 'degrees of freedom' (see Glossary) amongst which the energy has to be shared out. The pendulum of a clock only has two degrees of freedom for its energy – gravitational energy, when the pendulum is stationary at the top of its swing and – kinetic energy, when the pendulum is travelling with its maximum velocity at the lowest point of the swing. The forces of gravity and inertia act over the whole pendulum which responds in a coherent manner with a specific frequency. In any practical situation, the pendulum cannot have infinite coherence (zero spectral line width), if only because it must start and stop within the confines of finite time. There will also be small changes in its resonance frequency arising from random thermal vibrations affecting, for example, its length.

For an electrical oscillating circuit, the two degrees of freedom are the energy stored as an electric field in a capacitor and the energy stored in the magnetic field of an inductance. In each case, an energy of $\frac{1}{2}kT$ is apportioned to each of the two degrees of freedom of a system at a temperature of T K (K indicates the Absolute Temperature, k is Boltzmann's Constant). However, the magnetic interaction between the moving electrons gives a coherence to the whole circuit so that even though the conduction electrons are vibrating at random in the available six directions (simply described as North, South, East, West, up and down), if one measures the electric and magnetic fields over the whole of the circuit – the inductance and the capacitance – the circuit behaves as if it only has a single degree of freedom. Living systems, too, seem to be able to operate in this 'co-operative' manner. They may be able to choose between a broad-band, high data-rate, serial communication channel; or many parallel, highly coherent, narrow-band, low data-rate communication channels capable of parallel data processing. An example of the former would be a television appeal on behalf of a charity, an example of the latter, the individual contributions coming in.

Coherence

The concept of coherence is extremely important in understanding how living systems make use of electromagnetic signals. Highly coherent electromagnetic energy is very probably what is involved in many varied, popular descriptions of the unknown and intangible, such as 'vital energy', 'life forces', 'earth forces', 'energy bands' and so forth.

Given enough time to carry out a measurement, any signal, however weak, could be detected in noise provided that the signal persists for a sufficient length of time, i.e. that it is sufficiently regular in frequency and phase – 'coherent'. The note of an organ which sounds for as long as the key is depressed (or a cipher) is highly coherent, the note of a string instrument which decays within a second or so of being plucked has a short coherence time. The former is like the light from a laser, the latter like the light from the sun or a filament lamp. An experienced Morse Code operator can pick out his station and read its narrow-band (highly coherent) transmissions through extremely high levels of broad-band noise and interference because of the differences in their respective spectral power densities.

There is a fundamental limitation on the degree of coherence which can be achieved simultaneously in both time and space. This is a consequence of the Heisenberg Uncertainty Principle (Popp, 1979; Del Giudice et al., 1986). A light image builds up in a random manner as more and more quanta are supplied, but there is a greater probability that a quantum will arrive in a bright part of the scene than in the shadow. We are not aware of the 'snowstorm' effect which is a consequence of this in our ordinary vision because as light intensity decreases, our eyes lose resolution by just the right amount to blur over this quantum effect. If we take a precise, brief interval of time then the location of the spots of light forming the bright areas of the picture is uncertain; if we wait longer, a clear picture builds up but the instant at which the picture becomes visible is then correspondingly less certain.

It now appears likely that Nature is, more than previously suspected, using highly coherent electromagnetic signals within and between living systems. The range of frequencies involved extends downwards from the ultra-violet, where radiation becomes 'ionising', through to the sub-Hertz (seconds per cycle). The minimum intensity of the radiation may reach to the limits set by the chaotic noise background of the non-living, chaotic world – a signal-to-noise ratio of unity. The lowest frequency that could be meaningful to a living organism is the frequency corresponding to the reciprocal of its life-span (in the case of man: one divided by three-score-and-ten years per cycle). Such fine-tuning of frequency through the life-span of a living system carries with it the risk of sensitivity to and disruption by environmental coherent electromagnetic fields, just as there is a risk of chemical disruption of the genetic information stored in DNA by antagonistic chemical structures.

The fact that the living world is able to impose some degree of order on such a chaotic system is one of the mysteries of life. In the randomness of Nature, there are three types of statistics by which the randomness of three different systems of particles can be described. The idealised gas is made up of particles like miniature marbles whose velocities are given by what are called Maxwell–Boltzmann Statistics. Particles which have quantum properties either have Fermi–Dirac Statistics if each quantum state can only accept one particle, or Bose–Einstein Statistics if 'the-more-the-merrier' applies to a quantum state. The former apply to the electrons in a semiconductor (silicon chip) and these quanta are therefore called 'fermions'; the latter statistics apply to photons (quanta of electromagnetic radiation) and these are consequently called 'bosons'. This is the reason that photons can clump together in a co-operative manner to give the high intensity, highly coherent light of the laser. It is also the reason for many of the phenomena associated with Electromagnetic Man.

If a system is 'Boltzmann', if its energy distributions obey the Maxwell–Boltzmann Statistics corresponding to its temperature, then it is dead. By definition, a living system is one not in thermal equilibrium with its environment; it is also a so-called 'open system', one which can control the flow of energy through itself, just as a bank can control and make use of a flow of money, or cause it to build up for a major expenditure – a condensation of bosons.

The living world has evolved in an environment flooded with most electromagnetic frequencies, but these frequencies are only coherent over time intervals of less than about 10^{-8} s (spectral bandwidths of 100 MHz). This is due to the physical properties of the atoms which emit them. Thus, Nature would have been able to make use of all signals having higher degrees of coherence, narrower spectral bandwidths, for communication and control purposes during the evolution of life, without risk of interference from coherent signals in the external sunlit environment.

The near-quantum sensitivity of living systems to electromagnetic radiation makes it unlikely that their responses will be linear, that is, the magnitude of the response will not be directly proportional to the magnitude of the stimulus. It is more likely that there will be thresholds of sensitivity and an 'all-or-nothing' response, like the photoelectric effect. Weak stimuli below a threshold will give no response; all stimuli above the threshold will saturate or give a panic response.

Einstein and the photoelectric effect

In 1905, Albert Einstein pointed out the quantum nature of interactions between radiation and matter. When a light wave interacts and gives up its energy to matter (atoms and molecules) it must transfer one or more quanta of energy. He explained why the coloured spectrum of light from a sodium or mercury lamp appears as separate coloured lines and not as 'all-the-colours-of-the-rainbow'; it is simply that the energy of light is behaving as if it is packaged rather than behaving like waves spreading out over all space.

The energy of each quantum, or package of energy, was found to be determined by its frequency, given by the product of Planck's Constant, h, and the frequency v. The total amount of energy transfer (in Joules) must equal some whole number (n) of quanta. The numerical value of Planck's constant (h) is 6.6256×10^{-34} and is expressed in the physical units of Joule-seconds. Although this appears to be a very small quantity, the other numbers involved can be very large! The frequency corresponding to green light is $6 \times 10^{+14}$ Hz, so simple arithmetic shows that there must be about 2×10^{18} quanta, in a 1-Joule flash of green light energy.

This is roughly the amount of light energy in a powerful photographic flash, strong enough to bring 'after-image' spots before the eyes, yet our eyes have such a large dynamic range of sensitivity that when they have become used to seeing in dark conditions (dark adapted), they can almost sense the presence of a single quantum of green light. This ability to sense energy almost down to the level of a single quantum is an important characteristic of living systems and it combines with an ability to sense and respond over an enormous range of intensities to stimuli affecting the various sensory systems. This is only possible because living systems can make use of their own energy resources to get the necessary sensitivity. This must be done in the manner that a radio receiver uses its batteries to get the energy to amplify weak signals. Only the old 'cat's-whisker' sets derived all the power fed into the headphones from the energy picked up by the aerial.

The scientific evidence that light does actually behave in a discontinuous or quantum manner was subsequently provided by the discovery of the photoelectric effect by a number of scientists at the end of the nineteenth century and was eventually explained by Einstein in 1905. His explanation was not accepted until Niels Bohr had, in 1913, put forward his hypothesis that the energy (and the momentum) of the atom is quantised, and Millikan in 1916 had carried out his precise experiments which confirmed Einstein's theoretical predictions.

The photoelectric effect is as remarkable and unexpected as some of the phenomena in living systems. A quantum of light can travel from a distant star to a laboratory experiment on Earth and there and then eject an electron from an atom. This is as remarkable as it would be for a wave to cross the ocean and then pick up a single pebble from the shore and throw it to the cliff-top. If the frequency of the light is below a certain critical value for a given surface, no electrons are emitted whatever the light intensity. Intensity represents the rate of arrival of radiation energy; it is also the number of photons, each bearing its quantum of energy, crossing a unit area per second. (This statement ignores certain 'multi-photon' effects which occur when high-intensity lasers are involved.) If quantum effects rather than wave effects predominated on the sea, the corresponding situation would be that the large, long-wavelength, ocean rollers had no effect as they broke on the shoreline; but the small, short-wavelength ripples would be able to throw large stones about. The possibility of quantum effects which may be very frequency-specific and non-linear is of major importance when trying to understand the likely effects on Electromagnetic Man of various levels of environmental electromagnetic fields, and even possible phenomena beyond them!

The photoelectric effect gives a rather convenient way of measuring the energy of quanta. The energy required to remove an electron of electrical charge e (1.60210×10^{-19} coulombs) from an atom can be measured in terms of the electrical potential V (volts) required; this energy would then be equal to eV Joules. Conversely, an energy expressed in Joules may be converted into electron-volts with the advantage that much simpler numbers result. Thus a quantum of green light of wavelength 500 nm (frequency 6×10^{14} Hz), has an energy of 4×10^{-19} Joules or 2.5 electron-volts (eV). Table 2.1 compares the many different scientific terms which are used variously throughout the different branches of science to describe energy over the most important parts of the electromagnetic spectrum.

Quantisation, a property of electric charge and the energy of radiation, can also be a property of the magnetic field. Professor Herbert Fröhlich has pointed out that the quantised nature of magnetic flux was shown theoretically by Professor Felix Bloch in 1968. The quantum of magnetic flux is equal to Planck's Constant (h) divided by twice the charge of the electron. It comes to 2.07×10^{-15} Webers. Most man-made experimental systems are not sensitive enough to detect a single magnetic flux quantum. An exception is the SQUID (superconducting quantum interference detector). This needs to work at liquid helium temperatures and makes use of superconductivity to get the degree of ordering in the system, or coherence necessary for measuring such a small quantity. Unlike superconductors, living systems are thermodynamically 'open' and do not function well below the freezing point of water, let alone at the temperature of liquid helium (a few degrees on the absolute scale of temperature, or not quite $-273°C$), but it does not follow that they cannot detect and make use of magnetic flux quanta. If a living system can use its energy flow to generate the necessary coherence in the same manner that a laser generates its highly coherent radiation from the randomness of a gas discharge, then such a sensitivity to a magnetic flux quantum would be possible. A non-living, superconducting system is thermodynamically 'closed' – there is no energy entering or leaving. A living system is thermodynamically 'open' – energy flows through it like the water over the Niagara Falls.

Only specially prepared surfaces called photocathodes, such as are used in some television cameras and sensitive light detectors (photomultipliers), are able to emit electrons into a vacuum on exposure to visible light. Most metals and materials in general (including biological materials) will do this if quantum energy of the radiation exceeds about 5 eV (ultra-violet light of 250 nm wavelength). The quantum energy of visible (green) light is about 2.5 eV. Ultra-violet radiation is so called because in the spectrum of the rainbow it is found out beyond the violet, the limit to which the human eye usually happens to be sensitive, although some creatures, especially insects, can see in the ultra-violet. The fact that quanta of the shorter wavelengths of ultra-violet radiation and X-rays have enough energy to liberate electric charges from materials puts them into the category of so-called 'ionising radiation'. The ions are the positively or negatively charged atoms and molecules which arise when an electron is ejected or acquired. The loss of the negatively charged electron leaves the atom as a positive ion; if this electron happens to be captured by another atom or molecule, that becomes a negative ion.

All electromagnetic radiation for which the quantum of energy is insufficient to be able to liberate completely an electric charge from an atom is termed 'non-ionising'. This must not be taken to imply that it is necessarily without effect or non-injurious under all circumstances. For example, the non-ionising visible light can affect a photographic emulsion, infra-red (radiant heat) can start a fire, or trigger an exothermic chemical reaction.

Free radicals

In organic and especially in biological materials, ionising radiation can give rise to uncharged groups of atoms containing an unpaired electron called 'free radicals'. These are very reactive chemically. Living organisms need them to be able to use oxygen to get energy but have devised special ways of eliminating them when no longer required since they may be produced in the organism by chemical as well as electrical processes and give rise to unwanted chemical reactions, even leading to disease.

Levine and Kidd (1985) write of a 'Unified Stress Hypothesis' for disease causation and consider biological stress to include emotional factors, physical trauma, chemical toxicity, and infection, all of which can cause an increase in endogenous free radical production and possibly overwhelm the body's various antioxidant defences. The long-term consequences may include any of the inflammatory degenerative disease states which are often associated with immune system suppression or immune dysregulation, and carcinogenesis.

Free radicals are particular atomic or molecular species having a single unpaired electron in an outer energy level (orbital); the total of the electrons is usually an odd number. The presence of the unpaired electron makes the free radical extremely chemically reactive and interactive with electromagnetic fields. The free radical is able to propagate itself by taking part in chain reactions with other atoms or molecules. These chain reactions will continue until eventually neutralised by antioxidants, enzyme reactions or a chemical recombination giving a reaction product without the single unpaired electron. Free radical reactions are only destructive to the organism when they get out of control. This risk is the price organisms must pay for evolving beyond the anaerobic single cell by using oxygen to increase their efficiency in converting nutrients to available energy. Free radicals are essential to the oxidation processes whereby living systems generate their essential energy.

It is ironic that the reason why ionising radiation attracts so much attention because of its accepted carcinogenicity is the ease with which ionising radiation from a nuclear reaction within a single atom can be detected. This is overwhelmingly apparent following the Three Mile Island, and Chernobyl episodes and the continuing Sellafield saga. Yet, ionising radiation is only one way of generating free radicals in the body and which are only harmful when they get out of control. Our environment is polluted with many chemicals and electromagnetic fields which cannot be as easily or as sensitively detected as ionising radiation, but which contribute to the biological stress on the free radical regulatory systems.

The physical and chemical stress which a particular individual's constitution can tolerate can be represented as the capacity of a rain-water barrel. Rain up to the point at which it overflows represents an individual who can still cope with self-detoxication as represented by the normal draining of water from the barrel. The point at which the rain-water barrel overflows represents the maximum load of environmental stress that individual can tolerate under the particular environmental conditions at that time. If a cloud-burst 'rains' chemical or electrical stressors into the barrel faster than they can be removed, nothing obvious happens, until one day it overflows. The person is then diagnosed as having some clinically identifiable disease. This represents the absence of preventative medicine, i.e. the failure to notice or appreciate the rate of rise of water in the barrel leading to its eventual overflow.

Homeostasis

Control or regulation (homeostasis) is as old as the existence of purposeful behaviour and self-adapting beings. The situation of a regulatory system is akin to that of a resonator as shown in Figure 2.4. Near equilibrium, its response to stress is small and bi-phasic about a zero mean value; given a steady stress, the response to a further perturbation is

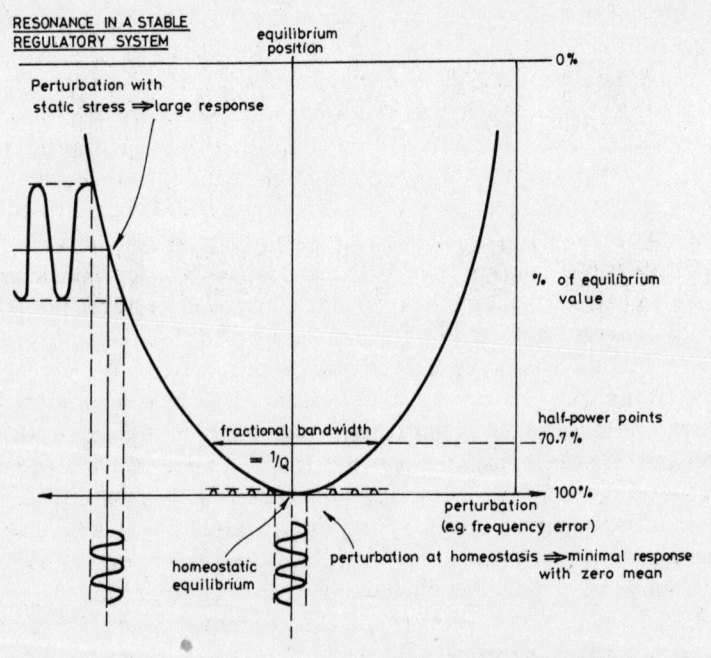

Fig. 2.4 *Resonance in a Stable Regulatory System* A stable system is represented as being at the bottom of a valley. Small perturbations cannot raise or lower it much. On the side of a steep hill, a small perturbation can initiate a precipitous descent. When a bio-regulatory system is stressed, it is pushed up the hill-side, and will give larger responses to a stimulus.

thereby magnified. Many control functions are automatic within the body; the control of heart beat, blood pressure, blood sugar, blood gas, the aperture of the eye-pupil, all take place without conscious awareness unless something goes wrong – unless there is a fault in the regulatory system. Control systems involve the use of feedback. This means that the quantity being controlled is also monitored and information is sent back to the control system to tell it whether it is meeting the criteria laid out for it, and if not, what action is required. The control systems of the engineers of antiquity were mainly concerned with water levels and hence flow rate.

To effect control, the signals must be coded with intelligence; dis-intelligence is typified by *The Sorcerer's Apprentice* fable. To transfer

Basic concepts 33

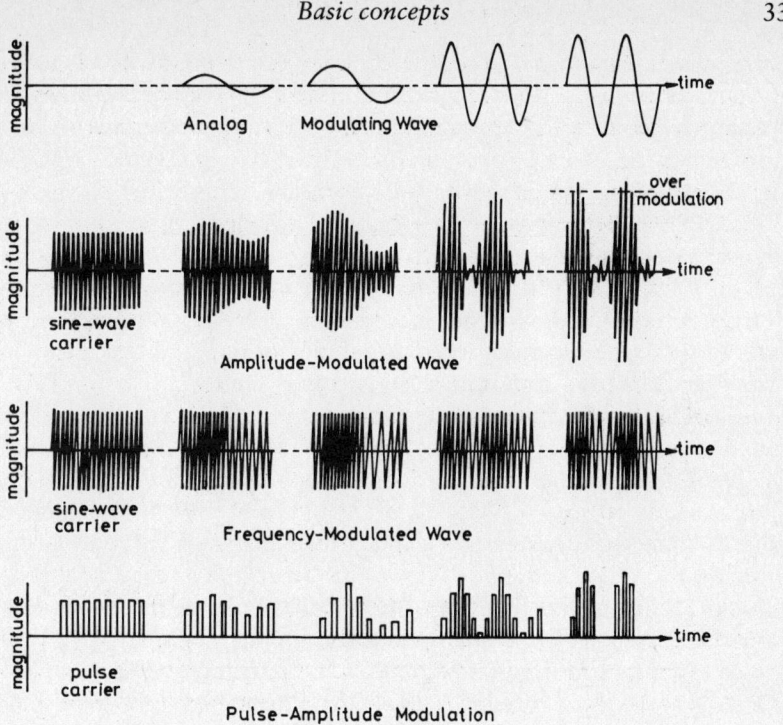

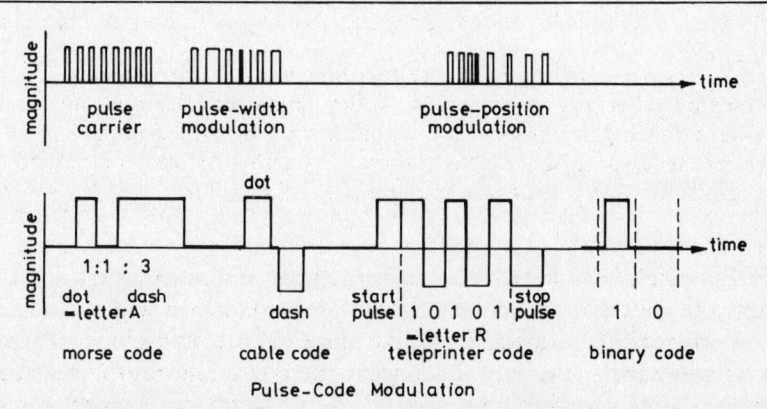

Fig. 2.5 *Information Transfer – Modulation* Oscillations and resonances happen in any structure, like rattles in cars. They only become useful when they are interrupted in a coherent manner to convey information. This process is called modulation. This figure shows the many ways in which the modulating wave at the top, can be impressed on a carrier oscillation. The carrier must be highly coherent so as not to change spontaneously during the longest modulation period. A train of pulses can also act as a carrier of modulation, and the pulses can be coded to transfer information.

the control signals from the point at which errors are detected to the point at which they are remedied requires a carrier for the information and modulation representing the intelligence. Various types of modulation used in electrical communications are shown in Figure 2.5. In chemical communication, the carrier is the molecule and the modulation is the particular arrangement of the atoms which gives it its uniqueness. A simple contemporary example of control is to be found in a domestic central heating system. If the temperature is too low, the thermostat switches on the circulating pump, the hot water raises the room temperature until the thermostat notices that it has become too hot and switches the pump off. This is a simple 'bang-bang' control; it is unlikely that living organisms will use such a crude system, refined versions with computed, non-uniform switching times are more likely (Chiabrera, 1986).

Although simple control feedback loops in living systems might be simulated and analysed, the scale of the problem for simulating the complete human regulatory system and pronouncing on the state of health or disease of a given individual is still far from being a practical proposition. In quantitative terms this means determining the probability of each regulatory system going outside its stability margins. To emphasise the complexity of the problem, it must be remembered that even something as basic to the organism as a single biological cell still has about 3000 enzyme systems in control of its chemical activities, and the human body comprises of the order of 10^{13} cells. The number of enzymes in the human body is thus of the order of 3×10^{16}; if their detailed reactions were simulated on a computer at the rate of one every 3 seconds, this would need computer time equal to the number of seconds that have elapsed since the beginning of the Universe, 10^{17}.

Living systems make much more precise use of physics than most man-made systems. This chapter shows how the commonly regarded limitations for all physical systems of a maximum velocity for electromagnetic radiation, a precise minimum, or quantum of the amount of energy that a given frequency can carry, and the order-within-disorder or coherence of an oscillation, can all affect the very structure and function of living systems. Highly coherent oscillations can act as carriers for modulation representing a control function for the regulation and maintainance of homeostasis in living systems. Certain groups of atoms called 'free radicals' are essential to the chemistry whereby oxygen-burning organisms generate their energy but they are capable of interacting strongly with electromagnetic fields as well as being highly reactive chemically. Figure 2.1 shows these physical quantities relative to all the scales of Man and his Environment, in space, time and energy. Only when we consider living systems at the boundaries set by physics will we see possibilities for interactions with them from beyond physics.

CHAPTER 3

The cosmic connection

> No clear boundary exists between the organism's metabolically maintained electromagnetic fields and those of its geophysical environment.
>
> Professor Frank A. Brown, Jr (1906–83)

The trouble with the cosmos

The trouble with the cosmos is that it is a long way off. Although man has walked on the Moon and space probes are opening up the planetary system even further, the idea that cosmic events can or do affect us smacks too much of astrology to be accepted easily by modern scientific minds and those conditioned thereby, this despite extensive evidence now available. (That there is even some reliable evidence in support of certain claims made by astrology, as discussed in Chapter 11, only serves to increase such reluctance and antipathy.) But pioneering research into biological rhythms has shown that solar radiation and lunar cycles, together with other cosmic events, do indeed have their influence on life on Earth in completely non-astrological ways; such phenomena have become established as an area of science known as cosmobiology. Playfair and Hill (1978), in *The Cycles of Heaven*, assessed the evidence from over 300 such studies out of a total now approaching 20,000. These cover such areas as planetary effects on the weather, to possible galactic influences on certain biochemical reactions. In the great majority of cases the basic mechanism of the influence is known or suspected to be electromagnetic in origin. The following sections describe the work of a number of researchers who have pioneered the study of cosmobiology.

Giorgio Piccardi

Giorgio Piccardi (1895–1972) was born in Florence, Italy, where for much of his working life he was an academic physical chemist doing conventional research in many different fields. However, during the last twenty years of his life he particularly concerned himself with investigating non-reproducible or fluctuating phenomena and their correlation with extraterrestrial and cosmic influences (Piccardi, 1962). Specifically, Piccardi studied the colloidal precipitation of the inorganic chemical bismuth oxychloride from a solution containing bismuth tri-chloride. From 1951, his various tests were carried out simultaneously by a number of co-workers around the world, every day, for approximately 10 years. They found, among other things, that the chemical reaction rate rose $3\frac{1}{2}$ times on days of solar eruptions and that it was also affected by strong magnetic storms and the 11-year sunspot cycle. Inexplicable annual variations were also observed, including a noticeable decline and a sudden enhancement in March, with another around the September equinox. Piccardi was forced to postulate that galactic forces were responsible for such effects through a combination of the Earth's rotation, its orbit around the Sun and its helical movement through space (at about 19 km/s) towards the constellation Hercules. Commenting on the variation of the Earth's helicoidal motion, which reaches its maximum velocity of 45 km/s in March and its minimum in September, Piccardi stated:

> During March, and only during March, the Earth is directed approximately, at maximum speed, towards the galactic centre – that is, along the lines of force of a radical field and perpendicular to the lines of force of a dipolar galactic field. This double condition will not be encountered again throughout the year. The conditions during March are thus quite exceptional. (Piccardi, 1962, p. 97)

Some have criticised Piccardi's findings. Kauffman and Beck (1987) criticise Piccardi for comparing his samples and controls pairwise instead of calculating averages for the test solutions and the controls. This is the correct procedure for averaging out variations about a mean to detect drifts in the mean value. If the mean is stable, this is to the credit of the experimentation. However, in many experiments involving biological systems the response to a stimulus is often what is called 'bi-phasic'; that is, it may change in either sense and there may be an equal number of positive and negative departures from the mean. Thus, comparing the means of the test and control will give a null result. There are other hypotheses that can be tested statistically: one, which is of particular importance in dealing with periodic events like planetary motion, is the hypothesis that there is a periodicity in the data about a mean of zero. Computer programs exist which can systematically do significance tests on a given set of data to determine whether any periodicity around a mean of zero correlates with that data (Baker and Smith, 1985).

Frank Brown

The late Professor Frank A. Brown Jr (1906–83) of Northwestern University, Evanston, Ill., found and, for many years, investigated, exogenous rhythms in plants and animals, especially lunar cycles. Brown (1962) showed how the metabolic activity of, for example, potatoes, carrots, earthworms and newts, as measured by oxygen consumption, depended on the lunar diurnal rhythm. Whereas Bradley, Woodbury and Brier (1962) and Adderley and Bowen (1962) confirmed that rainfall in both the Northern and Southern Hemispheres exhibits a lunar periodicity, Brown and Chow (1973) demonstrated that water uptake by bean seeds peaks significantly just before Full Moon. In perhaps his most famous experiment, Brown (1954) transported oysters in light-proof containers from the harbour in New Haven, Connecticut, to a darkroom in his laboratory in Evanston, Illinois, 1000 miles and one time-zone away. There he measured their activity in terms of valve opening. At first the oysters kept their valve opening and closing to the rhythm of the high and low tides in New Haven harbour. But, after two weeks, this rhythm had slipped back and re-phased to the exact times of lunar zenith and nadir at Evanston when the Moon would have caused high and low tides such as occur on the western shores of the near tideless Lake Michigan. Brown had shown that the oysters had responded to an exclusively exogenous, lunar rhythm.

Brown also investigated the effects of weak radiation upon various organisms and, with Park (Brown and Park, 1967), showed that mammals as well as marine life are influenced by pervasive, weak geomagnetic fields. He speculated that the receptive systems within the organisms can be anywhere, or indeed everywhere, within the body. Reviewing the evidence for extrinsic timing of internal rhythms in animals and plants, Brown (1972) concluded emphatically, 'No clear boundary exists between the organism's metabolically maintained electromagnetic fields and those of its geophysical environment.' In his last paper before his death, Brown (1983) boldly proposed that the long-standing controversy between proponents of an endogenous versus exogenous timing trigger for circadian rhythms could perhaps be resolved by taking plants and animals on an ocean voyage to reveal the details of how their biological clocks operate. Such a definitive test of his pioneering research and ideas should indeed prove decisive. The self-contained biological clock combines fantastic immunities to chemicals that influence metabolic changes – even to the complete paralysis of the organism's functions – and to temperature changes in its environment, with a high sensitivity to a specific stimulus or *zeitgeber*, which may be light or ELF electromagnetic field variations.

Harold Burr

Another who studied the effect of natural rhythms on living systems was Professor Harold Burr at Yale University, whose book (Burr, 1972) spans the years 1916–56. He studied the variations of the electrical potentials of trees and noted that they followed the lunar cycle and were also affected by the sunspot number (Burr, 1945). As early as 1935, Burr had expounded, with Professor Northrop, also of Yale, his Electrodynamic Field Theory of Life, postulating that all organisms possess an organising electrical field (of potential gradient, a so-called 'L-field') independent of local conductivity variations or ion currents in the tissues. Burr felt that electromagnetic fields had shaped the myriads of different life forms on the Earth. He and his colleagues claimed that an 'L-field' exists long before the organism is fully grown, can be picked up at a distance from the organism, and that, although normally steady, can be affected by external factors such as ELF waves and solar and lunar cycles. He later found that the 'L-field' changes in response to pathological processes and that monitoring such changes permits diagnosis of internal disease states, including cancers, long before they become manifest (Burr, 1972).

Leonard Ravitz

A pupil of Burr's, Dr Leonard Ravitz applied Burr's ideas to humans. He observed changes in electrical potential between head and chest of 10 subjects, which in all cases showed a 14- to 17-day cycle in rough correlation with the lunar phases (Ravitz, 1951) as well as longer periodicities. In a comprehensive review of the evidence for an Electrodynamic Field Theory, Ravitz (1962) reported that schizophrenic and manic depressive patients showed seasonal fluctuations and that many studies had shown a correlation between onset and change in psychotic episodes and different phases of the Moon. The most pronounced tides in environmental electric fields showed diurnal, 14- to 17-day, 28- to 29-day, seasonal and semi-annual variations. According to Ravitz, electromagnetic fields act as determiners of biological activity, rather than as epi-phenomena, patterning the nervous system and regulating every component part of it from within and without; they define living matter in terms of four-dimensional time-space and energy.

Very recently, a team of Soviet researchers has provided independent corroboration of Burr's and Ravitz's ideas. According to a *Times* report (Wiseman, 1987), the group led by Academician Yuri Gulyayev analysed electromagnetic radiation as well as audible and ultra-sonic sounds from the body. An imager recorded the infra-red radiation from 16,000 pixels on the body surface to an accuracy of $\frac{1}{100}$ deg. C at intervals of $\frac{1}{10}$ sec., while an extremely sensitive magnetometer, well protected from interference, measured the magnetic fields. Skin-glow, or bio-photon emission, was recorded with a photon counter. Besides measuring for the first time the strength and spatial distribution of fields around the human body, the Soviet team began to establish how people react to the fields generated by another person. They found that one person can sense changes in the infra-red radiation emitted by another, but that information transmitted by other radiation fields is ignored. They concluded that monitoring the various fields surrounding the human body can provide valuable clinical information about the condition of a patient's internal organs and general state of health. This demonstrates yet another unsuspected, subliminal diagnostic tool of the medical practitioner in doctor-to-patient contact. Such a potential tool is currently being explored in the UK by Dr Julian Kenyon in the Dove Project, a research project based in Southampton, investigating the subtle electromagnetic changes around the human body.

Aleksandr Chizhevsky

One of the first researchers to study the effect of solar activity on mankind was an historian in Russia, Professor Aleksandr Chizhevsky (1897–1964), who is considered by many as the father of heliobiology. Chizhevsky's main interest was sunspots, which he correlated with human activity. After collating data covering 2400 years, he claimed that it showed that the world's major mass movements, including all wars, uprisings and social movements, revealed regular cycles linked to the sunspot cycle (Chizhevsky, 1934, 1971). The peak in popular unrest coincided, in nearly every case, at or near the year of maximum solar activity. He claimed that mass excitability linked to each solar cycle could be divided into four phases – minimum, increase, maximum and decline – which matched the progress of each solar cycle. According to Chizhevsky, nearly 80 per cent of all major events in modern history occurred in phases 2 and 3 and only 5 per cent in phase 1. Some examples of the former include the French revolutions of 1789, 1830 and 1848, the commune of 1870, the two Russian uprisings of 1905 and 1917, and the outbreak of the Second World War (Playfair and Hill, 1978). More recent examples include the invasion of Czechoslovakia and the world-wide student unrest in 1968, the invasion of Afghanistan in 1979 and the Falklands War in 1982. The date of the next solar maximum is uncertain (Wilson, 1988) and may occur at the end of 1989 or early 1990; readers will be able to judge for themselves whether world events and tensions continue to be consistent with the above pattern.

Solco Tromp and Edward Dewey

Dr Solco Tromp (1909–83) was a pioneering investigator of all types of cosmic cycles. A former director of research of the Biometerological Research Centre in Leiden, the Netherlands, he published the first comprehensive survey of biometeorology (Tromp, 1963) which contains some 4400 references concerned with the effects of weather and climate on biological processes in plants, animals and man. His further reviews covered possible extra-terrestrial triggers of observed interdisciplinary cycles (Tromp, 1975a) and a very extensive *Biometeorological Survey* (Tromp, 1979). His main interest was the long-and short-term fluctuations of the physiochemical state of human blood and its possible geophysical causes (Tromp, 1967; 1973; 1975b), although his open-mindedness drove him to explore and research the whole area of dowsing (Tromp, 1949, 1972) in pursuit of a plausible scientific explanation, herein considered in terms of electromagnetic sensitivity (see Chapter 11). As editor of the *Journal of Interdisciplinary Cycle Research*, Tromp helped promote in Europe the prodigious work on cyclic phenomena of every kind gathered by the American, Dr Edward Dewey (Dewey and Mandino, 1972), who, in 1940, set up the Foundation for the Study of Cycles at Pittsburgh, Pennsylvania. Now affiliated to the University of Pittsburgh, the Foundation publishes the journal *Cycles*. Together, Tromp's and Dewey's life-long research contributed profoundly to the emerging sciences of chrono- and cosmo-biology and to persuading scientists to take an interdisciplinary approach to these and other areas.

The Sun and Moon, extraterrestrial ELF (1–300 Hz), and circadian rhythms

The ancient tradition that cosmic events influence the condition of man is said to be enshrined in the Italian word for influence which gives us the word 'influenza' – the influence of the Moon was considered to be the cause of 'flu epidemics. (An alternative and less romantic derivation for the word 'influenza' is from the Arabic for 'having a runny nose like a goat'.) The Moon has long been suspected of influencing mental stability. A 'lunatic' was said by Paracelsus to 'grow worse at the dark of the Moon'. Prior to 1808, Bedlam Hospital (London) inmates were beaten at certain phases of the Moon as a prophylaxis against violence (Gauquelin, 1982). Certainly, lunar influence has been confirmed in many biological systems, including plants (Sweeney, 1969; Kollerstrom, 1980), agriculture (Currie, 1988), fish (Bunning, 1964), rodents (Klinowska, 1972) and other animals (Downer, 1988).

Friedman, Becker and Bachman (1965) have correlated psychiatric hospital admissions and ward behaviour statistics with geophysical parameters. They find that there is an absence of a significant relationship between the total range of geomagnetic activity as measured conventionally, but that cosmic ray indexes relate significantly with both the above measures. Cosmic ray activity provides a quantifiable geophysical measure indirectly related to geomagnetic activity. This work is not yet at the stage of being able to suggest causal relationships with psychiatric illness.

Recently, Lieber (1979) published a collection of many studies purporting to show a reliable lunar influence on various areas of human behaviour, although Rotton and Kelly (1985), using meta-analysis, have fiercely contested this claim. However, whereas studies of social behaviour can be easily criticised for neglecting a variety of contributing variables, biochemical studies, like those of Rounds (1975), who has found a lunar periodicity in the concentration of neurotransmitter-like substances extractable from human blood, are more difficult to refute. Lieber suggested a theory of gravitational 'biological tides' as the possible mechanism of effect but the accumulated evidence indicates that an electromagnetic link is far more plausible.

The Moon is known to modulate the Earth's geomagnetic field during its monthly $29\frac{1}{2}$-day phase (synodic) cycle (Bigg, 1963). Bell and Defouw (1966) showed that this influence tends to peak at the Full Moon; the closer the Full Moon is to the plane of the ecliptic (the plane of the Earth's orbit round the Sun, i.e. to there being a lunar eclipse), the greater the effect. The celestial latitude of the Moon varies up to 5 degrees north and south of the ecliptic, in what is termed its $27\frac{1}{2}$-day 'nodal' cycle, after the two points of intersection, or 'nodes'. Bell and Defouw showed that when the Moon's position in its nodal cycle is within 1 degree of the ecliptic at the Full Moon (phase cycle), the effect on geomagnetic activity reaches its peak, and declines uniformly as it moves toward 5 degrees north or south of the ecliptic. Thus, any claimed effect of the Full Moon on human behaviour or other phenomena, for example, post-operative haemorrhaging (Andrews, 1961), may well vary in its intensity according to the Full Moon's celestial latitude in any given phase cycle. The conflicting results obtained in human lunar cycle investigations to date may be due to the neglect of the Full Moon's celestial latitude (nodal cycle position) and the actual geomagnetic variation produced by the Full Moon in each individual phase cycle under study. That is, rather than 'collapsing' the data from many lunar cycles on to a single plot, thus obscuring and averaging out individual cycle fluctuations, sequential analysis of each cycle by wave harmonic analysis should identify any subtle but consistent effects of lunar geomagnetic variability on human functioning. This is yet a further example of the importance of properly investigating fluctuations about a zero mean; the fluctuations may represent a highly coherent phenomenon. Time, as measured by observation of the transit of heavenly bodies, has a coherence of the order of parts in a hundred million. The findings of Bell and Defouw suggest that one should compare the effects of Full Moons within 1 degree of the ecliptic with those of Full Moons at more than 4 degrees from the ecliptic. One likely biosensor for any such effects is the pineal gland, which has been found to be extremely sensitive to changes in magnetic field and to ELF.

Living systems have a general facility for being able to sense very small changes in their environment without being overwhelmed by the large changes. This is an advantage to both predator and prey; no doubt those which could not sense food or an enemy failed to survive in the predator-prey confrontation. In dark adaptation the eye can reach the limitations set by finite numbers of light quanta, yet it can detect small changes in contrast, hue and movement in a bright sunlit scene. There is no reason to presume that living systems have not evolved appropriate ranges of sensors and sensitivities to the rest of the electromagnetic spectrum, including the Earth's magnetic field (Smith, 1986).

The existence of a magnetic field at the surface of the Earth has been known since ancient times. The first extensive review of the biological effects of the geomagnetic field (GMF) was published in Leningrad by Professor Aleksandr Dubrov in 1974 and subsequently translated into English (Dubrov, 1978). The GMF at the surface of the Earth has a steady component of about 0.5 Gauss (Oersted), 50 microtesla or 50,000 gammas (depending on the units of measurement). The actual value varies between 0.35 and 0.70 Gauss over the surface of the Earth. The direction of the local maximum field is inclined to the horizontal at the so-called 'angle of dip' of the compass needle. The GMF approximates to the field that would be given by an enormously powerful bar magnet about 400 km from the Earth's centre and inclined at about 11.5 degrees to the axis of rotation. Measurements on rocks show that the polarity of the GMF reverses every 10,000 to 100,000 years and has smaller variations over a period of 100 to 1000 years.

Superimposed on this steady field is a variable field component amounting to less than 2 per cent in magnitude but very important biologically. Under 'quiet' conditions, there are variations synchronised with the solar day and the lunar day, and there are also annual variations. Disturbances occur in synchronism with the 11-year sunspot cycle, and the 27-day period of rotation of the Sun about its axis. The Earth's orbit is within the outer atmosphere of the Sun and experiences a 'solar wind' of radiation and charged particles, as shown in Figure 3.1. These

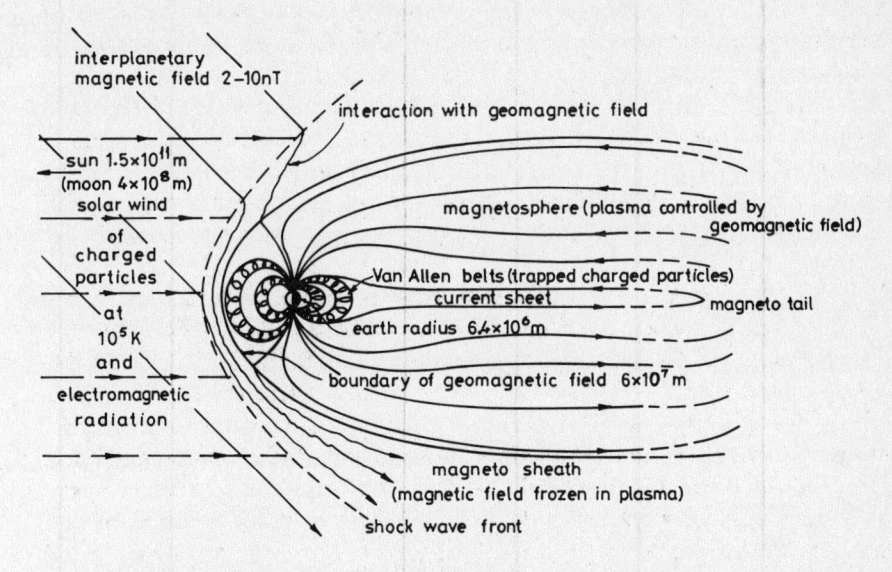

Fig. 3.1 *The Earth's Electromagnetic Environment* Our Earth is in the outer atmosphere of the Sun. This figure shows all the particles and electromagnetic fields which buffet us, protect us, and couple us to the tides and fields of the planetary system.

become trapped in the Earth's Van Allen radiation belts and give rise to the aurorae at the poles and to currents in the upper atmosphere which oscillate between the north and south poles. The Schumann Bands of ELF radiation (1–30 Hz) originate from resonances in the insulating cavity bounded by the conducting Earth and the conducting ionosphere. Magnetic storms are classed according to their magnetic field strengths – very strong, over 200 gammas; weak, 50 gammas (1 gamma (γ) = 10^{-5} Gauss = 1 nanotesla (nT) = 10^{-9} T). As we shall see later, such fluctuations are well above the theoretical threshold sensitivity of man and animals. These and the other phenomena depicted in Figure 3.2 combine to form Man's natural electromagnetic environment. Within the last hundred years, man has greatly added to these with the multitudes of electrical and electronic signals and noise producing the vast increase in the amount of electromagnetic 'smog' permeating his environment, as depicted in Figure 3.3.

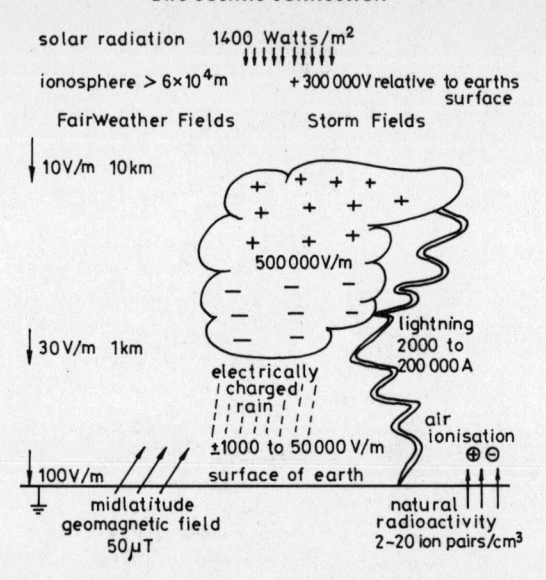

Fig. 3.2 Man's Natural Electromagnetic Environment We are warmed by the Sun, watered by the rain, and exposed to the electromagnetic fields generated by our weather systems. The thunderstorms keep us in touch with the state of the ionosphere by stimulating the Schumann resonances which are close in frequency to our brain-waves. Ions, blown through the magnetic field of the Earth are deflected and set up electric fields. Natural radioactivity from the core of the Earth, cosmic radiation and breaking water droplets, give the air an electric charge of ions.

In mammals, the pineal gland (Semm *et al.*, 1980) is a light-sensitive, time-keeping organ in which the cell activity is affected by magnetic field pulses of the order of the strength of the geomagnetic field. It is possible that the pineal gland in higher animals and man may have shifted its electromagnetic sensitivity away from a predominantly visible-light sensitivity, characteristic of the submammalian vertebrates. In these latter creatures the pineal gland, which is only covered with a translucent layer of skin, may have had the emission of radiation to attract food as its primary purpose – a sort of candle to moths.

A radio receiver can detect and amplify the one very specific frequency of the transmitter to which it is tuned (a coherent signal) and which can be present in its environment at an intensity far below the overall background of electromagnetic signals from the power supply cables, other and unwanted radio transmitters, and atmospheric electricity from thunderstorms. A simple calculation of the spectral power density (watts per cycle of bandwidth) will show whether, or not, the reception of

The cosmic connection

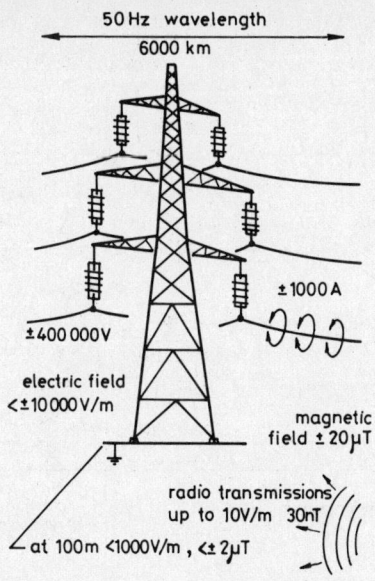

Fig. 3.3 Man Made Electromagnetic Environment It is just over 100 years since electricity generation started; 60 years since radio transmissions and 40 years since radar and telecommunications entered our environment. Like natural fields, man-made fields are limited by the physical properties of the environment; unlike natural fields, they are highly coherent and can interfere with our bio-signals.

a particular transmission is possible. The same calculation can be done in respect of the detection of electromagnetic signals by living systems.

For an organ of the size of a human pineal gland (Barr, 1979) to be able to respond co-operatively to changes in magnetic field, the following restrictions must apply. The coherent energy of the magnetic field within the volume of the pineal gland must not be less than the random thermal energy (Smith, 1985), which means that the minimum detectable magnetic field for the pineal gland is 0.24 nT or γ (2.4 μG).

The other fundamental limitation is set by the size of the quantum of magnetic flux. The strength of magnetic field which would give only a single magnetic flux quantum through a pineal gland comes out at 75 pT (0.75 μG). As this is the smaller, the energy or signal-to-noise limit is reached before the quantum limit. Honeybees (*Apis*) and birds are reported to be sensitive to magnetic changes probably less than 1 nT (1 γ, 10 μG) (Keeton, 1979), so that a limiting sensitivity calculated on the above criterion is not unreasonable both for humans with a 2-gram pineal gland and for pigeons with a 1.5-gram pineal gland. Apis should only be able to sense fields below 1 nT if all the insect is co-operatively involved in the field detection process. However, all these creatures should be quite able to detect the 'quiet' diurnal and the 'disturbed' variations of the GMF.

Experiments involving the shielding of living systems from the GMF have been carried out (Dubrov, 1978), but they are difficult and involve expensive shielding materials and techniques. In view of the extreme sensitivities discussed in the present book, it is doubtful whether many have achieved the degree of shielding necessary. Magnetic fields are very difficult to screen. A 1 mm thick shield of a high-permeability magnetic alloy will only reduce the steady field within the enclosure to about 50 nT (γ). The shielding of ELF magnetic fields presents an even greater problem; a 150 mm thickness of aluminium is required for a reasonable degree of shielding.

If the Earth's steady magnetic field is moving relative to the surface of the Earth, as has been claimed (see Chapter 11), the commonly used compensating arrangements of bar magnets or Helmholtz coils will not suffice to cancel moving fields, so that living systems would still be able to perceive them.

If the theoretical threshold for sensitivity to a magnetic field is proportional to the volume of the field sensing part of the organism, which may even be the whole of the organism, then the degree of shielding attained with high permeability magnetic alloys may still only be sufficient to screen effects from living systems up to the size of the larger eukaryotic cells 100 μm in size. Dubrov (1978) lists a wide range of effects obtained with magnetically shielded, 'in vitro' cell cultures, some of which did not appear until after many subcultures had been carried out. Plants shielded for a prolonged period from the GMF developed histological and physiological disturbances as well as peculiar tumours.

The senior writer and one of his students have found that geomagnetic changes at the surface of the Earth, and which can be synthesised in the laboratory, occurring when the dawn sunlight reaches the ionosphere, can trigger activity in plants so that they are ready for photosynthesis as soon as their dawn arrives, one and a half hours later, and so can make productive use of all their hours of daylight.

Definite alterations to the biochemistry, physiology and behaviour were found by Dubrov in a wide range of living systems ranging from insects to higher animals and man, following a high degree of prolonged total shielding. Of particular note are the physiological changes reported to occur among submarine crews who spend long periods shielded from the steady GMF by a thick steel hull and from much of the ELF by salt water. Whether those frequencies used to communicate with submerged submarines also have any physiological effects on their crews and on those who live in the vicinity of the land-based transmitters must remain a matter for debate (see chapter 10). In strategic matters, such things would be regarded as secondary to the national interest.

Equally important are the physiological changes in earth-orbiting astronauts who experience the complete cycle of variations in the GMF at each orbit of the Earth and the perturbations associated with the solar wind magnetic fields electrohydrodynamically 'frozen' into the plasma and carried along by its motion. To these effects must be added the possible consequences of altering the uniform velocity of the GMF as measured in the experiments of Charles Brooker (see Chapter 11) both in space flight and in East–West jet travel.

A number of experiments have been conducted involving persons living for prolonged periods in an underground dwelling, to some extent shielded by steel from the steady GMF and from the ELF, the soil adding to the shielding from the latter. Controls lived in a similar room with ordinary GMF conditions. Dubrov (1978) refers to some Russian work as well as the experiments on human circadian rhythms carried out by Prof. Dr Rutger Wever of the Max Planck Institute for Psychiatry in West Germany and which have been running for more than 25 years. In the course of these investigations involving human circadian rhythms, he (Wever, 1973, 1985) found quite unexpectedly that the human circadian systems had a remarkably high sensitivity to weak ELF fields. This was not sought directly but was found rather as a by-product of other work. He writes,

> Originally, the relevant experiments had been performed only in order to evaluate the dynamic properties of human circadian rhythms; and the ELF field had been applied only as an appropriate tool. It was subsequently, after the originally asked questions had been answered, that, in return, the properties of the tool became of increasing interest.

All his experiments were carried out in one of two underground isolation units. These comprised a living room with a bed, a kitchen and a bathroom. A double-door lock connected and isolated the control room from each unit. The units were constructed with double walls giving sound insulation; one unit also had 5 layers of continuous soft iron shielding to reduce the GMF. Electrodes and coils, invisible to the subjects, enabled any electric or magnetic field, steady or alternating, to be applied within the environment of the rooms. Over nearly 20 years, 325 subjects were tested; most subjects were isolated singly, but there were some group experiments. The period of an experiment was usually 4 to 6 weeks, but some lasted up to 3 months. Nearly all subjects felt positively well during the isolation and 80 per cent spontaneously asked for a repeat. The most relevant effect observed was the field-induced shortening of the circadian rhythm and systematic alterations in all the rhythm parameters.

In a constant environment without clues as to the local time, the sleep/wake activity and the deep body temperature periodicities tend to increase, for example, from a 24-hour day to a 25-hour day. It is remarkable that the human circadian rhythm was found to be insensitive to changes in the level of illumination, from total darkness to 1500 lux whether under voluntary or involuntary control. Thus, the dark/light cycle does not have the ability to function as a human *zeitgeber*.

In a number of cases, the phenomenon of internal desynchronisation occurred when the free-running circadian rhythm would abruptly alter its periodicity but, with the deep body (rectal) temperature retaining a 25-hour periodicity. This tendency was greater in subjects over 40 to 45 years of age than in younger subjects. Changes in the sleep/wake cycle of exactly half or twice the periodicity of the rectal temperature cycle were termed 'apparent desynchronisation' because the internal coupling was as great as in the case of full internal synchronisation with its 25-hour sleep/wake cycle. 'Apparent desynchronisation' is not related to the 10 Hz field (see below) or to the age of the subjects. Only with internal desynchronisation, where the different cycles are not in an integral relationship, does the 10 Hz field have an influence (Wever, 1985).

Early on, he was able to describe the circadian system in terms of a mathematical model. To check this out experimentally he needed a suitable stimulus to control the circadian rhythms. In various experiments with animal species, he found that regular changes in the intensity of light (electromagnetic radiation of frequency around 6×10^{14} Hz) was the most effective external stimulus. However, the human circadian rhythm was found to be remarkably resistant to attempts at using light as a timing stimulus (*zeitgeber*). This implied that a different stimulus was triggering the circadian rhythm in humans; this he found to be weak ELF fields. He was able to use as his 'standard' triggering field, a vertical electric field of 2.5 V/m (the field that would be developed by three torch batteries over a distance equal to the height of a man). This was applied between the floor and ceiling of the rooms in the underground units as a square wave at a frequency of 10 Hz. The rise time for the sharp edge of the square wave was less than 1 microsecond so that enough current would be induced to flow through the capacitance between floor and ceiling to give a small pulse of magnetic field. He considered that the possibility of this having an effect on the subjects could not be excluded.

The continuously operating, weak, 10 Hz square-wave electric field was able to prevent, or reduce, internal desynchronisation and affect the autonomous periods. When it was operated periodically, it could exert a *zeitgeber* influence and entrain a free-running rhythm into synchronism. The sleep/wake cycles and the deep body temperature cycles could be synchronised simultaneously to the weak 10 Hz field at a periodicity of 23.5 hours per day, for which there are no known natural or artificial *zeitgebers* in the environment.

Wever also reports preliminary animal experiments which showed that animal circadian rhythm had a similar sensitivity to weak ELF fields. It was noted that specially trained birds were able to differentiate between a 10 Hz field and a 9 Hz field. Evidence such as the above strongly supports the likelihood of interactions between coherent frequencies, circadian rhythms and their entrainment.

The electric field strength used in Wever's experiments was 2.5 V/m. The *natural* environmental fields at the corresponding frequencies have field strengths one thousand times weaker, of the order of 2.5 mV/m, although the man-made environmental fields are much greater. This is not necessarily a cause for concern because living systems are generally non-linear in their responses to electromagnetic fields, thus these thousand-fold differences in electric field strength may not be of any significance; if both exceed the threshold for the *zeitgeber* effects, both will be effective.

Jacobi (1979) found an effect on thrombocytes which could only be observed with 10 kHz 'sferics' after the 10 kHz had been modulated with the ELF frequency of 10 Hz. Previously drawn blood samples which were subsequently exposed to the same field did not show any effect, so it was the living subject that was responding. Furthermore, when the heads of these subjects were shielded by a cover of copper gauze during exposure to the field, no effect on the blood samples could be observed. The conclusion was that the head contains the field-sensitive region (it also contains the pineal gland).

In experiments on visual acuity (Cremer-Bartels *et al.*, 1983), a specific enzyme concerned with the synthesis of melatonin could be shown to react to weak magnetic fields. Melatonin is also linked with the generation of circadian rhythms. Melatonin and the enzymes responsible for its synthesis from serotonin have been identified in mammalian pineal tissue (Ganong, 1969). The likely involvement of the pineal in electromagnetic field effects has already been suggested. Melatonin has recently been implicated in jet-lag as a result of research at the University of Surrey by Dr Josephine Arendt (1986), from where in recent tests a group of volunteers travelled to San Francisco and stayed there for a fortnight. Before returning, half took melatonin and half took a placebo. After returning, their patterns of sleep and their mental and physical alertness were studied; the results showed that none of those who had been given melatonin had suffered from jet-lag. These results may show that taking melatonin reduces the body's need for synthesising it, and hence removes the *zeitgeber* effect of the changing ELF fields, which Wever has found to be effective in humans, during the return flight.

A recent newspaper reported described an unprecedented number of young suicides in Norway's northernmost province, near the Soviet border (*The Times*, 12 September 1987). There were suggestions that a shortage of serotonin in the brain, which appears to run in families, was correlated with the probability of suicide. However, it is also worth noting the possibility of two further biological stressors — the area may have been exposed to electromagnetic radiation from across the border, and that the geomagnetic field variations are greater in the northern latitudes.

The spectrum of the earth-ionosphere cavity resonance (Schumann Resonance) covers the 1 Hz to 30 Hz region (König, 1979). The 8 Hz component has been regarded as particularly important and generally beneficial to living systems; it also coincides with the brain's alpha rhythm (8–12 Hz). There is an equivalent power flux density of the order of 10^{-10} W/m^2 Hz in this natural Earth radiation (Gendrin and Stefant, 1964), which is greater than the threshold sensitivity for a 70 kg man and therefore strong enough to act as a potential *zeitgeber*.

Satellite measurements show that the radiation from the world's 50 Hz and 60 Hz power lines influence the magnetosphere more than 100 km above the Earth's surface (Luette *et al.*, 1979). This is another version of the 'Luxembourg Effect' which was discovered between the wars. When radio signals passed through the ionosphere above this very powerful long-wave-band radio transmitter, its transmissions became superimposed due to non-linearities in the ionosphere characteristics.

For some years there have been reports on other changes in the ionosphere, particularly that a hole in the ozone layer in the upper atmosphere has been growing for some years over the Antarctic region; as an indicator of other electromagnetic changes in the ionosphere, there could well be world-wide implications. In September 1987, scientists from 24 countries gathered in Montreal to sign an historic treaty entitled the *Vienna Convention on the Preservation of the Ozone Layer*, aimed at reducing damage to it. The ozone layer surrounds the Earth and protects living things from much harmful solar radiation, especially in the ultraviolet part of the spectrum. Scientists fear that increased penetration of such radiation would lead to a rise in the incidence of skin cancer, cataracts and a reduction in the strength of the body's immune system defences. Concern grew when it was observed that the ozone layer over the Antarctic was showing dramatic seasonal variations due, it was suspected, to the continual build-up in the atmosphere of man-made chlorofluorocarbons (CFCs) given off chiefly from aerosol spray propellants, plastic foam, and venting refrigerating plants to the atmosphere.

Research using infra-red detection for simple halogen compounds reported, and then confirmed (Farmer *et al.*, 1987) that CFCs were mainly responsible. In the first international control of a chemical emission, the Vienna Convention signatories agreed to a world cut in the consumption of CFCs of 50 per cent by 1999. It has been subsequently suggested this will be too little too late; also that there have always been wide variations in the ozone layer, but that the computers processing the data were not programmed to look for it. Following the discovery of a similar hole over the Arctic, a conference in March 1989 in London called for an international ban on CFCs by the year 2000. The implications are critical for living systems, which appear to be able to make use of all coherent frequencies from the ultra-violet downwards.

Dr Robin Baker, of Manchester University, has researched and written extensively on the sensing of magnetic fields by man and other primates (Baker, 1985a) and the possibilities for navigation and direction finding which this sensing ability opens up (Baker, 1984 1985b). He recounts how the idea of animals having an ability to sense magnetic fields and navigate by the Earth's magnetic field was ridiculed when suggested, in 1855, by a German scientist, Dr von Middendorf.

The location of magnetite deposits in bacteria and in the bone of birds, mammals and man suggests that an electromechanical torque sensor is involved and that the combination forms a magnetic compass. It has now been shown that bone is not piezoelectric as had been previously thought, but that the electromechanical potentials in bone arise through an electro-streaming process involving ions flowing through cavities. In living systems there are additional physical mechanisms which could give the extremes of electromagnetic sensitivity possessed by living systems when their regulatory systems permit, or when they malfunction. The presence of ferromagnetic materials in living systems may have direction-determining functions and Baker's work supports the idea that man and other organisms have a basic ability to sense weak magnetic fields. The whole area of magnetite biomineralisation and magnetoreception in organisms and man has recently been comprehensively evaluated (Kirschrink, Jones and MacFadden, 1985).

Dubrov (1978) notes that not only does the GMF exert its effects through a weak action, or extremely low energy threshold mechanism, but that it is one of the main causes of the rhythmicity in natural phenomena and of the dissymmetry which underlies the essential left-handed (laevorotatory) or right-handed (dextrorotatory) characteristics of all asymmetrical chemical structures, which must exist in one of two mirror-image forms, and whose effects on living systems can be very different.

Dubrov (1978) also quotes another Russian, Trincher, as stating that, 'water inside the cell is in a state of maximum order – in a state attainable in non-living systems only at absolutely zero temperature'. He discusses the possibility that the sensitivity of living organisms is related to biological superconductivity at the ordinary temperatures of living systems, a possibility which has been suggested by a number of writers (Cope, 1971, 1978; Ahmed et al., 1975; Smith, 1985). However, Professor Fröhlich has pointed out that it is not necessary to postulate biological superconductivity *per se* because, at a more fundamental level of physics, both the Josephson Effect in superconductivity and the near-quantum sensitive responses of living systems to coherent oscillations and electromagnetic fields can be accounted for by the fundamental quantised nature of the magnetic field (Fröhlich, 1984, 1985). (This is quite distinct from the recently discovered high temperature superconducting ceramics.) In biological systems any ambient temperature superconductivity is more likely to give rise to anomalous magnetic effects because the size of the biological cell is small compared with the Debye length and the coherence length of any such effects (Smith, 1985).

The Josephson Effect, which can occur in superconducting systems, but which does not depend on the presence of superconductivity – only the ability of the system to respond to the quantum of magnetic flux – does offer a possible physical connection between living systems and the weak electromagnetic fields of the cosmos in which they have their existence.

CHAPTER 4

Human biology and electromagnetic fields

> One must keep an open mind and admit that in Nature, the absurd
> – according to our theories – may be possible.
>
> Claude Bernard (1813–78)

This chapter tries to show how, and where, physics and electronics must get involved with biology and biochemistry in describing the structure, function and sensitivities of biological systems in general and Electromagnetic Man in particular. It assumes a reasonable knowledge of the various scientific disciplines. The layman may need to refer to Chapter 2, the Glossary and possibly some of the basic scientific texts cited in the references but a complete understanding of this chapter is not absolutely essential to appreciate the succeeding chapters. A summary of the essentials is given at the end of this chapter.

The serious application of theoretical physics to the problems of biology and medicine began in Paris some two decades ago. Professor Herbert Fröhlich, now Emeritus Professor of Theoretical Physics at the University of Liverpool, had been asked to give a physicist's view of biology (Fröhlich, 1969). Although what he had to say probably horrified the biologists, it delighted the physicists, as can be seen from the reported discussions which followed his talk. The importance of this meeting was that it first raised some very fundamental questions concerning the application of physics to biology.

In 1973 one of us (Dr Cyril Smith) started measuring the dielectric properties of biological materials in general and enzymes in particular and was co-operating closely with Professor Fröhlich. It was then clear that, from the point of view of theoretical physics, biological materials function in a most systematic manner even though they form extremely complicated chemical systems.

A common feature of the chemical reactions in the living cell is that they take place faster than would be the case if the reagents were just brought together in a test tube. It is well known in chemistry that certain substances, catalysts, can speed up the rate at which a chemical reaction proceeds merely by being present. They are not used up in the course of the chemical reaction. Catalysts of biological origin are termed 'enzymes'. The many chemical reactions that the living cell must perform in order to support its life and activity are controlled by enzyme catalysts. The rate at which the chemical reaction proceeds depends upon the concentrations of the enzyme and the molecule whose chemical reaction the enzyme very specifically controls, known as the 'substrate'. There are typically 3000 enzyme systems in a living cell (Smith, 1971).

Etymologically, the word 'enzyme' relates to yeasts. Historically, the study of yeasts gave the knowledge of the properties of enzymes. The production of wine by yeast fermentation emerges with the dawn of recorded civilisation from the East. There is an Egyptian painting of grape treaders under an arbour of vines from the tomb of an official who died in the fifteenth century BC. But it was not until Napoleon III, in 1863, asked Louis Pasteur to find out why so much wine went bad in transit that the role of oxygen in allowing the growth of vinegar bacteria was discovered. However, in Pasteur's day it was fashionable to think of a 'vital force' as only present in living organisms and as necessary for the synthesis of organic compounds. It needed Buchner's subsequent demonstration that sugar could be fermented by a yeast extract from which all living yeast cells had been removed for the way to the study of the chemistry and physics of enzymes to be laid open.

Detailed analysis of the chemical structure of enzymes revealed that all enzymes are proteins. Proteins are made up from a daisy-chain-like string of amino acids, of which there are twenty different commonly occurring types. Building proteins from amino acids is like building words and sentences from the twenty-six letters of the alphabet. Short chains of amino acids are referred to as polypeptides; when the chains have a length exceeding 50 to 100 amino acids, giving them molecular weights greater than 500 to 10,000, they are called proteins. By this stage, not only do the proteins have a specific sequence of amino acids along the daisy-chain, but the chain itself will take on a specific three-dimensional arrangement, with some parts flexible, others rigid, as determined by interactions between the different and adjacent parts of the chain. Molecular structure is very closely related to function.

Molecular biologists have established the detailed structure of many macromolecules and found that enzymes possess an active site where the specific chemical reaction catalysed by the enzyme takes place at a greatly enhanced rate. There is nothing in the chemical structure of enzymes to explain their enormous catalytic power, and there is no simple connection between molecular structure and enzymatic activity.

The specificity of enzyme action, which is not confined to living systems, has often been modelled after the mechanical 'lock and key' principle, but this still leaves many features unexplained, such as how the enzyme 'key' can find the substrate 'lock' and fit into it without jamming. Perhaps the 'key' can 'see' the light coming through the 'keyhole'.

When Fröhlich (1978) considered such a system in terms of theoretical physics, he represented it by two highly polarisable dielectrics capable of giant dipole oscillations which were separated by a distance greater than their dimensions. He showed that there would be a strong interaction if both oscillated at precisely the same frequency. For elastically bound particles of molecular dimensions he estimated this frequency to be of the order of 10^{13} Hz (corresponding to a wavelength of 30 μm). This is close to the frequency corresponding to the mean thermal energy which, at an ambient temperature of 27°C (300 K), comes to 6.25×10^{12} Hz.

He considers that from the point of view of physics, it would be naive to try to understand the catalytic role of enzymes in terms of their ground state molecular structures only and to neglect their excited states. High catalytic power requires a reduction of activation energies. Active biological systems are far from being in equilibrium. Although through the chemical structure of its active site an enzyme acts on its relevant substrate in a specific chemical way once the two are attached, i.e. in short-range contact, there is also the possibility of a specific long-range attraction between the enzyme and its substrate. These two possibilities are not exclusive but rather they are complementary.

In terms of electronics, an enzyme-substrate system can also be considered as an 'amplifier', if one regards the input signal as the amount of enzyme present and the output signal as the amount of reaction product formed per minute. The substrate consumption would be analogous to the current drain from the battery and the battery voltage analogous to the chemical potential of the particular reaction. Such an amplifying system might have a gain as high as 10^9 to 10^{10}. This can be deduced either from the enhancement of the chemical reaction rates or from the activation energy of the enzyme system. The input/output characteristics of such high-gain amplifiers are solely determined by any feedback arrangements provided from the output back to the input; the gain is unimportant so long as it is large, as it clearly is in this case. Such a feedback path or control-loop would form a regulatory system for controlling the amount of the particular reaction product and set up the condition of homeostasis. This is the point of divide between the chemistry of living and non-living systems.

It was the search for a physical characteristic common to most biological materials that led Professor Fröhlich to examine their dielectric properties (Fröhlich, 1975). The term 'dielectric' was coined by Michael Faraday in 1838 (Faraday, 1838). The simplest description of a dielectric would be to say that a dielectric is everything which is not a metal. The particular physical properties which are the concern of dielectric studies are the behaviour of non-metallic materials when subjected to electric fields, static or alternating.

The relevance of dielectrics to biological cells and tissues will be clear as soon as it is realised that there is a very high electric field across live biological membranes. This field is of the order of 10^7 V/m (ten million volts per metre), far greater than anything likely to be experienced by a person, even in the vicinity of overhead power lines. This field is strong enough to align all the macromolecules within a biological membrane relative to this field direction, thereby increasing their mutual interactions and their non-linear dielectric responses to eternal electromagnetic fields. Fröhlich modelled this situation mathematically in terms of oscillating dielectric dipoles. A dipole is the combination of a positive charge and a negative charge spatially separated, such as might occur on the surface of a macromolecule. It is the electrical equivalent of the magnetic compass needle, where the spatially separated North and South poles form a magnetic dipole. Fröhlich showed that non-linear, coherent excitations of these dielectric dipoles were theoretically possible and that this could lead to long-range interactions on a very frequency-selective basis, essential if one is to have a mechanism for the selective remote control of the chemistry going on in a particular cell of the body by some distant organ which has an overseeing function for that body's activities, or to provide the organism with sensors for external fields.

It is important to remember the duality which exists between chemical structure and a coherent frequency. Chemical bonds can be identified by measuring their characteristic vibrational, rotational and librational frequencies; without this duality, chemical analysis by spectroscopy just would not work. As a corollary to this, there must be as many refinements of observable frequency spectra as there are chemical structures. The electric field in biological membranes is sufficient to make the protein macromolecules in the membrane behave in a non-linear dielectric manner. These non-linearities could still further complicate the observed spectrum of frequencies. An array of dipoles ordered by the membrane field will show interactions between electrical and mechanical displacements, acoustic or surface tension waves, like the duality between a loudspeaker and a microphone.

At distances up to the thickness of a typical biological membrane

(10 nm) from a single electronic charge, its electrostatic field will be comparable to the cell membrane field, which provides a bias field ensuring that electric and mechanical forces arising from charge oscillations on the membrane will actually be at the frequency of the oscillation and not at twice that frequency. Two electron/positive-ion pairs on opposite sides of a biological membrane have an electrostatic energy of attraction greater than the thermal energy at 310 K (37°C), so they will remain stable against the dissipation forces of thermal diffusion.

The much-measured enzyme lysozyme is a compact globular protein with dimensions about $3 \times 3 \times 4$ nm. Its biological purpose is to attack invading cells by dissolving their membranes away. The whole of this enzyme and any substrate which may be in the active site would clearly be in a high-field, non-linear dielectric region due to all the electric charges present within the enzyme molecule and on the membrane of the living cell being attacked (lysed). An enzyme interacting with its substrate is the simplest component part of a living, working biological system but its role as a component in the regulatory system is often neglected. The phenomena and problems outlined in this section show the degree of complexity and sophistication present in these biochemical tools of the living cell.

Many enzymes can now be purchased with the biochemical preparation already done well enough for many purposes. They come, in vacuum compatible form, as freeze-dried (lyophilised) powders, rather like an instant coffee. As such, these preparations may, on measurement, give a value of dielectric constant (relative permittivity) little greater than unity, indicating few dipoles. Once the powder is allowed to become moist and the humidity exceeds a few per cent, the values of the permittivity and loss (conductivity) start to increase. At high values of humidity these values may exceed a million in the lower part of the frequency spectrum (Rosen, 1963). Dielectric measurements on aqueous materials are well known to be susceptible to errors arising from polarisation (the collection of charges) at the measuring electrodes. However, there are experimental techniques whereby such electrode effects can be eliminated (Shaw, 1942).

'Dirty effects'

There are some scientific advantages in not having air-conditioned laboratories and in working in a 'dirty old town'. In this context it is essential to study all laboratory artifacts which may arise and to understand them. Experience suggests that results from measurements on living systems which do not show evidence of 'biological variability' most probably represent instrumental artifacts.

In 1922 Flemming studied the effect of a substance that was later known as the enzyme lysozyme on an airborne coccus that came drifting into his laboratory; this led to the discovery of bacteriolytic enzymes. At the beginnings of nuclear magnetic resonance (NMR), as Professor Fröhlich often recounted, Bloembergen, in 1949, managed to detect NMR signals from Gorter's original 1936 sample of lithium fluoride with which Gorter had failed to detect NMR; this was because 'The Bloembergen Dirty Effect', as it became known, showed up the important point which Gorter had missed, namely that paramagnetic impurities could shorten NMR relaxation times so they became measurable. Looking at the lack of progress in the understanding of the ways in which living systems make use of electromagnetic fields and frequency, it seems that too much electromagnetic power has been used on too pure biological materials and, as we shall see later, with too little biological stress and too little patience to wait for the coherence time to elapse. Fortunately, many things in science are still not predictable.

From micro-dielectrophoresis experiments, the late Professor Herbert Pohl showed that the preference of a wide range of cell types for attracting polar particles in their vicinity is maximal at or near the time of the division of the cell nucleus (mitosis) and he attributed this to electrical oscillatory radiofrequency phenomena (Pohl, 1983). Because the polar particles used were probably also piezoelectric, these experiments may not differentiate between electric and acoustic oscillations. However, since the particles were counted at or near highly polar cell membranes where the electric and acoustic fields are equivalent, this is of no great consequence; but it would be interesting for this experiment to be repeated with high-permittivity particles that were not piezoelectric as this would separate the ranges of two possible types of coherent oscillation.

Non-thermal resonant effects have also been found in the growth of yeast cultures exposed to 42 GHz microwaves. The result was a biphasic dependence on frequency, with resonance bands of 8 MHz full-width-at-half-maximum (Grundler *et al.*, 1983; Grundler, 1985). It appears that the frequency of 8 MHz is a rather fundamental one for yeasts.

At a conference held at Nottingham University, England, to mark the retirement of Professor D.D.Eley in 1980, some raw data from dielectrophoresis measurements was shown by Professor H.A.Pohl. This contained an anomaly at about 2 kHz. Dielectrophoresis in this context involves the collection of biological cells from their suspension in highly de-ionised water or a non-ionic, isotonic medium or nutrient. The cells form as 'pearl chains' at the tips of point electrodes which give the necessary non-uniform field. Since the dielectrophoretic forces depend on the square of the electric field, they can be observed using alternating electric fields and thus distinguished from the forces of electrophoresis which are observed in steady electric fields. The other important parameter which determines the magnitude of the dielectrophoretic force is the difference between the permittivity of the cell and its surrounding medium (Pohl, 1978).

The appearance of an anomaly at a frequency of 2 kHz was very suggestive of a nuclear magnetic resonance interaction involving protons precessing in the geomagnetic field. This was confirmed and extended (Jafary-Asl et al., 1983; Aarholt et al., 1988). The simplest macroscopic demonstration of this phenomenon is obtained by setting up some 'pearl chains' by dielectrophoresis and then, with an externally applied magnet, slowly sweeping the ambient magnetic field through the proton NMR condition for the frequency being used to form the 'pearl chains'. Enough of the cells will repel each other to break up the chain formations. This can only happen if there has been a drop in the permittivity of these cells below that of their surroundings. This must be due to an increased lattice interaction of the magnetically resonant protons. That such a lattice interaction effect is possible may be demonstrated by measuring the permittivity of something as inorganic as the proton-conducting glass of a pH meter under proton NMR conditions.

The proton NMR condition represents a very sharply defined resonance condition whereby energy can be inserted into a living system in a very specific manner. When a bacterium was grown under proton NMR conditions, twice as many cells of half the size were obtained, although the total cell mass remained unchanged. In experiments on bovine eye lenses, it was found that subcapsular cataracts located in the posterior cortex of the lens developed particularly well when the microwaves were modulated so that the modulation frequency satisfied proton NMR conditions in the ambient magnetic field (Smith et al., 1987; Aarholt et al., 1988). In this case the microwaves would be merely acting as a carrier able to deposit the NMR frequency as the microwave modulation signal within the tissue, where the non-linearities would demodulate it. Since many microwave oscillators contain magnets, a technician moving about in the vicinity of such an oscillator would often be satisfying the necessary resonance conditions within his or her body tissues and thus increasing the risk of cataract formation or other disease.

Once the possibility of magnetic resonance phenomena in living systems is appreciated, it is clear that it could also be a source of highly coherent radiation. If a magnetic field pulse is applied to a living system, as in stimulated bone healing, the electric field induced by the changing magnetic field process can excite the spinning protons (or other particles having spin) and stimulate an increase in the proton population of a higher energy state; if the magnetic field is then reduced relatively slowly to zero in a time that is short compared with the spin relaxation times, the protons will not be stimulated to make the downwards transition back to the ground state. While the excited spin states relax in their own good time, all the tissues will be subjected to highly coherent spin relaxation frequencies containing all the information relating to the body chemistry which is contained in an NMR spectrum and hence its state of health or disease. Protons can also 'swop' energy states in such conditions by what is known as the spin-exchange process (Smith *et al.*, 1987).

Electrical phenomena in living systems

The history of the growth of an awareness of the various interactions of electricity with animals and man is described in the earlier chapters. The previous sections of this chapter indicate some ways in which individual cells may communicate electromagnetically. Because the high attenuation of water severely restricts the propagation of frequencies between the microwave and infrared parts of the spectrum, organisms need alternative paths for long-range communication. These are provided by chemical messengers (hormones) which provide a sort of postal system, and nerve cells which provide a 'hard-wired', telegraph network. Coherent oscillations along any chain of cells which have set themselves up to oscillate at precisely the same frequency can provide temporary, volatile, 'line-of-sight' communications networks like a 'bucket-brigade' or chain of semaphor signallers.

The basis of the body's 'hard-wired' telecommunications network is the excitable nerve cell. This is stimulated to give its action potential by depolarising the cell membrane with a destabilising pulse which exceeds the thermal energy of 25 mV. A current then flows externally to the cell; simultaneously, a net positive ion current flows into the cell through the membrane. This gives rise to a potential gradient around the cell which can be detected by external electrodes and can also trigger other excitable cells into producing their action-potential pulses. When the cell re-polarises, there is a positive ion current flow outwards from the cell membrane, giving a current in the reverse direction. It may happen that one cell triggers a whole group of nearby cells simultaneously (synchronous depolarisation); alternatively, a chain reaction may proceed through a group of cells as each cell triggers its adjacent cells (asynchronous depolarisation) until all the cells have been depolarised. In nerve cells the depolarisation may commence at one end of the long cell and then proceed as a travelling wave along the length of the cell.

Nerve fibres vary considerably in their size and the related velocity of the depolarisation wave. The larger nerve fibres in sensory and motor nerves are about 20 μm in diameter and have a conduction velocity of about 120 m/s, about a tenth of the velocity of sound in water. The smallest nerve fibres are of the order of 1 μm in diameter and give a conduction velocity of the order of 1 m/s.

As most bioelectric potentials are recorded from living organisms using extracellular electrodes, the results obtained represent the sum of the action potentials of many cells depolarising synchronously and asynchronously and will depend upon the number of cells involved, their shape and the type of stimulation applied, if any. It is important to remember that Nature provides these electrical potentials for a biological purpose, not merely to provide convenient waveforms for our research or clinical indicators for the body's state of health or disease. They are also a part of a homeostatic (regulatory) system and this may be perturbed by the application of measuring instruments.

Nature makes use of electricity in many other simple and elegant ways. A good account of these is to be found in the book by Becker and Selden (1985). Becker attributes his luck in his pioneering research on electrically stimulated bone fracture healing and tissue regeneration to his having 'spent far too much time on a few incurable patients whom no one else wanted, trying to find out how our ignorance had failed them'.

The remarkable ability of the salamander to regenerate lost limbs appears to depend on electrical effects. The skin produces a potential difference and a current flow around the injury location. Injury potentials occur widely and have even been detected in plant tissues. Frogs do not produce such large currents as salamanders and do not regenerate limbs, but even in the frog the development of bone, muscle and cartilage can be enhanced by implanting a minute electrical battery to enhance the injury potentials. Reversal of the battery polarity causes tissue degeneration.

This capability has not been completely lost in the progression of human evolution. Dr Cynthia Illingworth (1974) has over many years found that children with amputated fingertips are able to regenerate a new fingertip, even having the same fingerprint, provided that the injury is not sutured but just dressed and kept sterile so that the natural electrical potentials can establish themselves. Dr Tony Barker (Barker *et al.*, 1981; Barker and Foulds, 1983), using a vibrating probe measuring technique, found that the magnitude of the currents around wounds and their variation in time were identical to those produced by the amputated salamander.

Likewise, Dr Bjorn Nordenström has found out how to replace the injury potentials which should appear in the vicinity of tumour tissue by inserting electrodes, one into the tumour and the other into the surrounding tissue; he then applies the appropriate voltages from an external source. He has found that the electrical circuit for the resulting currents flows from an electrode, through the tissue to the capillaries which it enters through ion-permeable pores and thence through the blood plasma to capillaries in the vicinity of the counter electrode, from which it returns to the battery. He has had some remarkable successes with his technique in the treatment of inoperable tumours. He has written an account of his researches in a book which he has had to publish himself (Nordström, 1983); a short report of his work has also recently appeared (Taubes, 1986).

The mechanisms whereby the cell layers develop within an embryo to form limbs and organs are electrically controlled. Nerve cell growth cones migrate parallel to an electric field to innervate their target organs and can sprout outgrowths in fields of the order of $10\,V/m$ ($300\,\mu V$ across the cell width). Disaggregated muscle cells align themselves perpendicular to an electric field, thus maintaining the appropriate orientation of nerve to muscle cells.

Jaffe has investigated the possibility of electrophoresis taking place along potential gradients on cell membranes and considers that molecular separation is a possible mechanism (Jaffe, 1977). Working on the development of the egg of a brown seaweed (*Fucus*), Jaffe and his colleagues found that light triggered the flow of minute ion currents into the cell; these included a small component of calcium (Ca^{++}) ions which has subsequently been found to be an important controlling agent in living systems. In this case, the Ca^{++} ions control the asymmetrical development of the embryo so that the 'holdfast' root-structure develops on the dark side of the embryo where its anchoring rock will be. They also report patterns of ionic current through *Drosophila* follicles and eggs (Overall and Jaffe, 1985).

The eggs of the silk moth pump steady currents which function as a kind of self-electrophoresis. Once the embryo has grown to eight cells, seven become nurse cells and pump essential, negatively charged molecules into the egg cell. In frogs and fish, the developing egg cells are also electrically polarised during early stages of their development. During the contraction of the cytoplasm in cell division a current, which may be carried by Ca^{++} ions, enters along the region in which the furrow will form between the two new daughter cells a few minutes later.

The egg of the sea urchin makes use of electrical changes within a millisecond of the fusion of the first sperm to arrive in order to repel competing sperms, which would be fatal to it. This gives protection until the fertilised cell has had time to construct a protective membrane. By contrast, an amoeba will interpret a nearby current-measuring, vibrating probe as prey and move out a pseudopod in its direction.

The parasite *Leischmania*, which infests the mouth and gut of the blood-sucking sand-fly and is thereby passed on to cattle and humans, attaches itself to the walls of the sand-fly's gut with an amoeboid process which forms at the end of its cilium. It will not readily attach to the surface of a petri dish during 'in-vitro' culture; however, it will readily attach itself to scratches in the surface of a polystyrene petri dish (Molyneux et al., 1987). We found that if the surface of the petri dish is charged by electron bombardment, attachment may be enhanced. A preliminary explanation for this parasite regarding a negatively charged surface as a good place to take up residence is that the charge mimics the charge on the membrane of the live cells of its host and possibly gives it the correct microwave or infra-red reflection characteristics.

Theoretical limits to Man's electromagnetic sensitivities

The following is the non-mathematical description of a method of deriving a theoretical lower limit for the strength of an electromagnetic field or the power level of radiation at or above which any co-operatively acting living system may react.

(a) Take the equation for the energy per unit volume of the appropriate field;
(b) multiply this by that volume of the biological system which is co-operatively involved in detecting the radiation; assume that this volume is the apparent volume of the organism sensing the field;
(c) equate the energy calculated above to the ambient thermal energy (kT). This is equivalent to assuming that the system is operating with a signal-to-noise ratio of unity, i.e. that the signal is only just as strong as the background noise (Bell, 1960; Smith et al., 1987).
(d) the only unknown in the equation is the strength of the field which satisfies the conditions imposed for calculating the minimum field needed to trigger a response.

Just as radio-telescopes have large dishes to collect radiation, the larger the co-operatively acting biological system, the weaker the field which can be detected by it, as shown in Table 4.1. If the whole of a 70-kg man is, in effect, the antenna for the detection of an electric field, the above criteria would be met with a threshold electric field of 8 $\mu V/m$. This is of the order of the sensitivity of the most sensitive of the multiple-allergy patients we have tested (see Chapter 6), but it only occurred while the patients were in a reacting allergic condition. It corresponds to an incident power density of less than a picowatt per square metre.

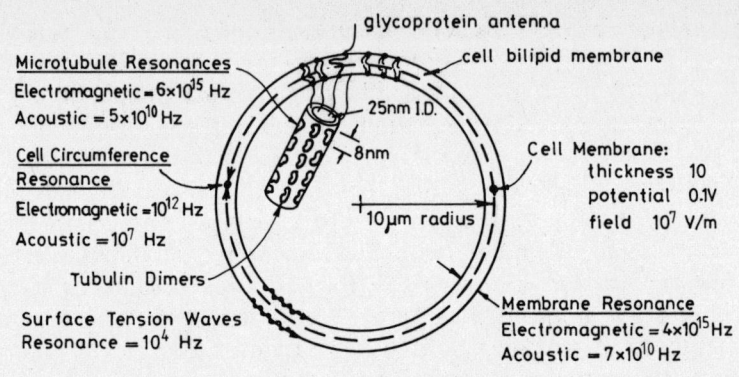

Fig. 4.1 *Resonances in an 'Ideal' Biological Cell* Like waves in a pond, the biological cell has its own resonances, and Q's. This figure is a physical model of an 'ideal' biological cell showing its possible resonances. Since most biomolecules are 'electrical dipoles' they will behave like microphones turning acoustic waves into electrical waves, and like loud-speakers turning electrical waves into acoustic waves so, the whole cell will act as an oscillating interacting entity.

Labels in figure:
- Microtubule Resonances: Electromagnetic = 6×10^{15} Hz, Acoustic = 5×10^{10} Hz
- Cell Circumference Resonance: Electromagnetic = 10^{12} Hz, Acoustic = 10^{7} Hz
- Surface Tension Waves Resonance = 10^{4} Hz
- Tubulin Dimers
- glycoprotein antenna
- cell bilipid membrane
- 25 nm I.D.
- 8 nm
- 10 μm radius
- Cell Membrane: thickness 10, potential 0.1 V, field 10^{7} V/m
- Membrane Resonance: Electromagnetic = 4×10^{15} Hz, Acoustic = 7×10^{10} Hz

Table 4.1 Electric and magnetic fields within the volume of the biological system which represent an energy of kT at 310 K

	Single cells			Hen's egg	Man
Size of system	1 μm	10 μm	100 μm	70 g	70 kg
Threshold (electric field)	3 kV/m	100 V/m	3 V/m	250 μV/m	8 μV/m
Threshold (magnetic field)	100 μT	3 μT	100 nT	9 pT	300 fT
Threshold (Poynting vector)	200 kW/m^2	80 W/m^2	80 mW/m^2	600 pW/m^2	1 pW/m^2
Fields for 1 flux quantum	500 μT	5 μT	500 nT	0.7 pT	0.7 fT

The lowest electric field that has been observed to evoke a response from certain fish is $1\,\mu V/m$ (Bullock, 1977), which is of the same order as the most extreme sensitivities of allergic subjects. Comparing this with the observed radiofrequency emission levels from yeast cells ($\simeq 0.1\,\mu V/\mu m$) and assuming that there is nothing particularly unique about yeasts in this respect, then it is clear that fish will have no problem in locating food, particularly if it happens to be some electrically 'noisy' plankton. The same ability might have applied to man in primitive conditions and may still be possessed by aboriginal peoples. Scouts and hunters in the bush and jungle may also unwittingly make use of it.

One of the common features of living systems in general is their ability to sense minute changes in the environment, and this in the presence of much larger irrelevant signals (Gamow and Harris, 1972). Such an ability is clearly to the advantage of both predator and prey alike. Living systems have many biosensors which are near to being quantum sensitive (Smith, 1986). To trigger a nerve impulse from a single quantum event requires an amplifier with a gain of the order of 10^9 to 10^{10} (this order of gain is also a feature of the reaction enhancement of an enzyme system). The characteristics of such an amplifier would be determined by its feedback network. If this goes open-circuit, then any signal above a threshold will give saturation, that is a 'panic reaction'. If the gain and phase-shifts at some frequency are correct, the amplifier will cease to amplify and will start to oscillate at that frequency. This behaviour is consistent with the definition of allergy as 'the failure of a regulatory system', and is an appropriate subject for the application of modern control theory, in order to measure the stability of a subject's regulatory systems – that is to determine how healthy that person really is.

By way of summarising this chapter, it may be said that enzymes enable and control the biochemistry of living systems and that there are about 3000 different enzymes in each cell. Electromagnetic phenomena are important for regulation even at this basic level of cell biochemistry. When one considers the biological cell, the electric field across a cell membrane is a good indicator that the cell is alive, when its electromagnetic activities may include the control of its enzymes to do its biochemical 'house-keeping' and information gathering or 'stock-taking'. It is likely that all electromagnetic frequencies from the ultra-violet to the life-time of the cell are involved in a highly coherent manner. Because many of the biomolecules are themselves electrically charged, acoustic vibrations and electrical vibrations are equivalent and interchangeable, the only difference being in their velocity of propagation. It seems that just as living systems are able to make use of single photons, they are also able to make use of single quanta of a magnetic field. If this applies, then they also have the ability to interconvert between frequency and voltage at the rate of 500 MHz per microvolt, that is they are able to make use of the Josephson Effect.

There are serious limitations to expressing measurements on living systems as a time-averaged frequency spectrum from which some mean value is derived. The time domain sequence of the signals from which the spectrum is generated is lost. It is not possible to recover the original speech, music or computer program from its time-averaged spectrum. If any observed features in a spectrum arise because Nature is using a series of time-sequential control signals like a computer program, there is no way of recovering the program from its time-averaged spectrum, although the information remains in the original raw data. Perhaps biological signals should be analysed by looking for repetitive sequences in the data and then determining the biological effects of applying such sequences as electromagnetic fields to living systems.

In the past, most bioelectric measurements have been concerned with the measurement of small, low-frequency or steady currents and voltages. Work on the radiofrequency and microwave effects in yeast cells strongly suggests that the Josephson relation (500 MHz/μV) should be applied to all experiments with living systems involving small, steady voltages, and that electromagnetic phenomena should be sought at the frequencies indicated. Any biological membrane is more likely to behave as a diode rectifier than a resistor. The interpretation of the results of existing bioelectrical experiments in terms of d.c. (direct current) is as difficult and as restricted as would be an attempt at interpreting the content of a television transmission or a computer program with nothing more than a 'cat's whisker' crystal set and a pair of headphones. Fig. 4.1 gives an 'electrical engineer's eye view' of a biological cell. Like a musical instrument or the waves on a pond, biological cells, and collections of cells, have their own resonances and sharpnesses of resonance (see Fig. 2.3, p. 23). It indicates possible electromagnetic couplings and modulation channels (see Fig. 2.5, p. 33) for communication between different cellular systems. The biophotons that cells emit in the visible and ultraviolet, the Raman resonances seen in active cells in the sub-millimetre, and the radiofrequencies found during cell division can all be observed experimentally. Any object having dielectric properties different from its surroundings, i.e. any cell will behave as a 'dielectric resonator' and thus will have an evanescent electromagnetic field in the space around it. This field does not radiate energy but is capable of interacting with similar systems. Here is a mechanism for the electromagnetic control of biological function. The opportunity for the much-needed, new approach to bioelectrical control mechanisms and electromagnetic effects in living systems literally dropped in with Dr Cyril Smith's mail, as described in Chapter 6.

CHAPTER 5

Electromagnetic fields in medicine

> The dynamic forces of mineral magnetism, electricity, and galvanism act no less homoeopathically and powerfully on our vital principle than medicines actually called homoeopathic, which overcome diseases when taken by mouth, rubbed on skin, or smelled. These other forces can cure diseases, especially those having abnormal sensations and involuntary muscle movements. But we still know far too little about the right way of using electricity, galvanism and the so-called electromagnetic machine to put them to homoeopathic use. At least they have been used until now only palliatively, with great harm to patients. The positive, pure effects of electricity and galvanism on the healthy human organism have not yet been thoroughly proved.
>
> Samuel Hahnemann (1755–1843), *The Organon of Medicine*, p. 286

There are some important landmarks in the history of electrical phenomena involving man in health and disease. By the end of the nineteenth century, physicists were actively engaged in the widespread application of the principles of the newly discovered electrochemistry and electromagnetism, many of which had been discovered by Michael Faraday in the first half of that century. These included applications in medicine and surgery which have always greatly benefited from the discoveries of non-medical scientists.

Wilhelm Conrad Röntgen, Professor of Physics at the University of Würzburg, discovered X-rays (Röntgen Rays) in November 1895 and published his results in the following January. These could be put to immediate clinical use because nearly every physics laboratory then possessed the necessary facilities. In fact, X-rays were around in the physics laboratories of that time awaiting discovery; this was narrowly missed on two occasions before Röntgen's work, because those experimenters were not prepared for the unexpected. The hazards of X-rays were not immediately appreciated and some 500 workers died as a result of overexposure to that X-radiation in the years that followed (Stead *et al.*, 1956). The extremely short wavelength, electromagnetic nature of X-rays was first suggested by the experiments of Walter and Pohl. Then, in 1912, von Laue, Friedrich and Knipping were able to measure the wavelength of X-rays using a crystal to scatter the radiation, and thereby provided one of the most powerful tools for the investigation of the structure of molecules which, in recent years, has been used to determine the structure of biological macromolecules.

The next important advance now applied to the theory of Electromagnetic Man was Hertz's development of the theory of electromagnetic radiation from a dipole. He experimented with what was, in effect, microwave radiation. He also discovered photoelectricity, which is the experimental basis of quantum theory and atomic energy levels.

Becquerel, Pierre and Marie Curie, Rutherford and Soddy all contributed to the discovery of radioactivity. Marie Curie died of leukaemia, the result of her excessive exposure to radioactivity; her husband died after a street accident in Paris. There was so much radioactive material dispersed in Soddy's laboratory that a book autographed by him and now in an American library still has radioactive fingerprints on the page.

Radioactive isotopes are unstable atoms, chemically identical to the corresponding stable atoms, which emit electrically charged particles (alpha- and beta-particles) and electromagnetic radiation (gamma rays) as they decay towards more stable energy levels and, incidentally, to different chemical structures. Radioactive materials make possible some very sensitive biochemical tests with great medical application. These allow the labelling of a specific part of a biomolecule or reagent with a radioactive element (e.g. tritium, sodium, iodine) which can then be followed through a series of chemical reactions, 'in-vitro' or 'in-vivo', in near-single atom amounts. Clegg (1983) has used radioisotope labelling techniques to investigate structure within the living cell, its properties and relation to metabolism. He has found evidence which strongly suggests that at least a large fraction of the total water inside a living cell is bound or structured in some manner which prevents free diffusion and that its electrical and other properties differ markedly from those of pure water.

All these historical events in the history of pure physics have now assumed great importance in clinical and research medicine. The parallel development of scientific instrumentation meant that from the end of the last century it has been possible to detect the electrical signals arising from the functioning of the heart. The first demonstration of the human electrocardiogram (ECG) was given by Waller in the 1890s using the capillary electrometer described by Lippmann in 1873. The next and more sensitive instrument, the Einthoven galvanometer, has long been replaced by electronic amplifiers. Merely connecting an ECG amplifier to suitable electrodes, appropriately positioned in related to the heart, gives electrical signals which when recorded on chart paper are termed an electrocardiogram. This is much used in clinical diagnosis, although practical considerations and safety precautions make the design of the apparatus and the clinical procedure less simple than might appear from this account (Strong, 1970; Green, 1968).

The largest of the electrical signals normally detected coming from Electromagnetic Man are those associated with muscle and nerve activity. The heart is the most important group of muscles in the body and the measurement of electrical signals arising from the heart is called electrocardiography. The measurement of signals arising from the 'striated' skeletal muscle contractions is called electromyography (EMG); other muscles, particularly the 'smooth' muscles surrounding major organs in the body torso, also give electrical signals which, although rarely monitored, give what is termed an electrogastrogram. The electrical measurement of small eye movements is termed electronystagmography. But the electrical activity of most sensory receptors on the body is too small to be readily, or usefully, detected; exceptions are the potentials in the middle ear when it is stimulated by sound and those stimulated in the retina by light.

These electromagnetic clinical techniques are briefly described in the following sections to emphasise the amount of detailed information that can be obtained concerning the biochemical and biological structure and functioning. The details of the regulatory control and feedback pathways are known in many cases; what is still missing is that sort of control information which enables one to determine, for a given patient, how well their control (homeostatic) system is working, how far it is from instability, and under what conditions it might be perturbed or stabilised either by chemical or electromagnetic therapy. Herein lies the possibility of obtaining an objective assessment of a person's state of health or disease.

Electrocardiography (ECG or EKG)

The most important muscle system in the body is the heart, and the mechanical events of the cardiac cycle are initiated by electrical stimulation. Between heart beats, there is a rest period (diastole) during which the heart fills to its maximum size, with oxygenated blood from the lungs going into the left upper chamber (atrium) and venous (de-oxygenated) blood from the circulation going into the right atrium. The onset of the pumping action (systole) is triggered by a bundle of pacemaking nerves (sinu-atrial node, or SA node) which generate electrical impulses that stimulate the contraction of the muscles comprising the two atrial chambers, forcing the blood into the ventricles beneath.

The spread of the atrial muscle contraction ceases at the fibrous septum between the atria and ventricles; here the contraction signal is picked up by the atrioventricular node and transmitted down the bundle of modified cardiac muscle, named after Wilhelm His, to the apex region of the ventricle, where it triggers a muscle contraction wave which spreads upwards and pumps the blood out through the valves into the blood vessels (aorta). After this, the heart returns to its resting phase, during which the electric potentials are restored (re-polarisation).

The de-polarisations and re-polarisations associated with the heart beat give characteristic action potentials of the order of millivolts in amplitude at the body surface. These potentials are what is measured in electrocardiography. The shape and timing of the waveform details of these de-polarisation waves may disclose clinically significant abnormalities in the heart muscles. Athletes can stress themselves to the point where their ECG appears to indicate 'heart failure'; the difference is that the trained athlete can come out of it again. A crack rifle-shot can learn to control the precise instant of heart beat so as not to affect aim.

Electromyography (EMG)

The basic unit of muscle function (the motor unit) comprises a motor nerve coming from the spinal cord, which branches into several motor end-plates, each connected to a single muscle fibre. A millisecond after the nerve electrical impulse reaches the motor end-plate, a chemical substance (acetylcholine) is released to bridge a gap between the nerve termination and the muscle (Fishman, 1985), causing a change in the motor end-plate potential. This leads to a propagating wave of muscle action electrical potentials and the contraction of the muscle fibre. After the acetylcholine has acted, it is destroyed by an enzyme (cholinesterase).

The arrow poison of the South American Indians (curare) reduces the motor end-plate potential changes to a value below that needed to trigger the muscle fibres; it is used as a muscle relaxant in surgical operations. Since it paralyses the respiratory muscles too, the patient must then be given artificial respiration for as long as the curare is allowed to be effective.

A single motor unit may comprise from 25 to 2000 muscle fibres and develop forces from 0.1 to 250 grams-weight. The motor nerves and the muscle fibres can only exist in two electrical states – polarised or depolarised (bi-stable – on/off – binary 1/0 – conditions). The potentials generated by the contraction of a single fibre go from $-90\,\mathrm{mV}$ to $+20\,\mathrm{mV}$ in less than a millisecond. The signal that is usually detected in EMG is the resultant of the action potentials of many fibres. This is likely to amount to about $10\,\mathrm{mV}$ and may consist of pulses lasting several milliseconds. It would be observed whether surface or needle electrodes were used.

The feed-back pathway of the motor-neuron system is through sense receptor cells (transducers) which may be sensitive to touch, mechanical movement or some other parameter, such as heat. The receptor system can respond logarithmically over a dynamic range of more than 10^7. This implies the presence of an amplifier having at least a gain of 10^7 which has been given a logarithmic response (transfer function) by the application of feedback (from the output back to the input) through a circuit element analogous to a chain of semiconductor (p–n junction) diodes.

The amplified signal from a bio-receptor produces trains of pulses in the sensory nerve fibres, at pulse repetition rates ranging from one to a thousand per second. These pulses are transmitted to the brain. The brain then responds by generating and sending back a control signal through the appropriate motor nerve to complete the feed-back loop. The sign and magnitude of this control signal will depend upon the 'error' between the actual and the expected signals.

Galvanic skin response (GSR)

'Galvanic skin response' is the variation in the normal electrical resistance of the skin. This may be due to changes in sweat gland activity, which in turn may arise from external stimuli or psychological stress. The measurement technique is very simple. It only requires a low level, normally imperceptible, voltage or current source and a measurement circuit, usually connected to a chart recorder. However, such an oscillator would still be more than enough to trigger allergic responses in a hypersensitive subject. The electrical resistance of the skin has a lower value within a few millimetres of the classical Chinese acupuncture points. The GSR is a very sensitive indicator that some change in the subject may have occurred; what that change is due to more often than not remains uncertain. The sudden ringing of a telephone can give a greater GSR response than pre-surgery anxiety. Attempts have been made to use the GSR as the basis for a 'lie detector'. However, as the secretary to a schools' examining board once remarked, 'There is no examination at which performance cannot be improved by application and the acquisition of skills by the student and the art of the teacher!' It would be surprising if it did not prove possible for some persons to learn to control their GSR, just as a marksman can control his heart beat.

Electroencephalography (EEG)

The brain provides Electromagnetic Man with the instrument for overall supervision and control, with a voluntary over-ride control for many of the feedback control loops that regulate body functions. The brain possesses both a long-term memory, which is thought to be contained in chemical modifications, and a short-term memory, which is thought to arise from electrical or electrochemical oscillations.

The development of modern digital computers through the development and applications of the formal binary-code analogies between brain and machine started with a discussion that John von Neumann had while waiting for a train at Princeton Junction railroad station. The human brain contains upwards of 10^{10} nerve cells, representing 10,000 Megabits of RAM (random-access memory). If each cell only stored a single 'bit' (binary-digit, 0 or 1) and acted as the brain's 'volatile' (non-permanent) memory, there still would only be enough memory capacity to store the information contained in every pixel (picture point) of 20 minutes of television pictures, assuming this was its only activity. The ROM (read-only memory) storage capacity of chemically stored 'bits' of information in the brain must be much larger but, even so, there is clearly a need for information processing to access and store all the data; after all, it takes many years to program the young human.

The brain structures nearer to the spinal cord evolved first and these affect the most primitive emotions and least easily controlled features of human behaviour. The outer brain structure (cortex) is allocated to the control of specific parts of the body; of all the species, it is most highly developed in man.

If an appropriate stimulus is applied to one of the body's sensors, its corresponding sensory region in the brain reacts with an electrical potential known as an 'evoked potential'. This can be detected and recorded externally on the scalp where, after passing through the bone of the skull, it has an amplitude of the order of tens of microvolts, but it requires very special interference-rejecting, differential-amplifiers for its detection. Such an instrument is known as an electroencephalograph (EEG). In brain surgery procedures, the precise location of the electrical signal arising from a particular sensor unit can often be located within the brain tissue to a precision of a cubic millimetre. However, the EEG does allow the non-invasive monitoring of the electrical activity of the brain (Hill and Parr, 1963). The EEG signals recorded are thought to be due to current flow in the cortex where synchronous interactions give oscillatory waves in the frequency band 0.5 Hz to 30 Hz. These have a spectral similarity to the geo-electrical Schumann Waves generated in the ionosphere, to which all organisms have been exposed throughout their period of evolution.

For the purposes of EEG analysis and clinical description, the frequency band has been subdivided into a number of so-called rhythms. The majority of normal adults can produce the 'alpha' rhythm, first described by Berger in 1929. This is within the range 8 Hz to 13 Hz and is the basic rhythm for a relaxed normal subject with eyes closed; it disappears with mental activity. The next most common frequency component is the 'beta' rhythm, which includes all rhythms faster than the alpha rhythm and is considered to comprise the band from 14 Hz to 22 Hz. The amplitude is usually less than 20 μV but is enhanced at the expense of the alpha rhythm by nervous tension. 'Delta' waves (0.5 Hz to 4 Hz) replace alpha waves in deep sleep and anaesthesia, but may also be due to eye movement artifacts. 'Theta' waves (4 Hz to 8 Hz) are prominent in the EEGs of normal children. Trains of spikes in the EEG waveforms are a feature of epileptic seizures.

It is in the clinical areas of brain abnormalities and disease, confirmation of clinical death, and sleep monitoring rather than in psychiatry that electroencephalography has found clinical application. The EEG responses may be modified in clinical testing for latent abnormalities by changing the brain's energy supply through changes in blood oxygen or blood sugar levels, and by rhythmic stimulation, such as flashes of light or sounds. Psychological phenomena have yet to be interpreted in the physiological terms of the EEG.

Electrical therapy

The therapeutic use of an externally applied electric current has long been an option available to the physiotherapist. Its clinical application dates back to antiquity if the use of electric fish (torpedo) is counted. Traditionally, the study and clinical practice of what is called 'electrophysiology' has been subdivided.

Clinical effects of steady currents

Body tissues are electrolytic conductors of electricity; that is, the charges are transported between the connecting electrodes by ions (charged atoms or molecules). In the process of electrolysis, material is transported through the tissues. This has been applied to the transport of ions and therapeutic materials from electrodes into the bulk tissue, as well as the surgical destruction of tissue (e.g. the removal of hair). It is also possible to carry out 'in vivo' electrophoresis, collecting the organic ions in a wick, washing them off, concentrating the solution and analysing them by thin-layer chromatography. These effects may also occur unintentionally if an electronic amplifier has an appreciable 'off-set', resulting in a small but long-term current flowing between the input terminals and the skin to which the electrodes are attached. This can give rise to irritation of the skin at the electrode sites.

Burns can be produced in cases of excessive or fault currents through the body, as well as the particular hazard of electric-shock-induced fibrillation (see below), if the current path is routed through the heart. Such hazards are taken care of in the design and regulations governing electromedical equipment. For this reason equipment not specifically designed for medical use, such as domestic appliances, must not be used for electromedical purposes.

Clinical effects of current pulses

A nerve impulse can be initiated by an external electrical stimulus, which can be used to stimulate muscles. If the pulse duration is longer than a millisecond, the current required is independent of the pulse duration. Pulses at one-second intervals give a muscle twitch at each pulse. Rapid pulse trains produce a tetanic contraction and, in the case of accidental electric shock, this tetany prevents the victim from letting go of the conductor. Even de-nervated muscle can be electrically stimulated with a current of sufficient intensity and a pulse duration greater than 100 milliseconds.

One of the reasons for the continuous monitoring of the ECG in an intensive care unit is that, should the heart get into difficulties, prompt action taken within minutes can save the life of the patient. If the heart suddenly loses its rhythmic muscle contraction and all the heart muscles begin to twitch in an unco-ordinated manner (fibrillation), blood will no longer be pumped around the body. The immediate and catastrophic result will be a shortage of oxygen in the brain. If not corrected within minutes, irreversible brain tissue damage will result. The heart can often be returned to normal operation (defibrillation) by using a large pulse of current (20 A for 5 ms) to produce tetanic contraction of all the heart muscles simultaneously. After the pulse, all the muscles will relax together and the heart will often be able to resume its normal rhythm and pumping action. This treatment is also applicable to cases where the fibrillation was induced by 'electric shock', provided the shock current has been turned off.

Some patients have a heart defect whereby the electrical triggering signals originating in the atria are not conducted to the ventricles which do the pumping. In this fault condition, the ventricles have their own 'fail-safe' system which can provide a heart beat at about 30 beats per minute, half the normal rate. This will support life, but it leaves the patient a semi-invalid. However, the appropriate triggering signal can now be supplied by an electronic 'pacemaker', which runs off batteries that last for a couple of years, and can be implanted beneath the skin so that there is no risk of infection entering the body along leads. There are hundreds of thousands of people wearing pacemakers these days and thereby enabled to live near-normal lives.

Clinical effects of microcurrents

Very weak, steady electrical currents and similar pulses of current induced by pulsed magnetic fields have been successfully applied for the past twenty years to enhance the healing of bone fractures, with success even after several years of non-union (Becker and Selden, 1985). These appear to be simulating the minute (nanoamp) injury currents which should occur naturally. The waveform appears to be particularly important. A sinusoidal wave is ineffective or deleterious; the successful waveforms resemble the output of the original, non-resonant 'Faradic Coil', which is a lower voltage version of a car ignition spark coil.

The steady current therapy for cancer developed by Nordenström (Taubes, 1986) should also be mentioned here, together with those for enhancing bone and tissue repair (Becker and Selden, 1985).

Clinical effects of high-frequency currents

The clinical use of high-frequency currents dates back to the end of the nineteenth century when both Tesla and d'Arsonval used them on the human body. In 1907, Nagelschmidt used the heating effects of high frequency currents (diathermy). In 1931, Lakhovsky (1939) brought out his first improved Multiple Wave Oscillator, which produced damped oscillatory electrostatic waves and was used in most European countries and America, with claimed success in cancer treatment.

The 'electric shock' risks are greatest when an electrical impulse coincides with the T-wave of the heart beat. This puts the electrical power supply frequencies, including most domestic supplies, in the most hazardous frequency range. Frequencies above 500 kHz do not stimulate sensory or motor nerves, neither do they cause electrolytic corrosive effects so long as there are no rectifying contacts, that is so long as the conductivity through the electrical connections does not depend on the polarity of the applied voltage. This would convert alternating (alternately positive and negative) voltages into steady currents able to produce the effects described in the sections above.

Because tissues do not conduct in a linear manner, the simultaneous application of two slightly different high frequencies will result in currents at their difference frequency. These may be in the frequency range for electrical stimulation, or other therapeutic effects, which would not be efficiently generated in the tissues if the difference frequency itself were applied directly.

The original high-frequency generators were high-voltage spark coils (Dudin's Resonator), the same, in principle, as the spark-gap and coil ignition system of the previous generation of motor cars. These were prone to cause television interference unless 'suppressed'. They generated trains of damped oscillations (like those from a plucked string instrument as opposed to the continuous sinusoidal waveform of the organ pipe) which caused a 'snowstorm' effect on the screens of television sets, blotting out the pictures. Electrically, the spark coils resembled the old 'spark transmitters' which remained in use on fishing vessels for many years because the wide range of frequencies emitted enabled emergency – 'm'aidez' ('MAY-DAY') – signals to break through any other transmission in the vicinity. For this reason their use would nowadays be prohibited, even clinically, because of the need to comply with regulations which restrict radiated electrical interference. For many years now, the whole of the available, but totally inadequate, electromagnetic spectrum has been allocated by international convention, and clinical devises must adhere to strict frequency bands.

An interesting device for generating radiation in the submillimetre region was devised in Russia in the 1920s, although there is no report that attempts were made to investigate any biomedical effects. Russian workers have been and remain in the forefront of research on the biomedical effects of electromagnetic fields. Dr Bill Guy, interviewed by *Microwave News* (1985, November/December) following a three-week tour of the Soviet Union, was reported to have said that, 'No one can say that they are not doing good science; they have brand-new equipment, they have adopted a good scientific approach and they work in large interdisciplinary teams composed of biologists, biophysicists and engineers.' The senior author visited Moscow and Kiev in January 1989 as the guest of the USSR Academy of Sciences and formed the same opinion.

Clinical effects and applications of ionising radiation

In the 'Preliminary Communication' describing his discovery of X-rays, Professor W.C.Röntgen (1896), of Würzburg University, wrote, '... if the hand be held between the discharge tube and the screen, the darker shadow of the bones is seen within the slightly dark shadow of the hand itself ...'. Within two decades, X-rays had become an important part of medical diagnosis and therapy. Immediately following Röntgen's discovery, several physicists examined natural substances to see whether any gave out radiations capable of penetrating metals and other optically opaque substances. Within a month, M.Henri Becquerel found a uranium salt emitted rays which gave an impression on a photographic plate enveloped in black paper. Mme Marie Curie examined the radioactivity of a large number of minerals and with her husband, Pierre, eventually isolated radium. This was shown to produce burns, like X-rays, and produce generally harmful biological effects (Rutherford, 1905).

The physical processes whereby these radiations are absorbed are well documented (Johns and Cunningham, 1969). They are energetic enough to ionise matter through which they pass and hence are termed ionising radiation. This includes ultraviolet light, X-rays, and gamma-rays. The latter was the name given to high energy electromagnetic radiation coming from radioactive materials before it was shown to be the same as very high energy X-rays. Other radiations from radioactive materials are alpha-rays (high energy helium atoms from which the electrons have been stripped off), and beta-rays (high energy electrons). Electromagnetic radiation is absorbed in matter by the physical processes of elastic scattering, photoelectric absorption giving rise to electrons, Compton inelastic scattering, and electron-positron pair production. The charged particles lose their energy by producing intense ionisation along their path. Neutrons, which are uncharged emitted particles lose their energy by generating protons (hydrogen atoms which have had the electron stripped off). At very high energies, other nuclear reactions become possible.

In living cells and organisms, these radiations can affect a number of cell functions. Trapped (solvated) electrons and free radicals (uncharged species containing an unpaired electron) represent the highly reactive chemical species formed by the radiation in the cell water; these can attack DNA and other important bio-molecules. Thus, heredity and the ability to reproduce are those functions most sensitive to radiation. This is the basis of radiotherapy for the treatment of cancers. The survival of cells is statistical and sigmoidal in respect of dose. It depends on the many conditions applying before, during and after irradiation; the environmental electromagnetic field is just one of these factors. Other conditions include the phase of the cell within the cycle of events leading to cell division, the level of molecular oxygen in the cell and the energy of the radiation.

The imaging of body tissues with X-rays dates to their discovery. What is seen is a shadow image formed by differences in absorption of the penetrating radiation in the tissues. This can be visualised on a fluorescent screen (fluoroscopy) or a photographic emulsion (radiography), and can be enhanced by television techniques to show movement in real time and relative safety. Sectional images of the body can be generated by computer techniques (computerised axial tomography, CAT scan) (Welkowitz and Deutsch, 1976). In principle, any penetrating radiation can be imaged in this way. Radio-isotopes (atoms with a modified nucleus having identical chemical properties but also radioactivity) can be used as sources of radiation without the need for a high energy accelerator, or as radioactive tracers to label molecules of physiological significance and by administration to the patient, follow their movements around the body with a gamma-ray camera. X-ray imaging is superb for visualising bones but, due to radiation scatter, it is not particularly satisfactory for examining soft tissues close to bone (e.g. the brain and spinal discs) and a contrast medium may need to be injected or ingested (barium meal); in this case nuclear magnetic resonance imaging is now preferable.

Nuclear magnetic resonance imaging

With nuclear magnetic resonance (NMR, see also Chapter 4) the magnetic moments of the atomic nuclei are measured and by computation can be made to give an image showing the state of all the hydrogen atoms whether in water or incorporated in other molecules. Phosphorus (^{31}P) and carbon (^{13}C) chemical shifts can also be used to provide direct measurement of metabolic processes.

NMR was originally conceived by Isidor Rabi in 1944 for investigating atomic nuclei, and then developed by Felix Bloch and Edward Purcell for studying the chemistry of a wide range of substances; all three received Nobel Prizes. It was then developed to analyse the metabolism of living cells and organisms without damage as it is completely non-invasive. In 1973, Paul Lauterbur suggested that NMR could be used to image biological tissues and built the first NMR imaging machine. The technique was first put to clinical use by Andrew Mansfield at Nottingham University and John Mallard at Aberdeen University and the Central Research Laboratories of Thorn-EMI. Commercial machines, which cost in excess of £1m, are invaluable for investigations in neurology and muscular disease, the diagnosis of brain damage and tumours, the detection of the sclerotic plaques of multiple sclerosis, Alzheimer's disease and for visualising the cerebellum and spinal cord (Bydder et al., 1982).

The technique (Young et al., 1982) involves the use of a strong magnetic field to align the magnetic moments of the protons, which then precess about it with a precise frequency determined by the magnetic field strength and fundamental physical constants (0.15 T gives a precession of 6.5 MHz). A receiver coil surrounding the area to be examined picks up signals from the precessing magnetisation which has been rotated by the application of a pulse of the radiofrequency and from the slice selected by an applied magnetic field gradient. The radiofrequency and gradient fields are pulsed. Different scanning sequences are used to show up different clinical features by imaging either the proton density or one of the precession decay times.

In Chapter 4, it was noted that certain biological effects were possible under NMR conditions. The NMR imaging technique only subjects one pixel at a time and not the whole organism, to NMR conditions and this for a time short compared with the cell mean generation times. The technique appears to be remarkably free from side effects, apart from some reports of memory effects and credit card erasures.

Diathermy

With the invention of the thermionic valve, it became possible to generate high-power (coherent) sinusoidal oscillations. With these it is possible to produce heating of bulk body tissues in a controlled manner, by the same physical principles as microwave ovens (Cameron and Skofronik, 1978; Clayton, 1958). The microwave cooker was invented by Professor Herman Schwan, now retired from the University of Pennsylvania, specifically for the purpose of cooking meals in submerged submarines. It is interesting that many allergic patients (see Chapter 6) tolerate microwave-heated or cooked food and water better than if these are heated with the 50/60 Hz power frequency current in a kettle or cooker. Microwaves cook more quickly and since patients have usually had less environmental exposure to the 2450 MHz microwave cooker frequency than 50/60 Hz, they are less likely to react against it. There have been several cases where the patient did not react against a coherent 2450 MHz, but did react against it when it was modulated at the sort of ELF frequencies which would be generated as the food rotated on the turntable.

Short-wave diathermy makes use of frequencies in the range 10 MHz to 100 MHz and usually uses non-contacting, capacitive electrode coupling to the body tissues to be warmed, although a length of cable may be wound around a limb. Whether the inductive or capacitive fields are used depends upon whether surface or deep-level heating is required. Long-wave diathermy uses a frequency around 1 MHz; because of the different tissue impedance at this frequency, the current is applied through electrodes in contact with the body tissues and the heating occurs along the current path.

Microwave diathermy developed following the availability of microwave oscillators at the end of the Second World War. A 'magnetron' oscillator feeds microwave power to a specially designed antenna, called an 'applicator'. The frequency allocated for this use, 2.45 GHz, is mainly of historical significance; a somewhat lower frequency, in the region of 900 MHz, would give more effective and uniform heating around bony regions of the body. It is used in the treatment of muscles and joints. The penetration depth into the body tissue is very dependent on the frequency and on the water content of the tissue; a 1-cm thickness of muscle or a 5-cm thickness of fat might both absorb half of that incident microwave radiation which is not reflected away at the body surface. The particular hazard with high-power radiofrequency and microwave sources arises from their ability to cause burns within body tissues, where there are no heat sensors to give an immediate pain warning. Such radiation is also a particular hazard to regions which do not have a blood flow to carry away excess heat – like the eye lens. These are what are termed thermal effects of non-ionising radiation. It has generally been assumed, or hoped, that these were the only effects. Theories of safe power densities and specific absorbed doses of non-ionising radiation are based on this premise. Nowadays, more people are less certain that this is the case (see, for example, the ongoing debate in issues of *Microwave News*).

Ultrasonic waves are also applied for the 'diathermy' of deep body sites, particularly in bone. Although these are waves of acoustic energy, and give up their energy as heat largely through mechanical dissipation processes, they may also exert therapeutic effects through pressure waves generated as they pass through body tissues, or kidney stones. Membranes have macromolecules, containing large and permanent electrical dipoles or 'electrets'. To vibrate these acoustically (or musically) is to generate an electrical oscillation just as a microphone does. Thus we cannot exclude ultrasonic diathermy in considering electromagnetic effects in humans, particularly if highly coherent acoustic waves are involved; this raises the unanswered question, 'Do coherent phonons give rise to coherent photons when they are absorbed in living tissue?'

Electrocautery and electrosurgery

In ancient times the bleeding of wounds in surgery was controlled by the use of hot oil and hot irons to sear (cauterise) the wound. This can now be carried out with a high-frequency arc struck between a fine wire probe and the body tissue to be treated; the probe will be connected to an oscillator giving voltages up to 15 kV, at a frequency higher than 2 MHz. When used to seal off small blood vessels it is termed electrocautery; when used to cut through tissue it is termed electrosurgery. The frequency is too high to produce muscle contraction and the power density is high enough to produce physical damage to the tissue within a millimetre of the probe. The ground connection to the oscillator is through a large-area lead plate ('Buttock Plate'), kept inside a cloth bag moistened with saline. This ensures a low electrical resistance at the place of contact with the body, preventing localised heating and burns at this site.

Electro-anaesthesia, electro-sleep and electro-convulsive therapy

Electro-anaesthesia can be induced by passing small currents through the brain. These would be of the order of a few milliamps, which for most persons only amounts to the threshold of current perception. The currents may be steady or alternating in the frequency range 100 Hz to 1500 Hz (Sances and Larson, 1970). The technique has advantages in cases where chemical anaesthetics cannot be given, but may have some of the respiratory and cardiac side-effects of electric shock. Slightly smaller currents, for example 1 mA at 100 Hz, can induce electro-sleep. Still smaller and very localised currents have been applied to the region of a tooth for dental anaesthesia.

Transcutaneous electrical nerve stimulation (TENS) devices are in widespread use for the relief of pain, particularly post-operatively. They greatly reduce the amount of chemical analgesics the patient requires.

The application of larger currents through the brain is used in the treatment of certain types of depression to induce a grand mal seizure. It is suggested that the seizure activity, rather than the other effects of the current, is responsible for the relief of depression. The treatment is carried out under anaesthetic and muscle relaxant. The currents applied would be of the order of hundreds of milliamps, since the method involves the application of an alternating voltage of between 70 V and 120 V for 0.4 to 0.6 s (Mayer-Gross *et al.*, 1969).

Dr Margaret Patterson (1978, 1986) has successfully used electrotherapeutic sleep and electroacupuncture (NeuroElectric Therapy) in the treatment of drug addiction and drug-related insomnia. When, in 1972, she was head of surgery in the Tung Wah hospital in Hong Kong, she used acupuncture techniques for pain relief and found that as a side-effect her drug-addicted patients reported that they no longer felt the need to take drugs. She has now developed an electro-acupuncture apparatus and electrodes which allow full mobility during the ten-day courses of treatment, but her work lacks support and recognition. As a *Guardian* headline (4 February 1986) put it, 'It beats cold turkey, but authority won't bite.' Government disinterest and lack of foresight in matters scientific is not new in Britain. Marconi was once told, 'The Navy has no need for wireless.'

Electrical safety

The bulk body tissues have an electrical resistance of the order of 500 ohms. If the skin is dry it may have a resistance of $1\,M\Omega$; if it is wet or just moist from (saline) perspiration, the resistance may be $1\,k\Omega$. In the former case, the domestic 240 V mains supply would give a current of 250 µA which would not be perceived by most persons; in the latter case the mains would give a current of $\frac{1}{4}$ amp, which is likely to be fatal. That is why there are stringent safety requirements for all electrical equipment and especially for electro-medical apparatus (Strong, 1970; BSI, 1979; Cameron and Skofronick, 1978). The availability of semiconductor devices known as opto-couplers has led to greatly improved safety. These allow signals to be passed from the patient-connected apparatus to mains-connected apparatus without any electrical contact being made between them; the information contained in the signals is converted into light or infra-red radiation which can pass through electrical insulation, capable of withstanding thousands of volts, and then be converted back into an electrical signal.

National safety standards

Hospitals in the United Kingdom are advised to purchase equipment which complies with the requirements of the appropriate British Standard (BSI, 1979). Non-commercial electromedical equipment constructed for clinical trials should also satisfy these requirements. Harmonisation of the standards of the EEC countries has been a major consideration and the decision was taken to use safety standards for medical electrical equipment prepared by the International Electrotechnical Commission (IEC) to supersede the earlier Hospital Technical Memorandum No. 8. While the following paragraphs indicate the scope of the safety measures, they are not to be regarded as quotations from the British Standard.

Electromedical Equipment is classified as follows:

Class I Equipment is run from an external power supply and has a protective earth ('ground' in North American parlance).

Class II Equipment relies on double insulation for protection; metal cases are not connected to the patient circuit; earthing is for functional, not protective purposes.

Class III Equipment relies on isolated 'Medical Safety Extra-Low Voltage Supplies' (<24 V AC, <50 V DC); any earthing is for functional purposes only.

Internally Powered Equipment either has no external connections to the internal power source, or the internal power source is spatially separated from the equipment during charging.

The equipment is further classified according to the degree of protection afforded against electric shock.

Type H is equivalent to domestic appliances and is not to be connected to a patient.

Type B is improved in respect of electrical leakage; if it has isolated (floating) patient circuits, it becomes Type BF, which is used where possible.

Type CF affords the highest degree of protection; it has an isolated patient circuit and is intended for applications where there will be a direct electrical circuit to the heart.

Some electrical equipment does, of its nature, give rise to leakage currents flowing to earth. Large permanent equipment with a permanent protective earth is allowed 10 mA of leakage current under normal conditions. Type CF Equipment is allowed 10 μA under normal conditions and 50 μA under 'single fault' conditions. According to the 'Basic Safety Concept', failure of a single means of protection shall not result in a safety hazard.

In the USA the electrical power supplies are at 110 V (220 V for large loads) and a frequency of 60 Hz; the earthing arrangements are also different. There, electromedical equipment must comply with the requirements of the Food and Drugs Administration (FDA). Criticism is voiced that any electronic circuit modification is treated as if it were a pharmacological modification resulting in a completely new drug. American underwriters require that no three faults occurring simultaneously shall result in a safety hazard. The saying there is that, 'Hell knows no fury like an attorney singed!' The American propensity for litigation means that many tests must be carried out on patients for the legal protection of the doctors and hospitals rather than for their diagnostic value. This practice of 'Defensive Medicine' has increased the demand for research into better instrumentation for objective clinical testing. Consumers' organisation reporting has raised the standard of hospital equipment, which is bought on the commercial market rather than through a government agency.

Electromedical apparatus in alternative medicine

There are many pieces of electrical apparatus associated with this area of medicine. Many are described by Kenyon (1983) and are also discussed in Chapter 7. They are based on standard electrical bridge circuits and oscillators and make use of the 'acupuncture points' of the body to access the various organs. However, this is not the whole story, because it appears that the operator as well as the patient becomes an essential part of the apparatus and that the apparatus functions rather as a refined 'dowser's wand', reflecting changes in the patient and the operator induced by electrical oscillations, chemical or therapeutic substances or disease conditions. If the sceptic needs convincing, he should take a chart recorder with high-gain DC amplifiers and tune an oscillator from 10 MHz to 1000 MHz nearby with no direct electrical connection between them. Enough of the oscillations will be picked up and rectified in the non-linearities of the amplifiers to send the pen all over the chart paper.

CHAPTER 6
Electrical sensitivity and allergy

> It appears that electromagnetic sensitivity exists as a definite clinical entity. Its recognition will aid in the treatment of the environmentally sensitive patient.
>
> Dr William J. Rea, in Dallas, 1987; appointed in 1988 the world's first Professor of Environmental Medicine at the University of Surrey, Guildford, UK

The following is an account of some problems which came the way of the senior author as a result of his work on the bio-medical effects of electromagnetic fields. In 1947, he started working in radar research; this involved electronics and the use of microwave oscillators. Later, in 1956, he moved up the frequency spectrum to ionising radiation and to the biomedical area when he worked on the intensification of X-ray images. In the early 1960s his interests moved from the surface of the Earth to the geophysical phenomenon of the sodium light from the twilight sky. In 1964, he joined Salford University and commenced working on electrical high-field phenomena in insulating liquids. Within ten years, his work had returned to biological materials and living systems, stimulated by the arrival of Professor Herbert Fröhlich FRS following retirement from Liverpool University. This particular research began with dielectric measurements on enzymes but was soon extended to include magnetic measurements. A number of the effects observed were found to be associated with living systems, so the investigations were extended to bacteria and yeasts. From 1979, the work began to acquire wider clinical and environmental implications. He then recorded a demonstration for a BBC-TV programme, *The Vital Spark*, produced by Dick

Gilling, in which he showed that the sort of magnetic fields used for the treatment of non-union in bone fractures by Bassett and Becker could also affect an enzyme reaction. As Hilary Bacon relates in Chapter 8, she saw this programme and wrote to Cyril Smith for assistance in understanding the experiences widespread in her Dorset village of Fishpond, which seemed to be related to the power lines which straddled it.

The next piece of the jigsaw came by serendipity. Following his unsuccessful attempt to get research funding from the New York State Power Lines Project, and no prospect of funding for such work from elsewhere, he wrote (Smith and Aarholt, 1982) that persons exposed to environmental electromagnetic fields could be experiencing body currents of the order of tens of microamps, currents comparable to those known to be able to produce electro-anaesthesia in dentistry, which in turn is associated with the stimulation of endogenous opiates, pain- and emotion-controlling substances manufactured in the brain and elsewhere in the nervous system (Patterson, 1986).

During the same year, endogenous opiates had also been linked with allergies in papers presented at two international conferences. This led Dr Jean Monro to contact him to seek help with the treatment of her electrically sensitive multiple-allergy patients. Since then, over 100 patients have been tested, first at the Wellington Hospital, then at the Nightingale Hospital and finally at the Lister Hospital, following the moves of Dr Monro's Central London facility. We also tested patients at her clinic in Hemel Hempstead and in Dr Bill Rea's environmental unit in Dallas, Texas. Most of these patients were found to have electromagnetic sensitivities which were critically dependent on frequencies over a range extending from at least milliHertz to GigaHertz, with less dependence upon the electric or magnetic field strength, so long as this exceeded a certain threshold value specific for the individual patients and their allergic state at the time of testing.

Dr Monro now directs her own hospital devoted to the care and treatment of the environmentally sick – the Breakspear Hospital, a former Catholic College, at Abbots Langley, Hertfordshire, England. There they have facilities for carrying out screening tests for chemical pollutants and electromagnetic sensitivities. There is a controlled environment unit in which the air is filtered and the construction is non-toxic and where patients can experience a period of withdrawal from common environmental pollutants.

Allergic responses

Allergy used to be concerned with skins and respiration, but in recent years allergic responses have been found to occur so widely that allergy may now be defined as 'the failure of a regulatory system'. The more severely allergic patients have acquired allergic responses to many chemical, environmental and nutritional substances; these may be counted in tens and even exceed a hundred in extreme cases. It appears that about 15 per cent of a given population function to some extent below their best performance capability due to a degree of allergy, that is one or more of their regulatory systems functions inadequately.

It seems that a new allergic response can be acquired, or transferred, by being exposed for a sufficiently long time to some hitherto innocuous substance while reacting strongly to an existing allergen. In such circumstances it seems that exposure to an electromagnetic frequency can sensitise the patient, so that their specific pattern of allergic responses is triggered on subsequently encountering that particular frequency. In general the pattern of allergic responses is the same whether the trigger is chemical, environmental, nutritional or electrical. In principle, such an accurate 'memory' for frequency is no different to the 'absolute pitch' facility that many musicians possess.

A therapy for chemical and nutritional allergic responses was originally described by Carlton Lee and modified by Miller (1972). There is good evidence from four double-blind studies that it is satisfactory in the treatment of food allergy and from a further double-blind study in respect of food allergy in migraine (Monro et al., 1984). Miller showed that the diameter of the weal on the skin of a patient following a 'skin-prick' (intradermal injection) test with an allergen depended upon the dilution of the allergen used. Furthermore, if a whole sequence of serially diluted allergens were applied successively, certain dilutions gave large weals but on further diluting there would eventually be a dilution at which no weal was produced. Still further serial dilutions would re-cycle through similar patterns of response. The dilution at which no weal resulted was termed the patient's 'neutralising dilution' because it could be injected to provide neutralisation of the symptoms due to that allergen and could provide prophylactic protection against subsequent environmental or nutritional exposure.

In the course of treating many extremely sensitive allergic patients, Dr Jean Monro and her colleagues found that such patients merely needed to hold a glass tube containing a dilution of the allergen for the symptoms or neutralising effects to become manifest. This even applied if the tube contents were still frozen following deep-freeze storage. The most sensitive patients could distinguish, double-blind, tubes of allergen from tubes of placebo if these were merely brought into the room. This led to the development of the technique of desensitisation using surface application to the skin of antigens in serial dilution. It paralleled the intradermal technique in provocation and neutralisation of symptoms (Monro *et al.*, 1984). This technique is much quicker to apply, because the drop of antigen can be merely wiped off the skin when the full allergic response has been observed; the patient is then ready for testing with the next dilution.

Electrically sensitive allergy patients

Based on the above techniques, a method of testing and therapy has been devised for the treatment of those electrically sensitive, multiple-allergy patients who experience symptoms which they can describe within a few seconds of being exposed to the allergen or electrical frequency (Smith *et al.*, 1985). However, the testing of electrically sensitive allergy patients must be regarded as a clinical procedure and not be attempted without the immediate availability of facilities and staff medically competent to treat anaphylaxis (a serious shock reaction arising from a hypersensitive condition of the body) should it occur. The most effective and rapid therapy for this is to place a drop of the patient's neutralising dilution of chemical allergen on the skin.

The procedure for testing and treating electrically hypersensitive patients is based on the provocation-neutralisation therapies of Miller (1972, 1987) and Monro *et al.* (1984). It appears that increasing a coherent frequency has the same clinical effect on electrically sensitive patients as increasing allergen dilution does on chemically or nutritionally sensitive patients. Thus, it may be possible to find particular frequencies at which the allergic reactions cease, just as a dilution of the allergen (neutralising dilution) which results in the cessation of the allergic reactions (neutralisation) is sought in the Miller Technique. In the electromagnetic case, it is the frequency and the coherence which is important; the field strength is less important so long as it is above a certain threshold, particular to an individual patient.

One is seeking, in this situation, to produce clinical effects by merely having the patient in the same room as the electromagnetic fields that leak from electronic equipment, such as ordinary laboratory oscillators or signal generators which can be borrowed from teaching and research laboratories. No electrical connection to the patient is necessary, nor should be contemplated for safety reasons. All that is done is to alter the environmental electromagnetic radiation by an amount well within the allowed limits for non-ionising radiation and comparable to the radiation leakage from a domestic television set, home computer, or other piece of electronic equipment. If the patient does not respond to this level of signal, then the patient has no problem with electromagnetic allergic responses. In general, the symptoms provoked on electrical testing are the same as those provoked on chemical testing.

An imaginary electrical allergy testing session

In response to many requests from medical colleagues to write an extended account of the testing procedures so far developed for investigating electrical hypersensitivities, the following is typical of what might take place during a testing session, but with nothing in this account relating to any actual person.

The consulting room, particularly if within an allergy unit, should be located as far as possible from the other patients in terms of the number of solid walls and floors separating them. This is important if allergic responses are not to be triggered in all the other sensitive allergic subjects throughout the building during the testing session. Distance alone is not a sufficient criterion because it is possible to choose a location which is a long way down the corridors and yet is only just across an open well in the building with windows looking directly into other rooms. The electrical and telephone wiring may carry the signals away from the testing room too. Even with these precautions we have had patients come into the hospital and say, 'When I came into the building this morning I felt just as I did when I was being tested electrically'. This was without being aware that electrical testing was being carried out in the basement at that particular time.

While it is possible to provide electrical screening to the practical limit of a ten-million-fold reduction in the ambient fields within a test room using wire mesh and metal sheets at frequencies above 10 kHz and below 1 Hz (Persinger, 1974), this may still not be enough to screen external fields from a person at the theoretical limit of sensitivity. The region between these frequencies presents especial screening problems and is why Schumann Radiation and power supply frequencies are so penetrating. However, screening also presents its own problems. When patients are reacting, they often emit electrical signals themselves; if these are reflected back to them by the very metal which is providing the screening, their allergic reactions may become more severe. We found this out when testing the patients in a chemically clean caravan lined with porcelained steel. We got round the problem by placing plastic buckets of salt water (about a handful of cooking or table salt to a gallon of water) at suitable positions inside the room to absorb electrical energy instead of having electrical resonances build up.

The room for testing electrically hypersensitive patients should be lit by daylight if possible, otherwise by filament lamps, not ordinary fluorescent lighting. Some doctors keep a fluorescent light available in their clinics to be able to switch it on to see whether patients react to it, providing a useful screening test for electrical sensitivities. There is some so-called full-spectrum fluorescent lighting which does not appear to give rise to these problems; this has been confirmed in cases where the tubes have been replaced over the weekend without the occupants being informed. It is also reported to make battery hens lay hard-shelled eggs and be more free from disease.

For testing purposes, laboratory oscillators, such as would be used daily in a university or school laboratory by staff and students, should be set out on a table near convenient power outlets. If available, battery-powered oscillators are preferable. There are safety advantages in having rechargeable batteries which must be removed physically from the instrument for re-charging.

Together, these oscillators should provide continuous frequency coverage from 0.1 Hz to at least 1 MHz and preferably cover a greater range than this in either direction (10 milliHertz to 10 GigaHertz). The types of oscillators in which the frequency is changed by the operation of a switch rather than by turning a dial are not satisfactory, since merely operating the switches can give rise to transients (electromagnetic impulses) which can affect the patients in an uncontrolled manner. Continuously variable (dial) controls both for frequency and attenuation are desirable since the switching operations at the ends of the ranges can also be troublesome. The level of the output signals is not critical but that typical of laboratory measuring instruments will suffice. Audio frequency oscillators usually have an output which can go up to several volts, radiofrequency oscillators usually have outputs extending to several millivolts, and low power microwave oscillators cover the microwatts to milliwatts range of output power. In all cases, no electrical contact is made to the patient. All that is done is to produce a controlled electrical environment.

The procedure is basically a question of controlling the coherent frequencies present in the patient's electromagnetic environment and observing any symptoms triggered. With the most sensitive patients, there may be sufficient leakage from the oscillator's case and power cord to produce the minimal symptoms sought. For the less sensitive patients, it is sufficient to trail a 1-metre length of insulated wire from the output terminal to the floor to serve as an antenna; this would be typically at a distance of several metres from the patient. For the microwave oscillators, a small loop antenna is better and more convenient. The signal level at the patient will be of the order of 30 nT or mW per square metre. There is therefore no likelihood of getting anywhere near the levels regarded as the limits of those safe to live and work in (see Chapter 9). If this arrangement produces no symptoms at any frequency, then either the patient does not have a problem with electrical sensitivity, or the patient has a delayed response and should be watched for reactions appearing up to 48 hours after testing. If the patient is thought to be

Electrical sensitivity and allergy

electrically sensitive from the case history, but does not respond to the frequencies from the oscillators, a more sensitive test is to make use of the techniques of kinesiology to assess changes in muscle response following each frequency change.

The tester sits at the table with the oscillators. The patient, who will usually be asked to sit or lie on a bed on the opposite side of the room, is unable to see the dials and knobs of the oscillators. The medical practitioner in charge of the case, who will have ensured that an oxygen cylinder and facilities for treatment of anaphylactic shock are readily available but out of sight, will be on the patient's side of the room so that the test is carried out 'blind' to both the doctor who observes and reports any symptoms and to the patient. Neither knows what frequencies, if any, are being radiated at any given instant. The tester records these along with any symptoms.

In general, the patients develop the same symptoms during electrical testing as they do during chemical or food testing, so that one usually has forewarning of the likelihood of an extreme reaction; in any case it is easier and quicker to switch an oscillator off, or change the frequency, than it is to remove an injected allergen. Patients with electrical sensitivities tend to have many (perhaps 10 or even 50) other sensitivities, which have usually already been investigated. If it has been possible to treat these other allergic reactions successfully, the electrical sensitivities are likely to have disappeared as well. In cases where the electrical sensitivities make it difficult to neutralise the food and chemical sensitivities, then the following protocol for neutralising the electrical sensitivities may help the other treatments to become effective. Electrical testing should not be attempted without adequate clinical facilities and staff because, for these patients, it is a clinical procedure and not a research investigation.

When setting up the room for testing, it is advisable to keep any microwave oscillators physically outside the room until one is ready to test in this frequency region. The old-fashioned, vacuum tube (valve) microwave oscillators are preferable because, having highly resonant microwave cavities, they emit a much more coherent oscillation than many of the inexpensive modern (transistor device) oscillators. However, the former do have highly resonant electrical circuits capable of a very coherent response to any incident radiation (in technical terms, 'High-Q' cavities). We have been able to trigger allergic responses by tuning such resonant cavities (connected to an antenna but without any oscillator functioning) in the vicinity of patients with extreme sensitivities in the microwave region. This is the reason for keeping these oscillators outside the room until needed. This shows that the limiting or threshold sensitivity of such patients is that level of radiation which they themselves emit. They seem to be able to 'zap' their environment electromagnetically and sense any resonances within it, rather like electric fish. Similarly, large metal reflecting surfaces near the patient can cause difficulties. That is why, when testing in an environmentally clean porcelained steel or aluminium-lined room or caravan, it helps to place a large, plastic bucket or glass jar filled with saline at about sea-water concentration, mid-way between the metal surfaces to damp the electrical resonances.

The testing session

This should commence with a few questions to get all the relevant information on one piece of paper: full name, age, the address, which should be that to which repeat prescriptions can be sent when needed. Also, the general sort of environment in which the patient lives – town or country, seaside, hills or vales, a new house or an old one, any nearby industries or electrical installations including electricity distribution sub-stations or transformers. Note that overhead power lines are marked on the 1:50,000 Ordnance Survey maps of Great Britain.

The apparatus is explained to the patient. It is conveniently described as a collection of electronic oscillators which together cover most of the electromagnetic frequencies the patient is likely to have met in the environment, while the strengths of the fields used are comparable to the fields which leak out of a domestic television set or a home computer; enough for the detector vans for unlicenced TVs to work off, or to enable snoopers to read what is on VDU terminals from outside a building, but not enough to be perceived by people who are not electrically hypersensitive. It is the electrical equivalent of a large reference collection of environmental, food and chemical allergens. During the testing, the oscillators will be slowly tuned through all the frequencies that the patient could encounter in the environment. What is wanted is for the patient to report any symptoms felt – if and when, or, as they come and go. Any symptoms are likely to be similar to those provoked when being tested for reaction to foods and chemicals.

The reason for asking the patient to sit or lie on a bed rather than in a chair is that the patient may lose muscle control and strength, so it will be easier for the testing and more comfortable to start off in a position from which the patients can lie down if they feel they want to. It is all rather like having eyesight tested – ultimately, only the subject can say whether they can read the line of letters on the chart clearly.

To estimate how electrically sensitive the patient is likely to be to electrical signals, it is worth finding out what neutralising dilutions are currently being prescribed. If the neutralising dilutions are all below five, there should be no great problem. If several are higher, do not first switch on any of the oscillators in the same room as the patient.

It is worth being forewarned of likely trouble by finding out what symptoms the chemical and food allergens trigger. These may be reported as: bad headaches with disturbances of vision which have persisted for years; sometimes the legs will not work, the patient gets stuck and cannot move; sometimes the patient becomes completely unable to speak; then again the patient may just get all 'zombie'-like and cannot do the simplest mental tasks; the patient may also get pains in joints, limbs, shoulders, head and sinuses, ears.

The patient's tolerance to water gives a good indication of possible hypersensitivity. Can the patient drink tap water? Must it be filtered to take out the chlorine, can the patient only drink bottled water in glass bottles? Does taking a shower, bath or standing bare-foot on grass or concrete have any effect?

The patient's comments on 'electrical things around the place' should be sought; do any cause discomfort? What about thunderstorms?

Typical comments are, 'I am no good with electrical things, the children switch them on for me if I need them'; 'The electric iron gives me a pain in the arm'; 'When I switch on the washing machine the programme goes straight to finish without doing any of the washing, the men say there is nothing wrong with the washer'; 'I cannot wear a quartz watch, it makes me go sleepy'; 'At work there are a lot of VDUs (VDTs in North America) in the office and I just do not like them'; 'The fluorescent lighting makes me bad, I turn it off and use a desk lamp'; 'Thunderstorms are not too bad when they break, I usually feel worse before they arrive'; 'Some people coming into the public part of the office make me feel ill as soon as they enter the door'.

These are all typical remarks from patients with electrical hypersensitivity. The dislike of fluorescent lighting is common; fluorescent tubes emit many frequencies throughout the electromagnetic spectrum and not just light. It is not clear why full-spectrum lighting should be better. Perhaps it is just because the increased spectrum makes it less coherent. Failure to make electrical devices work may be due to them triggering the patient into emitting quite strong electrical signals which in turn upset the electronic circuits, rather than the presumed ineptitude with things electrical. TV remote controls are often the subject of similar reports. There are electrical changes in the atmosphere some hours before weather fronts arrive and more so before thunderstorms. People can emit electrical signals which affect other sensitive persons; it is, of course, catastrophic if this situation arises between spouses or between parents and children.

It may be possible to find out what first started the hypersensitivities.

Did they start after getting sprayed with pesticide or herbicide? Does the patient have a lot of different metals in dental fillings? The amalgam of 'dental amalgam' contains the element of mercury which is highly toxic. Mercury metal is generally supposed to be difficult to remove from the amalgam, but there are reports that it does disappear from fillings and that electrical potentials can often be measured between different fillings in the mouth (Ziff, 1984). After chewing hot food or chewing-gum the breath may contain a high level of mercury vapour from the dental amalgam (BSCN, 1985). Kervran (1972) discusses the possibility of bacteria being involved in the removal of mercury from other biological systems and concludes that radioactive tracers should not be considered to 'behave biologically in a manner similar to stable isotopes'.

The patient has now been sitting in the same room as the pieces of electronic apparatus for some minutes; does the patient notice any smells coming off the paint or electrical insulation? Are there any cooking smells, traffic fumes getting into the room? Are there any unpleasant noises? Electrical and chemical reactions may give rise to hypersensitivity to sounds.

This gives an opportunity to find out if anything in the room, whether furnishings or fittings or any person, their clothing or their odours, such as perfumed soap, or tobacco, or outside traffic fumes, etc., are going to interfere with the testing. If there is any opportunity to get the testing room checked for geopathic stress before it is used, this should also be done so that all the patients' stresses will be due to the electrical oscillators and under full control. Geopathic stress may be located by dowsing (see Chapter 11), magnetic anomaly measurements, air conductivity measurements and background ionising radiation levels (Aschoff, 1986; von Pohl, 1987).

Reactions have been observed in sensitive patients which were triggered by the hospital paging ('bleep') transmission signals. If a portable radio receiver works in the room, then it is picking up transmissions which have penetrated its screening, and therefore other electromagnetic signals can also penetrate and interfere with the testing.

Still do not switch on any electrical apparatus inside the room with the patient, since you might get such a strong reaction, even from minimal fields, that it would take a long while for the reaction to wear off; meanwhile it would not be possible to detect any weak symptoms produced by other frequencies.

Keeping the fields to a level where the symptoms are just perceptible means that the patient will respond to a frequency within 10 seconds, and all the reaction that is going to occur will have happened within a minute. To determine this level for a given patient, the low frequency oscillator is taken about 10 metres down the corridor outside the room and out of sight of the patient and doctors. A number of tests with the oscillator on and off and at different output level settings will soon show whether the patient can detect anything. Experience shows that a frequency around 1 Hz is a good place to start. With some patients, there will be no obvious response at any frequency. A patient having many chemical sensitivities would be expected to be able to tell whether the oscillator is off or on at the maximum output setting, and at about heart-beat frequency when it is outside the room. They usually say, 'Something feels different, now', or, 'I don't like that!' when it is on.

In the former case, it is satisfactory to bring the oscillator back into the room and work systematically through all the frequencies using the minimum output setting (e.g. of the order of millivolts). If the patient reacts strongly to the oscillator outside the room, testing should be done with the oscillator at that distance, or the patient should receive treatment to reduce the level of sensitivity before the oscillator is brought into the same room as the patient.

Locating the neutralising frequencies

A cyclical occurrence of symptoms and their amelioration will be found to continue as the frequency is slowly increased. With some patients it can take three hours to go from Hertz to GigaHertz; with others there are decades of frequency in which there are no symptoms or no changes in the current symptom pattern and the tuning can be more rapid. The limitation is the 10 seconds or so that it can take for the symptom changes to appear; if the tuning is too rapid, reactions may be missed or attributed to a later frequency setting than that which actually produced the symptom. It is easy to check for this by tuning in the opposite direction – the same symptom should occur at the same frequency whether approached from higher or lower frequencies. With some patients this is easily done, with others there are so many delayed symptoms that accurate repetition is very difficult. If the patient is clearly uncomfortable or in pain at a particular frequency, it is much easier to tune quickly through this region than it is to make the equivalent change of dilution in food and chemical testing. It greatly enhances the comfort of the patient if a neutralising frequency can be quickly located so that when things get too uncomfortable, the oscillator can be quickly re-tuned there to give some respite.

The patient in the above example might have had the following frequencies free from all symptoms: 8.4 Hz, 450 Hz, 4 kHz, 25 kHz, 350 kHz, 20 MHz, 320 MHz, with all frequencies above 350 MHz producing symptoms.

The above frequencies represent the first attempt at finding the neutralising frequencies. It is now possible to go back to each of these frequencies to check that they really neutralise all the patient's symptoms; this is necessary because of delayed responses during the preliminary run through all the frequencies, but the patient should not have to put up with any more severe reactions because these have now been mapped and the frequencies can be avoided. The patients usually find this experience of having their symptoms turned on and off by an external agency quite comforting, particularly if they have been told by many doctors for many years that 'The illness is all in your mind' i.e. it's your fault!

We now have several frequencies which do not provoke any symptoms and which the patient says 'could be lived with'. The next thing to do is to expose a series of glass tubes containing saline, or other water the patient can tolerate, to a magnetic field produced in a coil connected to the oscillators set at each neutralising frequency for about 4 minutes.

The doctor will explain to the patient how to use the tubes to relieve any reactions due to environmental triggering: 'You should hold one of these tubes for a few minutes morning and evening to reduce the likelihood of environmental frequencies provoking a severe reaction, and told a tube if you are starting to get a reaction. The water will probably retain a clinical effectiveness for you for one or two months, but patients who hold a tube to quell a severe reaction report that the tube feels as though it has been drained. We know the frequencies to which the tubes have been exposed and can make a replacement and mail it to you when the first ones cease to be effective. This can usually be done satisfactorily if the glass tubes are well wrapped in aluminium foil and packed against breakage. The only times that we have had them arrive in a useless condition was when they were sent by rail, as packages are carried on an electrified railway line. Road and airmail, even across the world, seem quite satisfactory. You have tubes for several neutralising frequencies; I suggest that you use them in rotation like your foods so that you do not acquire a new reaction to any of them.'

Allergic responses to fabrics and electronic equipment

The results of some preliminary experiments to determine how reacting allergic patients would respond to a range of fabrics had suggested that the ultra-violet absorption properties of the fabrics might be an important factor (Smith *et al.*, 1986). This would be consistent with the preference of allergic patients for natural fibre materials which are untreated or only coloured with vegetable dyestuffs. This is also consistent with the reported widespread phenomenon of 'ultra-weak' photon (light) emission from living cells and organisms which is very probably coherent and extends into the ultra-violet part of the spectrum (Li, 1987). This emission is different from the emission resulting in general from chemical reactions and termed bioluminescence.

However, not only are these reacting allergic patients extremely electrically sensitive, they can also, when reacting allergically, emit electrical signals, rather like an electric fish. These signals can be large enough to interfere with electronic apparatus, as clinical case histories testify. The electrical signals which make it possible to eavesdrop on computers are sufficiently strong to trigger allergic reactions in sensitive patients who are then liable to feed 'garbage' back into the computer or other equipment. The subject area in electronics which deals with such problems is 'Electromagnetic Compatibility'. The problems which allergy patients have described are very wide ranging. One patient had a robotic system in a factory completely malfunction each time he stood near it. Another has had the electronic ignition system on successive new cars fail as soon as an allergic reaction was triggered by fumes from a diesel truck in front. There has already been a report of a computer-guided car failing each time it passed a microwave tower; the possibilities for 'zapping' electronics by allergic subjects are many.

One must hope that world peace does not depend upon the allergy-free status or otherwise of the strategic computer operators throughout the world's military installations. It is not inconceivable that a reacting allergic operator could set off a sequence of events like those in the film *The War Game*, but without the dramatist's ability to provide a 'happy ending'. A.J.P. Taylor has described the events leading up to the First World War in terms of the logical consequences of the railway timetables of Europe. We must ensure that the scenario of any future world conflict is not already written into computer programs throughout the world and merely awaiting the right sequence of fortuitous events to implement them. According to a recent report (Smoker, 1988), nuclear war is now reckoned to be more likely to be triggered by computer fault or human error than by deliberate action.

Unexpected effects in water

While it is possible for the patient to gain relief from the allergic responses by having an oscillator set to a neutralising frequency left on in the room, this is not a satisfactory or cost-effective solution, particularly in the microwave region. Furthermore, one patient's neutralising frequency is another's allergic trigger and in a crowded hospital or clinic, a multiplicity of personal oscillators would be as destructive of allergy testing as the presence of perfume.

When faced with this problem in respect of a patient who could only be neutralised at a frequency in the microwave part of the electromagnetic spectrum, Dr Smith and Dr Monro remembered that the homoeopathic *Materia Medica* lists potentised water exposed to electric currents, magnetic fields and X-rays. Dr Monro had already used dilution of water exposed to ultra-violet radiation as a therapy for hypersensitivity to light. A simple test confirmed that water which was tolerated by the patient and which was exposed to a magnetic field at the frequency which neutralised the patient's allergic responses was clinically as effective as having a microwave oscillator switched on in the patient's room. Water so exposed to electromagnetic radiation can be used as a neutralising dilution of allergen, and resembles in its effects a potentised homeopathic preparation (see section in Chapter 7). It is easier to keep a tube of such potentised water away from other allergy patients than to provide an electrically screened room to shield an oscillator from affecting them. It seems that such water retains this effectiveness for at least one or two months (Smith *et al.*, 1985), although the experience in Dallas is that it has a considerable shorter period of effectiveness (Rea, 1987).

When patients use a tube of potentised water to neutralise a strong allergic reaction the tube seems subsequently to have become ineffective. Superimposing a triggering frequency and a neutralising frequency on the same tube produces a tube of water which triggers allergic reactions rather than neutralising them. Patients and other persons are able to overwrite the water in their tube with their own electromagnetic emissions when reacting strongly. It does seem that an extended metal surface near a reacting allergic patient, acting as a mirror for the patient's own electromagnetic emissions, makes these reactions worse. A large glass container of salt water (approximately sea water concentration) near the patient helps to damp these effects. This may also explain the problems that some patients experience in cars and other vehicles of metal box construction.

Some years before this, Dr Smith's laboratory had found that the lysozyme solutions 'remembered' the frequencies and fields to which they had been exposed long enough for measurements to be carried out in a different building. Homoeopathic remedies based on electric currents and magnetic fields, as well as X-ray and ultra-violet and coloured light radiation, are well known amongst its practitioners; potentised preparations from tinctures exposed to these radiations appear in homoeopathic *Materia Medica* (pharmacopoeia). The action of homoeopathic remedies could be explained in physical terms if water, alcohol and lactose could be shown to take up some structure having the properties of an electrical resonator which matches electrical frequencies present, or missing, in the body. This would be the electromagnetic equivalent of the string or pipe of a musical instrument which 'remembers' the frequencies to which it has been tuned. Dr Smith (Smith *et al.*, 1985) has suggested that such a mechanism could provide a physical basis for homoeopathy. This is further elaborated in Chapter 7.

Homoeopathy is clinically effective at potencies or dilutions where no chemistry should remain. Potencies produced by serial dilutions beyond 10^{24} (in homocopathy, 24X or 12C potency) should have none of the original tincture molecules remaining. In allergy therapy using fivefold dilutions (1 + 4) this is equivalent to 5^{34}, or 34 dilutions; in physics and chemistry it corresponds to Avogadro's Number (in some countries it is called Loschmidt's Number), which is the number of molecules in one gram-molecular weight of any substance.

Although electrically sensitive patients react to frequencies in most parts of the non-ionising region of the electromagnetic spectrum, it is possible to do a lot of clinically valuable work with a high-quality oscillator covering a frequency range from 1 milliHertz to 20 MegaHertz. The testing of patients for electromagnetic hypersensitivity can be carried out using the field leaking from an oscillator. It appears that increasing the frequency of the oscillator produces a similar clinical effect to the serial dilution of an allergen. A frequency may be reached at which the allergic reaction is neutralised. The neutralising effect of this frequency can be transferred to a glass phial of water or saline which is known to be tolerated by the patient, by exposing the phial to a magnetic field at this neutralising frequency. Water treated in this way appears to be clinically effective for 1–2 months. This water can be used to prevent or relieve an allergic reaction by just having the patient hold the tube; it can also be applied sub-lingually, or extra- or intra-dermally.

Clinically, water seems to have a memory for past exposures to highly coherent frequencies which have taken place since it was last distilled. Apart from the clinical effects described above, some degree of laboratory demonstration is possible.

A capacitance bridge can be balanced with a test cell containing water, at a bridge frequency of, for example, 50.000 kHz, using chlorided silver electrodes to minimise electrode polarisation effects. If, without disturbing anything, the same oscillator is connected to a coil which exposes the water to an alternating magnetic field of about 1 Gauss at precisely the same frequency for some minutes then, on re-connecting the oscillator to the bridge, it will be found to have gone 'off-balance'. The bridge will measure the original capacitance value if the frequency is altered slightly; 50.020 kHz or 49.980 kHz will suffice if the bridge was originally balanced at 50.000 kHz. It will still be off-balance at 50.010 kHz and 49.990 kHz. There is no point in taking this experiment further unless it is possible to use an oscillator which can reproduce frequencies to parts-per-million.

In Paris, Dr Jacques Benveniste and his co-workers have followed immunological experiments through serial dilutions far in excess of Avogadro's Number (see Conclusion and Postscript).

The only other branches of physics which at present seem to be capable of probing the mysteries of water structure are convection, neutron scattering and X-ray diffraction. There have been reports from Russia that convection phenomena are affected by exposure of the water to electromagnetic fields.

In my own laboratory, work on ice formed by freezing water in a static or an alternating magnetic field shows an asymmetry in the crystals formed parallel or perpendicular to the magnetic field direction. X-ray diffraction patterns from this ice have been obtained.

Professor Mu Shik Jhon, from Seoul, South Korea (Moon and Jhon, 1986; Jhon 1987) has considered the importance of water structure in cryobiology and cancer and his medical co-worker, Dr Hidemitsu Hayashi (1988), from Kobe, Japan has been successfully applying an 'electric water reformer' in clinical situations. These devices electrolyse filtered but mineral-containing water in cells using electrodes which are also ferrite magnets giving fields in excess of 1.2 Tesla, and within which the anions and cations produced are separated by membranes. The anodic water is used externally for bathing, the cathodic water is used for all water ingested by the patients.

Electromagnetic emissions during allergic reactions

Objective tests for the existence of electromagnetic emissions from living systems are difficult to achieve. Radiofrequency emissions from dividing yeast cells have already been discussed.

Electromagnetic emissions in the audio-frequency part of the spectrum by reacting allergic subjects may be readily demonstrated by getting the subject to hold a plastic-cased tape recorder with the tape running and the recorder in the 'record' mode, but with no microphone connected. If the subject is reacting strongly enough, there will be sufficient interference passing through the plastic case to be picked up by the amplifier circuits. A wide variety of signals may be obtained on replay and these vary not only from patient to patient but differ on different occasions with the same patient. Sometimes there is a continuous sinusoidal oscillation, perhaps with distinct sidebands, on other occasions there will be a series of clicks; both these electrical waveforms have also been observed with species of electrical fish. The waveform of the clicks resembles that of a 'squegging' oscillator, for which the same piece of electronic circuitry can function both as an oscillator and as the highly sensitive, super-regenerative type of receiver which was in vogue in the early days of the wireless set, because it gave high sensitivity with a single valve.

The spectrum of the signals obtained from a reacting allergic subject holding a tape recorder can be analysed over a range of spectral resolutions on a commercially available audio spectrum analyser, so as to show the detailed frequency spectrum with all the complexity of the emissions. The spectrum analyser can be zeroed on the background noise level of a clean section of the tape, and checked for environmental electrical interference against a recording made with the recorder left running with nobody in the room. It has not yet been possible to determine whether the frequencies seen in the recorded spectrum correlate with those noted during the testing of electrically sensitive allergy patients. If tape recorder testing can be shown to have clinical value, a tape recorder is much more portable than a spectrum analyser, easier to use and, if battery-operated, electrically safe. However, some spectrum analysis facility would need to be available if the frequencies of individual patients are to be measured for clinical use. This still remains to be done, but there is electromedical equipment (e.g. MORA and BICOM), mostly originating from West Germany, which makes use of the patient's own oscillations for testing and/or therapeutic purposes; in such cases these are picked up, filtered, phase-inverted and then fed back to the patient. The patient's emissions are likely to be highly coherent so that quite coarse electrical filtering will suffice.

On the one occasion that it was possible to make a measurement using a spectrum analyser (HP-8553B) directly, electrical signals superimposed on the spectrum of the medium waveband radio transmissions were obtained; they ceased when the subject left the room. The measurements were made with the subject holding the 50 ohm impedance input lead of the spectrum analyser. A signal of 800 μV was obtained. The subject's measured d.c. skin resistance was 50 kohm so that, neglecting reactance, there should have been an open circuit voltage of 0.8 V available, enough to trigger the less sophisticated computer circuits (TTL-logic) and feed in false signals ('garbage'). The observed 'comb' spectrum of spikes extended to at least 2 MHz. In this case, ambient electrical signals were probably needed to trigger the allergic reaction in the subject because no emission was obtained with the subject and apparatus in an electrically screened laboratory. It should further be noted that most screened laboratories are not screened against the geomagnetic field or extremely low frequencies (ELF) below the power supply frequency. This particular subject was clearly sensitive to frequencies outside the ELF region of the spectrum.

A test for estimating the region of the frequency spectrum in which electromagnetic interactions are occurring requires a set of *metal* sieves or meshes graded in size, such as can be obtained from laboratory suppliers for grading powders and granules. The meshes must be metallic (good electrical conductors), nylon mesh will not do. To eliminate all but the ELF part of the spectrum, it should first be demonstrated that solid metal will screen off the interaction; then one should progress from the smallest mesh size to larger mesh sizes until an effect is observed. Dividing the velocity of light (3×10^8 m/s) by twice the mesh aperture measured in metres gives the lowest frequency, in Hertz, which can pass through each mesh. Thus, the first onset of the interaction can be bracketed between two mesh sizes, and hence two frequencies.

Edgar Brown and Kaye Behrens (Brown and Behrens, 1985) have used as pendulum bobs copper rods cut to half wavelength resonant lengths corresponding to the microwave region. They can, for example, say which foods react with the subject at which resonant wavelength. Following the suggestion that they should use metal mesh filters to check that the mesh size and the resonant length of the pendulum bob were consistent in giving the same wavelength, they were able to confirm that this was indeed the case. This experiment with metal meshes could also be tried using a muscle-test as described in the section on kinesiology in Chapter 7.

A metal mesh acts as a high-pass filter to electromagnetic waves. For example, the (1-millimetre) mesh on the door of a microwave cooker passes light waves (wavelength 0.5 micrometres), and the food can be seen inside. Very little of the longer wavelength (12 cm) microwave energy leaks out, so long as the door is not damaged; the energy is reflected back to cook the food. If any observed biomedical interaction is electromagnetic in origin, it should be completely screened by solid metal. One can only say 'should' because there are certain fields and frequencies (ELF) which need a considerable thickness of material (e.g. 6 inches of solid aluminium) or one of the special magnetic alloys (e.g. mumetal) for near-complete screening (Persinger, 1974). Thus, all frequencies, from those of ultra-violet light right through to the sub-Hertz of geomagnetic fluctuations and circadian rhythms, must be considered as being of possible biomedical significance, and be investigated.

Chemical and electromagnetic allergens

Every chemical bond has a coherent electrical oscillation which characterises it. This represents the duality which must exist between particles and waves, between chemical structure and frequency. If it was not for this chemical analysis by spectroscopy would not be possible. It may eventually become possible to show that the whole of the research effort put into the development of modern pharmaceuticals, which can be remarkably successful in acute conditions, has actually, although unknowingly, been directed towards the production of highly specific, electrical resonators at the biomolecular level. It is interesting to speculate how far one can go toward simulating a chemical effect by the electromagnetic frequencies characteristic of all the vibrational, bending, torsional and liberational modes of the molecule concerned. Can the right pattern of oscillations be created which will successfully mimic the corresponding chemicals? If so, we are on the way to 'Smelly-vision'! Phenol and formaldehyde are common allergens and simple molecules whose spectra could be experimented with in this way — would irradiating with their microwave spectrum act as a disinfectant, too?

Recent work by Dr Fritz Popp (1986) and his group has found that the oxidation of phenols and formaldehyde with hydrogen peroxide in the presence of homogenised (liquidised) plant tissue gives a great increase in their photon emission. Formaldehyde appears to be an effective biological stressor for the sensitisation of plants to other agents including homoeopathic preparations. If visible light is being emitted, then it is likely that other electromagnetic frequencies are also being emitted or are present as modulation and that these might be the triggers of allergic responses.

At the extremes of sensitivity of living systems, it is essential to realise that one is also at, or beyond, the state of the art of electronics equipment in its ability to detect signals in noise. Here, again, the remarked duality between frequency and chemical bonds appears. The effects of the macro-current therapies described parallel the effects of allopathic therapies, while the effects of micro-current therapies parallel the effects of homoeopathic remedies and other 'Alternative Medicine' therapies discussed in the next chapter. The reasons why both therapies work can be understood once the enormous dynamic range of the bio-sensor and bio-control systems of living organisms is appreciated. This is simply demonstrated by the dark-adaptation of the eye from sunlight to starlight, and the adaptation of the ear from pristine peace to the roar of a jet engine.

CHAPTER 7

Alternative medicine – the potential breakthrough

> We are accustomed to having men jeer at what they do not understand.
>
> Johann Wolfgang von Goethe (1749–1832)

A recent report by the British Medical Association (1986) was uncomplimentary about 'Complementary Medicine', yet when the Consumers' Association (1986) questioned nearly 28,000 *Which?* members, it discovered that one seventh of them had used some form of complementary medicine in the previous twelve months. This was sufficient to make the Association carry out a survey of the situation, the results of which emphasise the degree of antagonism still existing between complementary and conventional medicine in Britain. Of the one in seven who had visited a complementary practitioner in 1985, 81 per cent had already tried conventional medicine for their problem but were dissatisfied because they had not been cured, only got temporary relief or could not be treated; 82 per cent claimed to have been cured or improved, only 14 per cent thought that the treatment was ineffective, and only 1 per cent considered that their problem became worse. The types of complementary therapies most commonly used were: osteopathy 42 per cent, homoeopathy 26 per cent, acupuncture 23 per cent, chiropractic 22 per cent and herbalism 11 per cent.

At the first World Congress on Alternative Medicine, held in Rome in 1973, the provisional programme listed 135 different therapies. Stanway (1979) describes some 32 of these which he judges either have a distinguished past, a promising present or future, or are simply fascinating in their own right. For purposes of considering alternative or complementary medicine in the context of Electromagnetic Man, only those therapies are here discussed for which some involvement with the electromagnetic phenomena described in this book can be proffered.

Acupuncture

Acupuncture is a very ancient healing art; in China it dates back to 3000 BC. Little is known about the development of civilisation in ancient China because of the paucity of scientific archaeological excavations. What evidence there is suggests that technology then was similar to that employed in Western Asia. In the Middle East this period corresponds to the early dynasties; the beginnings of metallurgy with copper, tin, and gold; pottery and early writing on clay tablets; the wheel and the boat; quarrying and stone working (Hodges, 1970). It was said that soldiers wounded with arrows obtained relief from diseases at bony sites remote from the injury and that this led to the discovery of what appears to be some form of connection between internal organs and precise locations at the body's skin surface. About 1000 of these connecting lines, 'meridians', are described in classical Chinese acupuncture. Modern electroacupuncture techniques are finding still more. However, acupuncture is not an exercise in meridian plumbing; it is a philosophy of life that involves checks and balances which determine health or disease. The life forces, body energy or Chi (pronounced 'key'), are supposed to circulate through the meridians, day and night, 25 times in each. This is yet another of the circadian rhythms in the body. Wever (1985) has shown how the synchronism of some of these rhythms can be affected by environmental parameters and particularly by the very difficult to shield ELF environmental fields. These include the naturally occurring Schumann Radiation that is itself subject to the effects of tides and extraterrestrial radiation in the upper atmosphere, as well as all the man-made sources of ELF.

The art and philosophy of acupuncture cannot be understood in Western scientific terms (Kenyon, 1982a and b, 1983). Although there are a thousand locations on the body called 'acupuncture points', these are not distinguished by any observable structural features in the body tissues, although the electrical resistance of the skin does show a precise decrease within a few millimetres of the classical Chinese acupuncture points and can be used as an aid in locating them. Each relates to a specific and remotely situated body organ or function which can be affected by some treatment at the appropriate acupuncture point. The treatment may be the insertion of a blunt-ended needle of metal or ivory, which does not cause bleeding; alternatively, the effects may be produced by the application of weak electric currents or current pulses, or highly coherent radiation from a low-power laser (Trelles, 1985) or a microwave oscillator (Andreev et al., 1984).

Recent work by two doctors from Paris to test the validity of energy transport along the meridians has succeeded in visualising these meridians. Dr Jean-Claude Darras and Professor Dr De Vernejoul injected a radioactive tracer (solutions containing one of the radioactive isotopes: technetium, mercury or xenon) at an acupuncture point and found, using a gamma-ray camera, that the radioactivity travelled along the acupuncture meridian with a velocity of 3–5 cm/min. This is of the right order of magnitude to give 25 circulations per day or night. It was found to be slower in the case of diseased organs. They confirmed that the radio-isotope did not diffuse appreciably if injected other than at an acupuncture point, and that it did not enter into the lymphatic system or the blood circulation. It penetrated a tournequet preventing circulation. It only diffused towards the target organ if injected at an acupuncture point a part way along a meridian. The diffusion was not due to electrophoretic forces because a non-ionic radio-tracer (xenon) was equally affected. The rate of diffusion along the meridian was increased when the acupuncture point was stimulated, whether by a needle, electrically or by a helium–neon laser (Darras and De Vernejoul, 1986).

There is a report from China that the acupuncture points can also be sites of luminescence. The emission of radiation from acupuncture points, whether in the visible or lower regions of the electromagnetic spectrum, is compatible with the experiments of Egely (1986) on rotation of water in a petri dish when a subject's hands are positioned above, but not touching it; likewise, with a report (personal communication from Dr Monro) that a reacting allergic subject being examined in the night by the light of an all-metal-case torch was able to make the torch bulb glow more brightly by pointing at it.

A physical process which could offer an explanation for the properties of the meridians would be to assume that there is an electromagnetically rotating field maintaining a pressure in the direction of the target organ. The sense of the screw pitch and the direction of the rotation would be critical. Among the modern techniques of acupuncture (Kenyon, 1983) is apparatus which distinguishes dextro- (right-handed) and laevo- (left-handed) rotation of the plane of polarisation of electromagnetic waves other than by measurement of the optical activity. This is usually measured with a beam of light that has its vibrations confined to a single plane by passing it through a polarising filter, the equivalent to polarising sun-glasses. It is then passed through the solution and finally through another polarising filter. A solution of optically active molecules is able to rotate the plane of the polarisation of the light through electromagnetic field interactions, and the measurement is made in terms of the angle between the two polarising filters when no light passes. Blood is normally dextro-rotatory, but urine is normally laevo-rotatory and so is a pathological specimen of blood. This is what would be expected if the direction of flow of waste products is to be reversed, that is to flow away from the target organ, under the influence of a common, rotating, electromagnetic field.

With any needle, metal or ivory, inserted at an acupuncture point some electrical contact potential will be set up. This may be small, but the body is capable of extreme electrical sensitivity. The practice of rotating the needle may be to effect the removal of a 'Helmholtz Double-Layer' from a polarised needle and restore the original electrochemical potential.

Modern acupuncture (Kenyon, 1982a, 1982b, 1983) now makes extensive use of electrical devices which are used in many ways, both for diagnosis and therapy. When one walks around an exhibition in which all the various manufacturers are displaying their wares, the clear impression is that the operator and the patient form an essential part of the apparatus and the measurement procedure. Some of the features of the apparatus seem to be arranged so as to optimise electromagnetic coupling between nearby persons and the apparatus. The relevant biocommunication signals may not travel in apparently obvious directions. For example, an electrical output from the apparatus may trigger allergic responses in hypersensitive subjects and their subsequent electromagnetic reactions may affect the electrical resistance as then measured at the acupuncture points of the patient or at the acupuncture points of the person testing the patient. If it is remembered that a reacting allergic subject can identify a tube of an allergen merely brought into the room, then the ability of these pieces of apparatus to determine the correct potency of a homoeopathic preparation should not be cause for surprise.

Although, in many cases, the pieces of apparatus are clearly versions of that school physics experiment known as Wheatstone's Bridge, or else high-gain, low-frequency amplifiers and filters, this need not imply that they are actually responding to the low frequencies for which they were designed. Most commercial chart recorders will produce all sorts of complicated traces on the chart paper, with no connections at all made to the input, if an oscillator on the other side of the laboratory is merely tuned across a band of frequencies from perhaps 10 MHz to 1000 MHz. These frequencies travel around the laboratory space and the power wiring and become converted to small steady voltages by the high-gain amplifiers in such pieces of equipment – not a feature intended by the designers! Living systems can also emit such frequencies and at a sufficient intensity to affect electronic equipment. This, indeed, is the basis of one piece of apparatus which detects the patient's own oscillations, processes them electronically and feeds the resulting signals back to the patient as a therapy. This apparatus comes the nearest to being able to re-stabilise a patient's regulatory feedback loop. However, the filtering is so broad-band that the signals must merely be determining which of some very much more coherent modes of oscillation in the patient are to be enhanced by an additional flow of energy.

At the present state of the art, some clinicians are able to get useful results on some patients with the various types of apparatus involving the use of the acupuncture points; why is still not understood. For a comprehensive account of modern techniques of acupuncture, the reader is referred to the three volumes under that title by Kenyon (1982a, 1982b, 1983).

Bach remedies

Bach remedies represent a system of herbal remedies devised by a medical practitioner, Edward Bach (1880–1936). He had convinced himself that warmed dew taken from plants had absorbed their clinical herbal properties. He then found that the same result could be more conveniently obtained if the appropriate flowers were placed in a glass bowl of pure spring water in strong sunlight for a few hours. These observations are now relevant when considered in the context of the emission of electromagnetic oscillations by living systems, including botanical, probably spanning the whole spectrum from the ultra-violet to the sub-Hertz, and of the ability of water to 'remember' frequencies so far as clinical effects with allergic subjects are concerned.

Biofeedback

Biofeedback uses some form of instrumentation, usually electronic, to display to the patient or subject the value of some body function parameter, for example blood pressure or an EEG wave. The task is to optimise this parameter by any means possible, whilst having the values being achieved continuously presented as feedback. Biofeedback aims to train a person to control, at will, body functions usually regarded as involuntary. It demonstrates the power of the mind over the body in states of health and disease, and gives a method of affecting regulatory systems. It should be possible for a person to learn to enhance, or diminish, sensitivity to electromagnetic fields.

Colour therapy

Colour therapy, too, dates back to antiquity. The colour of a person's environment may have therapeutic effects or it may result in emotional or behavioural disturbances. The colour of material objects is associated with their chemistry; colour is merely the selection of particular frequencies of electromagnetic radiation in the visible part of the spectrum. But it should be remembered that selective absorption and reflection of radiation occurs throughout the electromagnetic spectrum and not just in the visible region. If our eyes were sensitive far beyond the visible, into the ultra-violet or infra-red, we would describe clear window glass as 'coloured'. Coloured dyes may give rise to clinical effects due to properties associated with spectral absorption characteristics outside the visible part of the electromagnetic spectrum. In common parlance, these effects would still be related to the perceived colour.

Coloured light therapy makes use of an intense, full-spectrum light source and three quite broad-band (50 nm), optical glass filters for the primary colours. In one apparatus the light is directed through fibre-optics light-pipes at specific points on the patient's skin. In another apparatus, the light is not applied to the patient but is directed to photodetectors, the output of which is amplified and the resulting signal fed to a treatment probe. The techniques are reported to be clinically useful; but existing scientific descriptions are useless for determining the mode of action. Either colour is a convenient label by which to characterise electromagnetic signals in some other part of the spectrum, or quite broad-band illumination is sufficient to stimulate much more highly coherent oscillations in the body. Backward children respond well to brightly coloured clothes and surroundings. It is not necessary to 'see' the light to be affected by its colour; a blind person can respond to colour and people can learn to distinguish colours with their fingertips. The effect of colour can also be acquired through water exposed to sunlight in coloured containers. The large areas of intensely coloured flower crops growing in fields have been reported to trigger allergic responses in some persons; these were successfully treated by homoeopathic preparations from tinctures of that particular colour.

Stanway (1979) cites a trial in which patients with pain were treated with different placebos. It was found that red placebo tablets were more effective than the real pain-killing tablet which had been included in the trial. There is a great need for the placebo effect to be properly investigated as a legitimate therapy instead of being written off as just an effect, since 35 per cent of the physically ill and 40 per cent of the mentally ill respond to placebos.

A recent example of what may prove to be another example of colour therapy is contained in a report of a clinical trial of a transcutaneous electrical nerve stimulator. Two groups of twenty male patients recovering from surgery for hernia were given these instruments for pain relief. However, one group had instruments which were inactive even though they still displayed the red lamp indicating that they were functioning. The results of comparing the pain scores of the patients and the quantities of medication taken showed no difference between the two groups. The workers concluded that the presence of the glowing red light must have exerted a powerful placebo effect even though there was no electrical stimulation of the nerve fibres. Further work would be needed to determine whether a red LED (light-emitting diode) can be clinically effective and to eliminate the possibility that the instruments were emitting ELF in the 8–10 Hz range, which is supposed to be generally beneficial.

Healing

Healing by the 'laying on of hands' is very ancient; it is particularly associated with priesthoods and the founders of religions, but many ordinary people also have the ability and may be practising it, consciously or unawares. There may be activity going on at many levels, spiritual and material, in both the healer and the patient. So far as Electromagnetic Man is concerned, it must be made clear that the electromagnetic sensitivity of a hypersensitive allergic person can be several orders of magnitude greater than the electromagnetic signals emitted by the muscle activity of the hands and arms. If a healer is able to sense the necessary electromagnetic frequencies and generate these through a biofeedback process, perhaps involving synchronous muscle or metabolic activity, then there is no reason why the patient should not respond with a cure, in seconds, as fast as the neutralisation of an allergic response by any other technique. If the healer is able to thought-transfer state of health information back to the patient, then healing could be effected through the patient's biofeedback mechanism, even without the presence of the healer. Biofeedback represents yet another way of correcting a faulty body regulatory system; could it possibly help to correct a faulty spiritual system as well?

Herbal medicine

Herbal medicine involves the use of plant materials for therapeutic purposes; however, it really extends from such dietary items as that ubiquitous infusion of the tea plant, to the 13 plant drugs which are defined as prescription-only medicines, encompassing some 5500 herbal products available as pharmacy medicines, or by general sale (Consumers' Association, 1986). The properties of plants that are of present concern are those associated with the electromagnetic oscillations of living systems, including necrotic radiation, as living plant material is absorbed whether as food or medicine. Referring to the section on the Bach remedies, one also needs to consider any electromagnetic frequency effects which can be imparted to water from herbal products. The efficacy of these aspects of botanical materials will not be properly tested by clinical trials and biochemical assay so long as the physics of coherent oscillations is ignored.

Homoeopathy

Homoeopathy originates from the work of a German physician, Dr Samuel Hahnemann, born at Meissen in 1755. He became highly critical of the current medical prescribing of his time. He found that when he, as a healthy person, took small amounts of a remedy for malaria, chinchona bark, he produced a malaria-like fever in himself which persisted until he ceased to take the chinchona bark. Malaria, known as the ague, used to be endemic in Europe – this included the marshes around London. The bark of the chinchona tree became so named after the Countess of Chinchon, wife of the Viceroy of Peru, who was supposed to have been cured of malaria by this bark of the Peruvian Indians' 'fever-tree', discovered in 1600 by a Jesuit missionary, Juan Lopez, who had been cured of malaria by an Indian tribal chief.

Hahnemann proposed and used as self-evident two axioms contained in his 'Law of Similars' – Like Cures Like. This assumes, first, that every medicine produces a pattern of symptoms in a healthy person resembling the symptoms of a disease which the medicine will cure in a sick person. These symptoms and therapeutic effects will be produced even when the medicine is highly diluted. Second, the remedy which produces effects in healthy persons most nearly matching the total symptom picture of the patient will exert the greatest curative effect; the required dose is the minimum necessary to evoke the symptoms.

Homoeopathy, like the medically acceptable immunisation, stimulates the body to do its own fire-fighting. Allopathic medicine and surgical intervention are seen to have become necessary only if the fire has been allowed to get out of control, perhaps because the body's own regulatory system is unable to cope or has been damaged.

The scientific problem is to relate Hahnemann's axioms to the criteria of modern science. In 1811, Avogadro deduced the principle that equal volumes of all gases at the same temperature and pressure contain the same number of molecules. The actual number of molecules per mole (the molecular weight in grams) was measured by Loschmidt in 1865 and in the German literature it is known as Loschmidt's Number, according to the usual custom in science; elsewhere it is known as Avogadro's Number. Its value has been determined with precision and is given as 6.0232045×10^{23} molecules per mole with an uncertainty of 5.1 ppm

(CRC, 1976). It is the same for any substance. This implies that when a homoeopathic preparation has been serially diluted 24 times, each by a factor of 10 (24X, 24D), or 12 times each by a factor of 100 (12C), there should be none of the original molecules left. Yet, clinical results (and veterinary and horticultural results) are claimed for homoeopathic preparations at dilutions far higher than the above, and these are supported by research studies (Reilly *et al.*, 1986). Recently, Benveniste (Davenas *et al.*, 1988) and his colleagues in Paris have demonstrated clearly that it is possible to serially dilute an aqueous solution of an antibody virtually indefinitely without losing its biological activity – and indeed showed rhythmic fluctuations in that activity. This finding prompted a baffled editorial in the same *Nature* issue and amazement in the scientific fraternity, which has been placated, temporarily. Some of the most recent developments are discussed in the Postscript.

It is clear that physics and not chemistry is the science from which to seek an explanation. There are two problems: What sort of bio-information is contained in a homoeopathic preparation? How does it interact with a living system to produce a clinical effect?

The preparation of a homoeopathic remedy is basically as follows. If the material for the remedy is a solid, it is ground up (triturated) with the diluent, usually lactose. Then, one part of this intimate mixture is again ground up with a further nine parts of lactose to give a one-in-ten dilution. This dilution process is repeated successively. If the material is soluble it is diluted in alcohol (ethanol), or water and alcohol, and 'succussed' – shaken vigorously against the palm of the hand. Dilution on its own will not necessarily produce an effective remedy. There are machines which will carry out the succussion. A high-pressure jet of water will also succuss effectively. It is probably the generation of shock waves in the liquid which is effective. The whole process of preparing a homoeopathic remedy is known as 'potentisation'.

Brucato and Stephenson (1966) suggested that the process of potentisation induces electrochemical changes in the diluent: Callinan (1986) discussed a number of possible structural changes in water in connection with the mode of action of homoeopathic preparations. Dr Cyril Smith (Smith *et al.*, 1985) has proposed a helical structure in water which is capable of 'remembering' frequency. This developed from electrical frequency measurements made on allergy patients who showed a rhythmic pattern of stimulating/inhibiting responses to increasing frequency, which resembled those found with increasing homoeopathic potency (Callinan, 1985) and with increasing allergen dilutions (Miller, 1972).

Various electrical measurements by Mishra and co-workers on homoeopathic preparations have shown similar rhythmicities with potency in respect of capacitance, pH and electrode potential (Jussal *et al.*, 1982) and pH and enzyme activity (Jussal *et al.*, 1984). Frequency resonance measurements have been made on homoeopathic preparations as a function of potency by a number of workers. Ludwig (1986) gave the principal frequency for Arnica 1000X potency as 9.725 kHz and 300 Hz for phosphorus 6X. Another worker's set of measurements over a range of potencies of sulphur covered the whole of the audio-frequency region with frequencies being specified to 0.01 Hz.

Slawinska and Slawinski (1986) have measured ultra-weak photon emission from living plant tissues treated with various homoeopathic preparations and potencies. Sacks (1985) has done NMR spectroscopy of homoeopathic remedies.

The mechanism for the action of homoeopathic potencies must lie in the regulatory systems of living organisms. Whereas allopathic preparations are used in sufficient quantity to replace or swamp the body's own chemicals, there is no chemistry in homoeopathy, apart from that little in potencies below 24X or 12C. The most important result came from the work with electrically sensitive allergy patients as described in Chapter 6; a sealed tube of water which produced no clinical effects on a patient would, after being exposed to a magnetic field at one of the patient's allergy neutralising frequencies, function as an allergy neutralising dilution for purposes of that patient's therapy. Thus, a potency has been induced into the water by a purely physical means. Furthermore, the water is able to retain the effect of the frequency for a period of time, which may be weeks or months. The alcohol used in homoeopathic potentisation is said to stabilise the preparation; this has not yet been investigated in respect of frequency-treated water.

The term 'homeostasis' was coined in 1932 by W.B. Cannon to describe 'the various physiologic arrangements which serve to restore the normal state, once it has been disturbed'. Many of the homeostatic systems in physiology are negative feedback control systems, characterised by having a sensor to detect deviations from the normal or required value of the system output and a feedback path to convey this information to a regulator which adjusts the system accordingly. With any negative feedback system, the phase shift around the feedback loop must be controlled to prevent instability; oscillations will build up at any frequency where there is the particular combination of a 180-phase shift in the loop and a net loop gain greater than unity.

The simplest and most general, precision, negative feedback, analogue control system in electronics is achieved with negative feedback around a high-gain amplifier. In the case of enzyme-catalysed reactions, the gain of the enzyme as an amplifier has been determined, although it is not usually described in these terms by chemists. If the gain is taken as the ratio of the rate of reaction – molecular turnover – when catalysed by the enzyme to the uncatalysed reaction rate (Callinan, 1985), then the gains can be suitably high, as Table 7.1 shows. Note that electromagnetic radiation corresponding to the activation energy would be in the infrared.

Table 7.1 Enzyme reactions as high-gain amplifiers

Enzyme	Gain	Activation energy ($V = kT/e$)
Carbonic anhydrase	3.6×10^6	0.38 Volts
Catalase	3.6×10^8	0.49
B amylase	1.7×10^9	0.53
Kinases	3.2×10^{10}	0.60

It can be shown mathematically that so long as the open-loop gain of the amplifier is very high, its precise value does not matter. This is because mathematical approximation makes the closed-loop gain become effectively equal to the reciprocal of the feedback factor; for example, if 1 per cent of the output is fed back to the input, the closed-loop gain will be 100, if 0.1 per cent is fed back the closed loop gain will be 1000, and so on. Thus any fault in the feedback path which decreases the amount of negative feedback will make the closed-loop gain tend towards the open-loop gain. Then, either the control system will fail because it saturates in the permanently 'on' state, or in the permanently 'off' state, or else, if the above gain-phase criteria are satisfied, it will oscillate. It can even do both, but in either case it will cease to exert a controlling function.

Living systems can maintain homeostasis over a wide dynamic range of perturbations. They usually show a logarithmic response to a stimulus. These properties imply not only the presence of a high-gain amplifier but also non-linear elements like diodes in the feedback circuit to generate the necessary logarithmic characteristic.

The obvious way of influencing a homeostatic system with a homoeopathic remedy is to have it affect the magnitude and/or phase of the feedback factor. Even though there is probably nothing more tangible than frequency-structured water in the remedy, this must convey the information contained in the original tincture molecules, precisely modified by potentisation.

The theory of homoeopathy must be able to explain how clinical responses can occur within seconds. Cases have been described where an exact diagnosis and correct potency have relieved the particular condition in seconds, as quickly as an allergic response can be neutralised by the correct dilution of allergen. The time taken for the hydrogen bonds in water to rearrange themselves is about 10^{-11} s; the distance that a hydrogen atom has to move in order to be considered a part of an adjoining atom is 7.6×10^{-11} m. Thus the maximum velocity with which any rearrangement of water structuring could propagate through the body water of a living system is a few metres per second. This is just fast enough to affect all the water in the body in under a second and to be consistent with the action of homoeopathic remedies and allergy neutralisations.

Watterson (1982) has already considered the effects of structure waves in water. In order to account for magnetic field effects and a memory for frequency (Smith *et al.*, 1985) it is desirable to think in terms of a helical structure in water, so that the structure waves would occupy those electromagnetic and acoustic modes of propagation appropriate to a helix. These must be capable of being set up in water by the spectrum of coherent oscillations, which uniquely characterises the chemical bonds comprising the original tincture molecules; or, in the case of electromagnetic potentisation, by the frequencies of the electromagnetic fields applied.

It does not matter whether the structure waves are electromagnetic or acoustic because biomolecules are mostly large dipoles and will behave as transducers (energy and signal converters). Control must be considered at each level of organisation in the living system. The most basic is the control of the cell and body chemistry through the enzyme systems. The basic characteristic of an enzyme reaction, with its substrate to form a product, is a dependence of the 'velocity' (rate of formation of the product) on the substrate concentration, directly proportional at low substrate concentrations, but reaching a maximum velocity at high substrate concentrations. Classically, this is described in terms of Michaelis and Menten's derivations, with the assumptions removed by Haldane (Gutfreund, 1977). However, this relates to a situation not involving the homeostatic control of a living cell.

To be able to relate the action of a homoeopathic remedy to the theory of control systems, and apply it to an enzyme-controlled reaction in a living system, it is necessary to postulate a feedback loop from the enzyme's product back to the enzyme. For present purposes this must be so conceived that a homoeopathic remedy can affect it. Since the living cell is to be involved, one should consider that the presence of the remedy alters the natural spectrum of oscillations of the cell in a manner which is characteristic of the electromagnetic spectrum of the original tincture material. The greater the concentration of the reactants, the stronger – and possibly more coherent – will this negative feedback signal need to be. A frequency-selective path through structured cell water might be able to couple these stabilising oscillations back to the enzyme (probably located in or on a membrane). Finally, the oscillations reaching the enzyme must then be able to control its activity. If the enzyme control fails, only the limitation of insufficient substrate will prevent the reaction from running at its maximum velocity. What would be required of a homoeopathic potency is to supply, on a self-propagating basis, the missing negative-feedback path through the structured water of all relevant cells in the living system concerned, or a target value.

This is a tall order, but at least the above hypothesis provides a map for buried treasure, containing specific features which can be tested against reality. How could one test it? First, separate the living cell from an enzyme reaction, get the cell to regulate the enzyme, and interpose electromagnetic filters to determine the frequency of interaction. Dr Eugene Celan (1986), in Bucharest, has, in principle, carried out this experiment already, but only between two different types of cells. He has taken a culture of tumour cells growing, in darkness, in a pendant drop beneath a quartz cover slip, placed on the upper surface of which is a drop of actively dividing yeast cells. He has shown that radiation from the yeast cells which passes through quartz, but not through glass, will kill the tumour cells.

The second requirement is to show that homoeopathic potencies can restore communication between a cell and an enzyme reaction that it is controlling. Homoeopathic potencies can affect the coherent optical photon emission from cells whose homeostatic system had been pre-stressed by the poison formaldehyde (Slawinska and Slawinski, 1986). This involves optical frequencies and, as Dr Fritz Popp remarks, 'A living cell needs the bandwidth of an optical communication link to function in real time'. If cells are using coherent light as the carrier frequency for communication, then the modulation may extend even to the low frequencies associated with homoeopathic remedies when potentised electrically. For example, Dr Wolfgang Ludwig (1986, 1988) finds the frequency of 9.725 kHz associated with Arnica 1000X. If this is a modulation frequency component on an optical frequency carrier, the latter must be coherent to 1 part in 10^{15}. This is the sort of precision physics that will be needed to demonstrate the scientific basis of homoeopathy.

Hydrotherapy

Hydrotherapy is concerned with the use of water from natural sources which are reputed to have healing properties, for various therapies including drinking it and bathing in it. The spa towns of Europe in the last century reflect past popularity. The possibility of electromagnetic effects in water adds a further dimension to what appears to have been a diversion for the wealthy, but which is regarded as a cost-effective therapy for workers in Eastern Europe. From what has already been written above, it seems that water is able to take up therapeutic effectiveness from plants, light and potentised tinctures of any chemical substance. Therefore it is not surprising that the source of the water is of importance. Kervran (1972) writes:

> To show that chemical analysis is inadequate in determining the biological properties of a substance, let us have a look at the case of activated water. All specialists in hydromineral treatments know that it is dangerous to consume excessive quantities of the gushing water from the spring of a spa ... water flowing underground acquires special properties. Yves Rocard, Director of the Physics Laboratory at the École Supérieure in Paris, has shown that water sets up an electromagnetic field which can be detected by a very sensitive magnetometer. It is this property which permits diviners to detect water running between particles of rock in the ground. ... We know nothing of the physical disposition of molecules in 'activated' water. It can be produced empirically by various methods; for example, by electromagnetic fields of very low frequency (about 10 Hz), but sometimes fields of higher frequencies (3–4 kHz, 10 kHz) but superimposed on frequencies which differ very little, in order to obtain a low frequency impulse.

'Activated' water was studied by Piccardi (see Chapter 3). When heated, it de-scales boilers, converting the insoluble scale into a colloid. The alga *Chara foetida* loses its normal calcareous membrane by precipitation in 'activated' water. The behaviour of colloids in 'activated' water, particularly those containing organo-metallics, has been the subject of much research.

Kinesiology

Kinesiology makes use of an effect whereby, if an allergic subject is confronted with one of the substances to which he or she is allergic, there is a sudden drop in the available force from the voluntary muscles. This empirical observation has led to a number of testing techniques for assessing allergic responses. Dr Hugh Cox has developed this technique to the point where he is able to test several allergens a minute on a routine basis (Cox, 1985). Effects of muscle reactions in one triggered allergic subject can be propagated through a chain of passive 'third parties' to a person whose muscle response is actually measured by the tester; this effect is made use of in the testing of infants and small children.

An electromagnetic explanation is the only really plausible one for such effects.

Certain allergic subjects are able to use a dowser's wand or a pendulum to assess their likelihood of developing allergic responses, particularly in respect of foods about to be eaten. It is likely that the dowsing phenomena (see Chapter 11) are electromagnetic in origin and are probably associated with small involuntary muscle movements such as those measured in the kinesiology tests and which the wand or pendulum merely amplifies.

The resonant rod experiments of Brown and Behrens (1985) could be extended to kinesiology by successively joining the thumb and index finger between various sections of copper rod, cut to a range of lengths from, say, a millimetre to the maximum handspan of perhaps ten centimetres and carrying out a kinesiology response test for each length of rod. For example, the tester might take the index finger of each hand and attempt to pull the subject's thumb and finger apart so that the rod falls out. The strength of the thumb-finger grip is greater than the force the tester can apply with two index fingers, unless the subject experiences an allergic response resulting in a sudden weakening of muscle tone.

Kirlian photography

The Kirlian photographic technique was developed in Russia in the late 1890s. At a photographic exhibition of the Russian Technical Society in 1898, Yakov Narkevitch-Todko, an engineer and electrical researcher, exhibited 'electrographic photographs obtained with the help of quiet electrical discharges'. Remember that this was only a couple of years after the discovery of X-rays by the German physicist, Wilhelm Conrad Röntgen, of Würzburg; at this time all physics laboratories were experimenting with electrical discharge apparatus.

Dr Semyon D. Kirlian and Dr Valentina Kh. Kirlian of the Kazakh State University, USSR, devoted much of their working lives to the photographic and visual observation techniques by means of electrical discharges, which are named after them (Kirlian and Kirlian, 1961). The techniques record the pattern of the luminous Tesla discharges in the air surrounding an object which is subjected to a high voltage at a frequency which is too high to be perceived. There are a number of pieces of electromedical apparatus for recording such images, typically from the fingers and toes, and the pads of animals. These are used for clinical diagnosis. The observed Kirlian patterns change with the person's mental and physical state and have been used as a qualitative indicator of the efficacy of a particular course of therapy and for certain diagnostic purposes. It is interesting that the acupuncture points of the body can be observed in this way (Mandel, 1986). Kirlian pictures taken of blood and other tissue samples have also been used for diagnostic purposes. The precise physical mechanisms involved in the formation of the Kirlian image are not known. Ionisation is a dark process; the light comes from recombination processes and in moist air these are extremely complicated.

There is much empirical clinical evidence on the efficacy of Kirlian photography as a diagnostic tool even in its present stage of development (Mandel, 1986). In the UK Oldfield and Coghill (1988) have recently described case studies and advances in diagnosis and technique.

Naturopathy

Naturopathy makes use of the natural power of the body to heal itself, perhaps with some assistance. Kirlian photography is used to diagnose illness, even in the pre-clinical stage, and to monitor the progress of healing. Hippocrates (400 BC) was aware of the body's powers of self-healing; Paracelsus distinguished doctors who healed miraculously from those who healed through medicine; Mesmer referred to these powers as 'animal magnetism'; Reichenbach distinguished them from the forces of chemistry, electricity or magnetism; Lakhovsky attributed them to electromagnetic resonances in the cell which was capable of emitting and absorbing electromagnetic radiation. This is getting quite close; the great difference between the life forces, healing forces and all the other forces in living systems is probably to be found in their degree of *coherence*. It is this which makes laser light so different from sunlight.

Negative ion therapy

Negative ion therapy corrects the imbalance of air ionisation which occurs particularly in urban environments but can also occur in association with geological and meteorological conditions. The only almost clean air left in the whole world nowadays is to be found at the foot of a glacier; the contamination condenses out on the cold surfaces. In the country, the air may contain 300–1000 negative ions per cubic centimetre. These will be mostly negatively charged oxygen. This is the environment in which evolution took place. Civilisation, with pollution and air-conditioned buildings, reduces this concentration and may even create an excess of positive ions. These are associated with the restlessness, anxiety, irritability, depression, headaches, nausea and eye troubles of the 'sick-building syndrome', although additional factors such as sensitisation by high levels of formaldehyde are also involved. In certain parts of the world there are winds that come off the deserts bringing with them a ten-fold drop in humidity, a rise in temperature, and an increase in positive ion concentrations. In Israel it is the Sharav wind; in California it is the Santa Anna; in Canada the Chinook; in Austria, Germany and Switzerland it is the Föhn; in Argentina it is the Zonda. In Israel, Professor Sulman has shown that these symptoms can be triggered by an endogenous chemical – serotonin – and that these winds give raised serotonin levels. The symptoms could be cured by drugs which are antagonistic to serotonin, or by breathing air with enhanced negative ion concentrations. Apparatus is available for generating negative ions indoors. Figures for patients' obtaining relief by this means range from 40 to 80 per cent (Hawkins, 1981). However, with multiple-allergy patients, there is a risk that excessive use of any treatment will turn it into another trigger for allergic reactions. In Nature negative ions are generated by water-drop formation – springs and fountains, mountain weather – and by vegetation. The early negative ion generators also produced the toxic oxygen compound ozone. The more modern ion generators should not give off any ozone during operation. Unfortunately, when ion generators first came on the market, they were so 'oversold' in the USA that the FDA banned them in 1961. Even now in Britain, only minimal medical claims are allowed to be made for them in advertisements, despite the growing evidence for their efficacy in certain conditions.

Orgone therapy

Orgone therapy was the brainchild of Dr Wilhelm Reich (1897–1957), one of Freud's pupils, who broke away from the Master and eventually set up his laboratories in Orgonon, USA, in 1934, for research into Primordial Life or Cosmic Orgone Energy. He too claimed the presence of an energy distinct from electromagnetic energy, as he knew it. He was eventually defamed and discredited by conspiracy, on the grounds that orgone energy does not exist, and finally died in jail.

His 'orgone accumulator' consisted of layers of wood and metal in a box, or a stack of metal pipes; he directed this energy through a tube and used it for healing purposes. He found that he got an adverse reaction with radioactive materials and termed this Deadly Orgone (DDR). What he thought he had done is of less concern than what he actually did. First, any metal/insulator structure will resonate at some electromagnetic frequency. Allergic subjects can be affected by such resonators because of reaction with electromagnetic radiation which they emit themselves. His accumulators resembled laser resonators, so one should consider whether his apparatus was capable of using air ionisation (natural or enhanced by radioactive materials) or water vapour as an energy source for the generation of coherent oscillations in the centimetre, millimetre or sub-millimetre wave part of the spectrum. The honeycomb matrix used in many electrodiagnostic devices may well function as an orgone accumulator and affect the operator.

Osteopathy

Osteopathy involves the manipulation of the body, particularly the spine. The possible connection with electromagnetic phenomena lies in the fact that bone has electromechanical properties rather like the crystal in a record player pick-up. These are now considered to be due to electro-streaming of ions rather than piezoelectricity, but the effects are similar. Manipulation will generate electrical potentials, but it remains to be shown whether these are clinically effective. If the natural streaming currents generated by functional activity in connective tissues influenced the tissue, then the currents produced by the natural mechanical oscillations of the loaded bone may be very significant (Collier and Donarski, 1987).

Pattern therapy

Pattern therapy relates shapes to biomedical effects. This encompasses such phenomena as the ideal shaped containers for making yoghurt and brewing beer, to the shape of psychiatric hospital wards. As already mentioned, allergy patients have been triggered by passive microwave resonators in their vicinity; they also react against certain regular metallic structures in the environment, such as railings. Pattern is coherence in space rather than in time, and as such it only needs to be scanned in the manner of a record or tape player to be converted to a coherent frequency. Many effects of structural geometries and buildings on people, animals, foods and even homoeopathic remedies are listed by Stanway (1979).

Pyramid healing

Pyramid healing is also based on shapes having an effect on living systems, but in this case it is exclusively concerned with pyramid shapes having the proportions of the Great Pyramids of Egypt. Structures having these geometrical proportions have been described as 'generators of energy' (Ostrander and Schroeder, 1979). Any electromagnetic rationale behind such propositions must derive from similarities with the geometries of acoustic and electrical resonators.

Radiesthesia

Radiesthesia is the French term for the use of dowsing for medical diagnosis and the selection of remedies. The history and broader aspects of dowsing and man's environment are discussed in Chapter 11. Regarding the clinical, allergy, nutritional, and environmental testing applications of dowsing, Brown and Behrens (1985) give a full account of their 'Humonetics' Testing Procedure, which appears to use an electromagnetic interaction between the tester and the person or substance being tested as indicated and interpreted from the motion of a pendulum held by the tester. The work of Haylock Fidler (1983) on the quantification of the dowsing response should also be noted.

The radiesthetist (clinical dowser) (Stanway, 1979) uses the pendulum with the patient or a 'witness' which may be a piece of hair, nail clipping or a blood specimen. The radiesthetist takes a clinical history from the patient and then mentally concentrates on questions relating to the condition of the patient, while observing the pendulum, and then interprets its response. The pendulum can be calibrated against known clinical specimens (Turenne witnesses) positioned relative to the 'witness' on a rule or chart. The rule is usually placed East–West with the radiesthetist facing North or South. Possible remedies, for example homoeopathic potencies, can then be selected for the patient in a similar manner. The technique is clearly at the interface of mind and matter because radiesthetists can operate remotely from the patient, for example using a 'witness' in the absence of the patient or with the patient on the telephone. Such topics are discussed in Chapter 11.

Radionics

In radionics, another technique that is difficult to comprehend, the operator seems to be an essential component of the instrumentation. The origins of radionics go back to the beginning of the present century and an American physician, Dr Albert Abrams. Using percussion on the abdomen of a patient with cancer of the lip, he found a change of the percussion sound occurred only when the patient faced to the West. He was also able to elicit the same change in percussed sound from a healthy patient, but only when a tube containing a piece of malignant tumour was placed on the forehead.

Abrams developed a piece of apparatus described briefly by Stanway (1979) and in more detail by Day and de la Warr (1957), writing in collaboration with George de la Warr, who had developed the original radionics techniques and instrumentation of Abrams in England. After Abram's death, the radionics techniques were picked up in America by a chiropractor, Ruth Drown; she eventually fell foul of the medical profession and the FDA, was tried in 1951 and eventually served a jail term for fraud and medical quackery. She died shortly afterwards.

Radionics instruments are not described in detail even in books on the subject. They do not contain conventional electronic circuitry and are not usually powered from the mains. If it is remembered that ordinary electronic components, such as variable resistors and lengths of wire, have very different properties in the microwave region, and that, as noted for pattern therapy, persons can respond to electrically resonating configurations, then one sees radionics equipment as a tunable resonator excited by electromagnetic signals emitted by the patient, with the resonances sensed by the operator or some form of electronic circuit. It must be remembered that electronic circuits will often respond to oscillations at frequencies outside the range intended by the designers; this is the sort of thing that electronics engineers discuss under the heading 'electromagnetic compatibility'.

De la Warr succeeded in photographing patterns which related to radiations associated with objects and pathological specimens. He made a number of models of his cameras, which functioned in some manner as an aid to the operator's 'extra-sensory perception'. The camera is said to have photographed, in the course of over 10,000 exposures, only what the operator knows or is deliberately thinking. The technique gets one close to the area of interaction between mind and matter, the spiritual and the natural worlds, inasmuch as changes were produced in the radionic photographs of Oxford tap-water following the ceremonial blessing of samples of the water by two priests; furthermore, a remarkable radionic photograph was obtained from a reliquary of St Ignatius.

It seemed to be necessary for a suitable operator to load the photographic plates into the holder as some form of preconditioning. To obtain a developable photographic image pixel, it is only necessary to cause a pair of electrons to transfer from a silver halide crystal to the gelatin matrix.

When it came to having to submit funding applications for his laboratory (Delawarr Laboratories) and convince academic and medical authorities, insurmountable problems arose. De la Warr could not explain how his apparatus worked using the language of the conventional sciences, even though he could readily demonstrate its effectiveness under test conditions. He remained largely unbelieved by the scientific establishment and, although taken to court for fraud, in his case the judge dismissed every allegation. De la Warr continued his work until his death in 1969, having founded an organisation to continue his research.

Sound therapy

Sound therapy covers the techniques whereby sounds are used for therapeutic purposes. It extends from music and speech, the healing prayers and mantras of religions, to the use of specific frequencies to mimic the natural resonances in bones which, due to injury, are no longer generated during ordinary movement. Manners (1986) has evolved a system of applying audible sound directly to the body for healing applications.

It must be realised that all sounds other than noise (waves on the beach sound), that is sounds which have a more or less well defined pitch, are coherent oscillations. Since water and many biomolecules are electrical dipoles, to produce a mechanical or acoustic oscillation is equivalent to producing an electrical oscillation and conversely. Hence one should expect such an interconversion based on frequency. Some allergy patients react similarly to sounds of the same frequency as electromagnetic oscillations which trigger reactions. The ability of a musical ear to pick out one 'wrong note' from a large number of players and singers is an example of the selectivity in coherence which man can achieve.

Current research

As far as ongoing research in the above areas in the UK is concerned, the Dove Project, coordinated by Dr Julian Kenyon at the Centre for the Study of Alternative Therapies in Southampton, is probably the only project involving an investigation of the body's electromagnetic fields and the possibility of monitoring them for advance warning of impending disease or dysfunction.

The Centre for Complementary Health Studies was established at the University of Exeter in July 1987 with the aim of initiating 'an integrated and scientific exploration of the phenomena of complementary medicine'. It will support interdisciplinary postgraduate study in many areas, including the theories of health and illness underlying complementary medicine. It is setting up a bibliographic and research data information service in collaboration with the Scientific Information Centre of the London-based Research Council for Complementary Medicine, which has access to all major medical and scientific databases throughout the world.

In West Germany, there is the Essen-based Zentrum zur Dokumentation für Naturheilverfahren and, in the United States, there is the California-based (Sherman Oaks) World Research Foundation providing information and data services. The latter has the motto 'Only with knowledge can one decide the merits of any idea. Free choice is not free – it must be pursued, defended and utilised.'

The teaching seminars at the Exeter Centre for Complementary Health Studies will include discussion of models for legislation for the provision of complementary therapies and their integration with orthodox systems. This is timely because there was for a while a pending EEC Directive which would have demanded that, by 1989, alternative therapies should be able to show convincing scientific evidence for their efficacy or face prohibition, a scenario likely to lead to outrage and large-scale non-compliance in many EEC countries. Presumably such things as psychotherapy would have fallen under its strictures. The current state of play seems to be that the Directive may have disappeared, like the 'Cheshire Cat'.

To keep abreast of developing research and theories in this field, the reader is recommended to monitor the *Journal of Complementary Medicine*, published by the Institute of Complementary Medicine, the journal *Complementary Medical Research*, published by the Research Council for Complementary Medicine, and the *Journal of Alternative & Complementary Medicine*, published by Argus Health Publications, all of which are based in London. To keep up with developments involving exclusively electromagnetic phenomena in living systems, the reader is recommended to *Microwave News*, published in New York (PO Box 1799, Grand Central Station, NY 10163, USA).

CHAPTER 8

Electromagnetic environmental pollution

> Whatever hasn't happened will happen and no one will be safe from it.
>
> J.B.S. Haldane (1892–1964)

Part 1 Fishpond – the history of a campaign

> When the Present has latched its postern behind my tremulous stay,
> And the May month flaps its glad green leaves like wings,
> Delicate-filmed as new-spun silk, will the neighbours say,
> 'He was a man who used to notice such things'?
>
> Thomas Hardy (1840–1928)

While many cities in England are falling into their crumbling network of Victorian sewers, the *cloaca maxima* in Bath (Aquae Sulis) is still as functional as when the Romans left it. Although we know how to provide cities with clean water and to remove wastes, the will to put this knowledge into effect against competition for resources and without a damaging impact on the environment is not always so apparent. The Danube (Donau) cities of Germany, Austria, Czechoslovakia, Hungary, Romania and Bulgaria are required to take in their water downstream from their point of waste discharge; but even this rather strong measure appears to have been ineffective in protecting their common interests. At the present time the world is not becoming a healthier place in spite of high technology medicine. Certainly, more can be done for those who present with illnesses, but why are so many people still becoming ill? Unlike the chemical and biological pollutions of man's environment, the need for an electromagnetically acceptable environment is not appreciated or not admitted. Even if it were, it is still not known how to provide an electromagnetic pollution-free environment compatible with modern demands for frequency allocations in an already overcrowded electromagnetic spectrum.

Man, like all life on Earth, has evolved in an environment flooded with electromagnetic radiation of most wavelengths and varying degrees of coherence. That he feeds and breathes is due to plant photosynthesis. The frequency spectrum with which living systems are concerned probably extends from the ionising ultra-violet radiation through non-ionising, visible, microwave, radio and audio frequencies to the sub-Hertz, perhaps even to the frequency corresponding to the reciprocal of the lifetime of the organism itself, which clearly has a coherence in space and time throughout its existence. The low-frequency Schumann radiation from the upper atmosphere appears to be of particular importance in relation to biological rhythms and has a frequency spectrum which resembles that of the human (EEG) brain-waves. In electrotherapy, the frequencies 27.5 Hz, 55 Hz, 110 Hz, 220 Hz, 440 Hz and 880 Hz are said to be extremely effective. In interferential therapy (Savage, 1984), frequencies 0–5 Hz affect the sympathetic nerves, 10–150 Hz affect the parasympathetic nerves, 10–15 Hz affect the motor nerves, 90–110 Hz affect the sensory nerves, 130 Hz affects the nociceptive system and 0–10 Hz affects unstriped muscle. The musically inclined may not need reminding that orchestras tune to A-440 Hz and it is interesting to speculate what beneficial effects might have accrued by now if 55 Hz, instead of 50 Hz or 60 Hz, had been chosen as the power supply frequency on either side of the Atlantic. The frequency of 5 Hz is usually regarded as being depressive, while the range 8–10 Hz is associated with well-being and general alertness.

In this chapter, Hilary Bacon tells of her battles to survive an electrically polluted environment. In years to come the general public will have cause to be very grateful for the ability and determination of campaigners such as Hilary Bacon and to contemplate with amazement some of the ironies of coincidence which have characterised her attempts to elucidate an infinitely complex, hardly understood but vitally important biological truth. The discovery of that truth stems from the concept of electrobiology which, as Dr Robert Becker points out, can be considered to have originated with the work of Albert von Szent-Gyorgyi, a Hungarian physician and biochemist who won a Nobel Prize in 1933 for his work on biological oxidation mechanisms and vitamin C. In 1941 he postulated that the atomic structure of such biological molecules as proteins was sufficiently organised to function as a crystalline lattice, so that such phenomena as semiconduction could exist not only within metals but also within living systems (Becker and Marino, 1982). In his later years, he focussed his research on cancer in what he termed quantum biology, and in 1978 published *The Living State and Cancer* in which he outlined his theory that cancer is, fundamentally, a submolecular, electronic disturbance.

Dr Szent-Gyorgyi died in 1986. Much of his most important work was done at the Marine Biological Laboratory, Woods Hole, Massachusetts, where for many years he was joined each summer by Professor Ron Pethig from the University College of North Wales, Bangor. Mrs Bacon was married to the grandson of Dr Frank Lillie, founder of the Woods Hole Institute. Two of Dr Lillie's great-grandsons became unwitting guinea-pigs in circumstances which finally began to bear out, however distressingly, the truth of Szent-Gyorgyi's bioelectric theory. However, by the time Mrs Bacon began her campaign she was no longer married, and in fact had no knowledge of Szent-Gyorgyi's work or indeed of any physics or biophysics at all; her career had been almost purely literary, beginning with an MA in English Language and Literature from St Hugh's College, Oxford, then studying French and German in those countries, and finally lecturing at two universities in the United States. Perhaps it is appropriate that she should begin her account with speculations about the earliest written traditions of civilisation.

The sensitivity of all living systems to the earth's natural electromagnetic field must have been recognised and put to adaptive advantage, in whatever fashion, since ancient times, as it still is by primitive peoples and by animals today. The highly developed early civilisations – Egyptian, Arabic, Chinese, Eastern and American Indian – almost certainly codified this awareness into a working body of knowledge. But the great library of Alexandria, which contained much of it, was pillaged and finally burnt many centuries ago; the records of the Mayans and the Aztecs were destroyed by the Spanish conquistadores; China was isolated, India subjugated, and their respective esoteric teachings eventually became regarded in the West as weird curiosities – although often inexplicably successful, especially in healing. Such knowledge as has survived has done so in the forms of shamanism, ritual medicine, faith-healing, acupuncture, dowsing, tales of the sixth sense, all considered by Western medical and scientific establishments to be distinctly 'fringe' concepts and practices. As a result it has been extraordinarily difficult for even accredited scientists and doctors to re-discover and apply this cardinal biological fact of human electromagnetic sensitivity. For ordinary people, the involuntary re-discovery through their own reactivity has been nightmarish because of its indescribable strangeness.

The experience of living or working in artificial electromagnetic fields superimposed upon the natural background electromagnetic environment is, in evolutionary terms, extremely new to humans – perhaps no more than 40–50 years old as far as extensive industrial and domestic exposure is concerned. The radiation frequencies in question span the extremely-low-frequency (ELF) electromagnetic waves of the Earth's Schumann field superimposed on the Earth's more or less steady (geomagnetic) field of about $50\,\mu T$ (0.5 Gauss) which directs our compasses – to which, of course, all biological systems have adapted as they have developed, or indeed by which, perhaps, their evolution was originally moulded. Because these electromagnetic frequencies and fields are so low and do not demonstrate any dramatic thermal or ionising effects, such as those produced by nuclear devices, there has, until very recently, been a commonly held fallacy that they must therefore be harmless. Even radiations such as X-rays and microwaves were not initially investigated closely for potentially harmful bio-effects – probably because they were technologically or medically so useful. In 1956, 60 years after the discovery of X-rays a memorial to the 500 Radiation Martyrs, including many British, who died as a result of overexposure to X-radiation in the course of their research or clinical work, was erected. Two recent but still pioneering investigators, Dr Alice Stewart, at Birmingham University, working on the effect of X-rays on unborn children (Stewart et al., 1956, 1958), and Dr Milton Zaret, of Scarsdale, New York, investigating microwave-induced cataracts (Zaret et al., 1963), met with enormous difficulties in getting their early work on the public's behalf accepted or even published: their findings indicate that radical changes are necessary to ensure the safety of the high-tech world we have built up at such speed. The same is equally true of the ELF electromagnetic earth frequencies to which we are attuned through evolution, and which work on us so subtly that, in general, their effects are difficult to detect except over an extended period of time. The main stumbling-block to acceptance or even investigation in this area seems to be that such ELF frequencies are now so widespread. They occur directly or as modulation of a higher frequency, coherent, carrier oscillation in the transmission of information and electrical power, in many industrial processes and domestic appliances such as microwaves ovens, and in computers, with the increasingly widespread use of visual display units (VDUs) and electronic information systems of many kinds.

There are two highly salient aspects of the discovery of ELF electromagnetic bio-effects by the general public. The first is that it is only recently that such a possibility has even been suggested in the official literature, let alone become current in the public domain, so that the peculiar symptoms and experiences reported could not have been suggested from elsewhere. Second, these effects are time-related and cumulative, so that, as time has passed, the claims of ill-health have been increasingly voiced and confirmed. However, this has meant that it has become correspondingly more difficult for the sufferers to pursue their search for the truth about their conditions in such a hostile climate. What is, perhaps, the clearest example of this discovery in Britain illustrates the difficulties – and also the excitement – so well that I feel it is worth telling in some detail.

It all started because of the construction of one small section of the National Grid over the tiny village of Fishpond, in Dorset. This was erected in 1967, but it was not until 1973 that the villagers began to report effects which they hardly knew how to describe. The lines dip sharply down over their fields and houses in two fairly massive circuits, which run parallel to the village and, because of the steep hillside, almost level with the houses. One circuit was energised at 400 kV (400,000 volts), the other at 275 kV but with the in-built capacity to be up-rated. Fishpond lies at the head of a steep and narrow valley rising dramatically from the coast nearly a thousand feet below. It is extremely beautiful; in fact the valley now belongs to the National Trust, and in former years the Impressionist painter Camille Pissarro and his son Lucien, also a painter, spent much time there; one of Camille Pissarro's Fishpond paintings, called *The Gap in the Hills*, is in the collection of the Tate Gallery. The earth is iron-bearing (the head of the valley is flanked by two Iron Age forts) and the whole area is riddled with underground streams and earth faults – in fact it is part of the well known and treacherous Dorset coastal slide. Further, strong south-westerly gales and heavy sea mists are funnelled up from the English Channel below. All these environmental factors seem to render the area highly susceptible to electromagnetic interactions, though none of the authorities seem to have taken that into consideration either when planning the route or later after receiving complaints, nor in similar situations elsewhere, and the villagers were certainly not aware of it.

I can tell the story of this search in some detail because, as a resident there from 1973 to 1984, I myself felt the effects and embarked on the search – although to describe the full extraordinary sequence of events in this discovery would take a whole book certainly longer than the Tales of a Thousand and One Nights. However, the simple outline of the story shows that the gulf between science and ordinary life is not as great as has been suggested, and that it is imperative for medical doctors of every discipline to learn again to consider all aspects of illness in relation to the whole environment.

When the HV (high voltage) lines were first set up over Fishpond, the villagers not only objected on aesthetic grounds, but feared that the unsafe terrain posed serious dangers (about 20 out of a total of 30 people lived within 100 metres of the lines). Almost immediately they discovered another unpleasant aspect of this technological barbarity: that is, the buzzing or singing of the lines in misty weather and the howling or clashing of the conductors in high winds. Separators were installed which alleviated the clashing, but not the howling, which often reaches banshee-like levels and produces a relentless throbbing throughout the body.

When I moved to Fishpond in 1973, to a house immediately under the lines, I knew nothing of this; I thought the lines hideous, but the valley was so beautiful and the nearby school for my sons so good that I felt I could accept them. We moved in during a spell of unusually hot weather, during which I seemed to feel more than usually exhausted by the heat, in fact too tired to explore the lovely valley at all. I decided to paint most of the rooms of the house, which I did, but lost my voice for over two weeks. I attributed this to some viral infection, especially when my voice came back after a cracking thunderstorm in which the hot weather broke and the pylon above our garden burned with blue flame. But as the autumn drew on, I found that I still experienced strange lassitude, headaches which I had never had before, and an odder feeling which I had difficulty in describing even to myself. It was as if I had some kind of a mental barrier between my thoughts and myself so that I found it hard even to write a letter. Since I was working as an editor and proof-reader, I found this mental block very disturbing and decided it must be due to the South Coast weather, as it always seemed to be more pronounced on wet, windy or misty days. Later I discovered that another villager, who had been born and bred there but had never experienced this strange feeling before the lines were erected, described it far more graphically as 'like being caught in a net'.

Gradually, as I began to get to know the other villagers, I found that many of us, as different as we were, shared the same unusual mixture of debilitating symptoms – headaches across the eyes, exhaustion, sleeplessness, loss of appetite, even occasional dizziness, or palpitations of the heart, with trembling – especially in extremes of wet, windy, very cold or very hot weather. Although I come from a medical family I have no scientific or medical training and therefore thought of this as simply a response to prevailing weather conditions, though extreme and somewhat unfortunate; and, until fairly recently, that is the way in which far better informed people have also considered it. But later in that same year I happened upon an article by an electrical engineer describing the effects upon office and factory workers of abnormal ionisation of the air caused by central heating or air-conditioning. These effects – headaches, eye-strain, exhaustion, dizziness – tallied so exactly with ours that I suddenly wondered if it might be not just the weather – which was common to all of Fishpond, and indeed to all the south west of

England – that was causing our symptoms, but possibly also the other factor we shared in common, namely the overhead power-lines, producing abnormal ionisation of the air. This question has been very difficult to resolve because it has proved so difficult to measure such subtle changes in the open environment and, moreover, the measuring equipment itself is affected by the electromagnetic fields radiating from the power-lines. Nevertheless, it did lead us into the gradual understanding of these fields, hitherto unknown to almost all of us.

A retired electrical engineer, formerly an inspector of factories, who moved to Fishpond in 1976, dismissed the idea of ionisation or other effects, but did theorise that the unpleasant throbbing or pulsing which we felt in high winds might be attributable to subsonic harmonic oscillations generated by the lines. In 1980 Dr Cyril Smith first visited Fishpond. Then, and on several subsequent occasions, he took seriously the symptoms that we all experienced and measured the electric and magnetic fields around Fishpond. But at the very beginning of our inquiries, in 1973, none of us had any notion of such things. It proved almost impossible to pursue even the idea of abnormal air ionisation; the electrical engineer, Mr Cecil Laws, said he could not help us; the Central Electricity Generating Board (CEGB) said that nobody else around the country had complained so therefore there couldn't be anything in it; the DHSS said the work quoted by Mr Laws (done by Dr Albert Krueger, in California) had been disproved by subsequent research elsewhere – which later turned out not to be the case. Finally, in desperation, we tried the telephone information service and, by great good luck, found a friendly and sympathetic operator who recognised our plight and looked through the London directories until she happened upon the Institute for Occupational Health and Safety. This was a major breakthrough for us because in its files we discovered the first indication that anyone in the professional world was considering possible power-line health effects.

The study in question was carried out in France in 1970 on the health of people living within 100 metres of HV lines (Strumza, 1970). These subjects did not appear to be more unhealthy than a control group living at a distance, but they did pay more visits to consultant specialists. Although this report may appear vague and inconclusive at first sight, it is in fact very important, for at least two reasons (besides the simple fact that anyone had decided to do it). First, it was undertaken fairly soon after HV power-line systems were erected throughout Europe, and not then normally at the present high voltage levels; it is now known that ELF electromagnetic health effects are time-related and cumulative, depending on the length of exposure. And, second, although the people did not appear to be significantly more 'ill' than the control group, their local doctors were baffled enough by their variety of symptoms to refer many more of them to specialists. In the light of what has been discovered since 1982 by Dr Cyril Smith and Dr Jean Monro about the relevance of the allergic responses of sensitive individuals to the particular bio-effects produced by ELF electromagnetic fields, the evidence from this early report is far more than merely circumstantial – or, as the authorities prefer to describe it, 'anecdotal'. However, neither we nor, it appears, anyone else appreciated this at the time.

On a later visit to the Institute for Occupational Health and Safety we found far more conclusive evidence for clinical effects from such fields; but, in the meantime, visitors from the United States remembered reading about a US Navy ELF communications project which had to be abandoned because the electromagnetic fields produced by the wires buried underground radically disturbed the earthworms and therefore the composition of the soil (see Chapter 10). This, of course, sounds laughable at first, but we quickly became accustomed to being laughed at (and worse); in fact, like this study, much of the earliest accepted evidence came from studies on bees and birds rather than on humans. In the mid-1960s a study from Germany (Wellenstein, 1973), which showed that bees subjected to ELF electromagnetic fields stopped making honey, sealed up their hives in mid-season and therefore committed social suicide, was accepted by bee-keeping associations throughout Europe within a few years and indeed was quoted authoritatively by a local inspector to a Fishpond villager whose bees had become so savage and unproductive that they had to be moved to a farm twenty miles away – where they thrived once more. Again, in the early 1980s HV power-lines near bird sanctuaries and pigeon-breeding communities in Gloucestershire were buried underground because of their acknowledged disorienting effects. It remains one of the mysteries of bureaucratic arcana – or economics – that such effects on humans are still not officially accepted, at least in Britain. What makes this even more ironic is that the first Public Inquiry presenting the question of these effects on humans was also held in Gloucestershire, in the village of Innsworth in 1978 – but the question was dismissed.

Fishpond took part in that Inquiry because by that time we felt that we had more then enough material to back up our case. Our friends from the University of Chicago had sent us not only two US Navy Reports to the White House (1973 and 1974) about the ELF communications project (code-named Sanguine), but also an article published in the American *Sierra Club Bulletin* (Spring, 1973), a strongly environmental journal, by an American biophysicist, Dr Louise Young. She also wrote *Power over People* (Young, 1973) and '*Pollution by electrical transmission*' (Young, 1974). The former was the first book published in the West specifically on possible power-line hazards; in it Dr Young not only cautioned the authorities and the public in some detail, but also gave us one of our greatest tools in our campaign – for she explained how the presence of the electromagnetic field, due to corona discharge from the lines, can be demonstrated by holding up an unconnected fluorescent light tube beneath them. This then glows in an eerie, almost uncanny way, wavering only with the wind, like a candle. Of course, this in itself proves nothing except that there is an electric field and enough current passing through the person to ground to produce the light intensity observed. But it was enough to attract attention from the media and also from people who previously had only laughed at us, so that we finally felt bold enough to ask our Member of Parliament, Mr (now Sir) Jim Spicer, for help. He was immediately sympathetic (and has always remained so) and encouraged us to find whatever other material we could.

So we went back to the Institute for Occupational Health and Safety, and this time discovered two studies, from Italy (Meda et al., 1969) and the USSR (Danilin et al., 1969), on the health of workers in 500 kV electrical substations. Both studies, quite unrelated, reported effects on the cardiovascular system, the peripheral nervous system and the leucocyte count (which was raised). These effects tallied so exactly with unexpected findings in a recent medical check-up I had had that we felt certain, at last, that we could substantiate our claims. Had we known how long this would take (and is still taking) we would not have rejoiced quite so early – but at least we had now aroused public attention, although originally that had never been our aim; and it was from a member of the public that we received our next vital help.

In 1975, a London librarian, Miss Winifred Whiteman, heard of our story, and because she had been researching this subject as a result of an extraordinary electrically-related accident suffered previously, sent us a list of all the scientists in the West who were working on ELF electromagnetic bio-effects. The list was dauntingly long – and equally discouraging was the fact that none of those scientists was working in the UK. But we divided the list up among ourselves to contact; and as it happened, the very first letter I wrote struck gold. This was to Dr Andrew Marino, a biophysicist, who at the time was working for the US government together with Dr Robert Becker, an orthopaedic surgeon. They had been asked to study bio-effects of ELF electromagnetic fields (possibly as a result of the findings of Project Sanguine) and in their laboratory work on rats and mice had found stunted growth and decreased fertility within three generations. More than that, both Dr Marino and Dr Becker were at that moment testifying on behalf of the public at a long and very acrimonious hearing held by the New York State Public Service commission concerning a proposal to run 765 kV power-lines across the State to connect into the Canadian system. The decision to testify was taken entirely by Dr Becker and Dr Marino themselves as responsible medical scientists, and it cost them not only years of work and time but also professional slander and even the security of their jobs; and, in Dr Becker's case, possibly also a Nobel Prize, for which he was being considered because of his work on mending difficult bone fractures and reducing oedemas with externally-applied ELF electromagnetic fields. Indeed, it was because of this work that Dr Becker decided to testify at the hearing; he had seen how, almost miraculously, such electromagnetic fields helped damaged cells to repair themselves and re-grow in their biological formation, but he had serious doubts about similar effects on normally healthy tissue subjected involuntarily to these fields – doubts which are now being vindicated. After the New York State hearing, he wrote a book on electromagnetism together with Dr Marino, the most comprehensive and scientifically based book published up to that time (Becker and Marino, 1982) which carries further Szent-Gyorgyi's theory of semiconducting crystalline lattices in biological structures; later, he published a second work (Becker and Selden, 1985), which is the testimony of his life's work as a pioneering doctor and in which he proposes a biological theory (which he also substantiates) that will almost certainly bring about fundamental changes in our understanding of the origins and workings of life on Earth.

When Dr Marino answered my first letter, he enclosed copies of Dr Becker's testimony (which warned unequivocally against the random subjection of healthy systems to ELF electromagnetic fields) and of his own as yet incomplete cross-examination, which was not only illuminating but also brilliantly argued in the face of deliberate hostility. Much later, when I finally met Dr Marino, I commented on this and he told me that he had taken an extra degree in law because he felt, as a biophysicist, that there were so many dangers in our present environment that someone should be fully qualified to argue on the public's behalf. To know that we had people of such calibre behind us was an almost miraculous step forward for us.

Unfortunately, the authorities in Britain, like those in the United States, did not see it in the same way. In 1976 our MP had arranged a private meeting between Fishpond residents and the CEGB to discuss our concern; when we presented the material we had gathered with such difficulty one senior official put his head in his hands and groaned, 'This is what comes of public education'; Dr Becker and Dr Marino were dismissed as 'troublemakers'. It was this attitude which decided us to help the villagers of Innsworth in their Public Inquiry, and although this turned out to be a bitter and in the end a losing battle for us, once again coincidence and good science both came to our aid.

During the summer of 1978 I had read an article (quite literally in the paper wrapped round the fish) about the work of Dr Leslie Hawkins at the University of Surrey, in Guildford, who was studying abnormal ionisation of the air and its effects (Hawkins, 1981). We wrote to ask if he might come to Fishpond and measure ionisation levels under the power-lines. He replied that he would indeed be interested, but did not know exactly when he could come. As it turned out, he found he could come only in early October, after the Innsworth Inquiry had begun. I therefore left the Inquiry and returned to Fishpond to meet him. Dr Hawkins' findings were so unusual, even on a still and sunny autumn day, that he felt they should be re-confirmed in case his measuring equipment was being affected by the fields. What he found were not only abnormal balances of air ions, tending especially toward a preponderance of positive ions, as before a thunderstorm or one of the world's debilitating winds such as the Mistral or the Santa Ana, but also the extraordinary phenomenon, immediately below the HV lines, of a total absence or cancellation of positive and negative ions, a condition in which laboratory animals had been found to die within three months. Although Dr Hawkins had once built a theoretical model of a situation like Fishpond's without knowing it existed, it was this result which startled him and made him wonder about the power-line effect on his meter. In fact, even today no one can be certain of the performance of their ionisation meters in such an environment. Funds to continue such studies have been promised by bodies such as the National Radiological Protection Board (NRPB), but then, mysteriously, never materialised.

However, on the day of Dr Hawkins's visit to Fishpond (without which I would have been at the Public Inquiry in Gloucestershire) I received a telephone call from a physicist, Dr David Smith, at the University College of North Wales in Bangor. He had earlier heard a BBC radio programme about our dilemma, in which Dr Marino was interviewed, as was also an Electricity Board official who attributed our symptoms to fanciful fears of the pylons dominating our village. Dr Smith became interested and in fact began a correspondence with the CEGB on the subject; then, when he saw a very small mention of the Innsworth Inquiry in the national press, he rang to ask if he might testify in corroboration of our evidence because he felt that a very important factor was being glossed over by the authorities. This is called electric field enhancement and is known to all students of physics, though not normally to the general public. The electric fields under the lines at Fishpond has been measured as reaching 6 kV per metre at their maximum (which was already above USSR safety standards for living in the vicinity of HV lines). But these measurements were made at ground level, with a meter on a very long handle. In a sense, therefore, they were theoretical rather than practical for, as Dr David Smith explained in his testimony, a field so measured would be described as 'unperturbed' – that is, it has no objects within it. As soon as an object is placed within an electric field, the field behaves rather like a curtain and drapes itself in close folds over the object, leaving a clear space beneath. The field so folded can reach values up to a hundred times that of the ambient, unperturbed field. In ordinary working or living conditions, such an object might be a car whose top is at head level for the person standing next to it, a gate or a piece of equipment similarly placed at the level of the heart, a child's climbing frame, or a pram with a baby inside. The possible biological implications of such field enhancement are considerable.

Although Innsworth lost this Public Inquiry, in the sense that the power-lines were up-rated and moved closer to the houses and the school, and also in the sense that it developed into a battlefield of personal harassment quite unexpected by the protesters, it proved an important stepping-stone for other reasons. The most important by far was the personal and intellectual aid offered by Dr David Smith; but we also received many letters of corroboration and support from other people in similar situations who, like ourselves, could not imagine what was happening to them. Some additional interesting points emerged.

In the spring of 1978, six months before the Inquiry, at least four people in Fishpond had experienced strange and distressing blackouts within the space of one week – one of these people was a visitor who blacked out while riding his bike under the lines, fell off and broke his ribs. Another was my fourteen-year-old son, who had never experienced anything like it before, and indeed did not tell me until we discovered that we had all suffered in the same way but without telling each other at first because it seemed so weird. For another villager it was a series of spells of dizziness. For myself, it was an almost indescribable episode in which the light seemed to go black (although I could still see) and I was completely disoriented; even though I was in my own garden, I could not tell which way the house was, nor even which way was up or down. This, of course, occasioned much jocularity amongst the opposition when I described it at Innsworth; but later in the Inquiry we learned, from an engineer, who had not been present on the day I testified and obviously had not read my statement, that it was at that time that the lower 275 kV circuit at Fishpond had been up-rated to 345 kV — without anyone being told (Best, 1981).

The Innsworth Inquiry, which did not include a single independent medical assessor, ended in December 1978, with no decision made by the two Inspectors (one each from the Departments of Energy and the Environment) for two years, and even it was both equivocal and too late – the HV lines had already been moved closer to Innsworth. The

Inspector's report on the Innsworth Inquiry contains a number of errors; for example, in Section 25.51 it is implied that only three villagers besides myself had sent letters reporting effects, whereas in fact a letter was signed and presented by 20 villagers attesting various complaints. In Section 25.52, the Inspectors state that I denied my medical history to them, whereas I told the CEGB Medical Officer, Dr Bonnell, through the Innsworth lawyer that they were welcome to see my medical records so long as they requested them also from everyone else who complained.

It was late in 1978 that a judgment was reached on the New York State Public Service commission hearing. Despite the divisive and occasionally even libellous nature of the proceedings, the final New York ruling ordered the electrical utilities to leave a 350-yard corridor around the lines, and to contribute $5 million toward an independent research project, subsequently entitled the New York State Power Lines Project, on ELF electromagnetic bio-effects (Marino and Ray, 1986). Although Becker and Marino's early findings concerning lowered growth rates, lowered fertility and reduced life expectancy were hotly contested, independent research appears to be confirming them; by September 1986, at a Toronto conference on 'Health Effects of ELF Fields: Research and Communications Regulation', Dr Richard Phillips, who used to head research in that area at the Battelle Pacific Northwest Laboratories in Richland, Washington State, confirmed that such fields appear to be biologically active – and when asked from the floor if he would choose to live even along the right of way of HV power-lines never mind under them, agreed with Dr Marino that he would not (*Microwave News*, September/October, 1986, p. 9). In 1983, a Swedish study found fewer normal pregnancies among the families of HV switchyard workers on account of more congenital malformations (Nordstrom *et al.*, 1983); Dr Jose Delgado, working in Madrid, observed malformed and aborted chicks from eggs which had been exposed to ELF radiation (Delgado *et al.*, 1982) – as did farmers in New York State, who reported in a 1984 Channel 4 Central TV documentary, *The Good, the Bad and the Indefensible*, that their hens living underneath 765 kV power-lines laid, as it were, 'scrambled' eggs. Other elements, too, were beginning to enter the debate.

Quite independently of the scientific controversy, a general practitioner in Staffordshire, Dr Stephen Perry, had begun to notice unusually high levels of depressive illness and even suicide among those of his patients who lived near high-voltage lines. Like the Fishpond discovery and others corroborating it, this observation was completely spontaneous, made without any prior knowledge of possible effects. Most unusually for an ordinary GP, Dr Perry's group practice gave its members a regular six-months sabbatical every few years and he used his to complete a study of these findings. What was more unusual was that his results appeared for the first time to implicate the magnetic component of the power-line electromagnetic fields (Perry *et al.*, 1981). This is so low – lower by far than the Earth's own extremely low magnetic field – that it had been mutually agreed at the Innsworth Inquiry to be negligible. However, Dr Perry's study was one of the first to suggest that the importance of the magnetic field lies not only in high-power strengths but also in extremely low-power alternating fields with frequencies which resonate with, and reinforce, biological wavelengths. The reason why his patients living near the invisible underground HV lines suffered the same distressing depressive and suicidal effects as those living near visible overhead lines, of which one cannot fail to be aware, has to be a question of the basic physics of magnetic fields. However, Dr Perry's study was perhaps the first to suggest that magnetic field bio-effects depend not only on the strength of the field but also on its frequency if, as in the case of that generated by the majority of the power-lines in the UK, it is alternating. Once again, as with the electric field, it is a matter of biological frequencies. And, quite apart from the tragic aspect of Dr Perry's findings, which were by their nature retrospective but are still being corroborated by personal reports I have received, his study is of great importance in doing away with the quasi-intellectual superstitution which often attributes hysterical self-suggestion to electropollution sufferers; for it shows quite clearly that depressive illness and suicide were found to be statistically increased just as much among patients living near invisible, underground HV lines, of which they were unaware, as among patients living near overhead lines.

His findings, and subsequent related work by Dr Cyril Smith (Smith and Baker, 1982), seem relevant also to the earlier and more generally accepted studies on bees and homing pigeons, both of which are known to have receptors which are able to sense the Earth's magnetic field and its variations, which they use to help direct their survival behaviour. My own extraordinary first experience of complete dis-orientation below the lines may also be relevant; I had never experienced this before, though I have done so since, most notably after I had held up a fluorescent tube for over an hour, to be photographed under the lines; the next day, after a distressingly sleepless night, I found what looked like a burn on that shoulder.

Meanwhile, other oddities had begun to manifest themselves, perhaps unremarkable on their own but, in such a small community as Fishpond, worthy of note. One child born in the village had already suffered a rash which amazed the specialists; another, who had often been left out in her pram under the lines crossing her grandparents' garden (before we began to research our suspicions), developed severe rashes and later a mild epilepsy. Another older child, who had always lived in Fishpond, developed a similar form of epilepsy. In the end, I myself developed a more severe form of epilepsy triggered by flickering light, which resulted in a serious car accident and a partial loss of sight. Already in the letters we had received after the Innsworth Inquiry there had been an account of seizures, especially when the weather was wet or misty. Our headaches and rashes were further intensified in patterns which did not necessarily appear to depend on the weather; for instance, two years running, at roughly the same time in May, I developed severe skin rash, swelling of the face and inflammation of the eyes, which I did not at first connect with the power-lines — nor did I connect with them a newly-developed allergy to cow's milk and cheese. Yet it now seems more than likely that both were triggered by the electromagnetic field — if not directly, then synergistically, interacting with some other feature, possibly chemical (pesticide or herbicide) sprays, possibly the local water which was all well-water, possibly chemicals getting into the wells. (Not until 1982 did most of the houses receive mains water, and then by no means all.) This latter form of interaction may well be the cause of a striking development in Innsworth since the lines there were moved close to the houses; in the row of houses a few yards from the 400 kV lines at least seven people have now developed thyroid trouble. One of these sufferers, Mrs Stella Ross (who, despite severe and painful eye problems associated with her thyroid imbalance, has long been Innsworth's most dedicated campaigner), wrote to Dr Becker early in 1984; he replied that he had noted thyroid disturbances of various types in people exposed to HV power-lines in the United States. It should be noted that Innsworth is the home of an airfield with all the accompanying radar and communications equipment; thus it may well be an example of yet another synergistic interaction suggested by Dr Becker in a letter to the *New York State Journal of Medicine* (Becker, 1977). (For further discussion of the effects of radar, see Chapter 10.)

By the mid-1970s it was already becoming apparent to many that microwave radiation can be biologically harmful; Dr Milton Zaret was demonstrating clearly (despite the now customary hostility from the authorities and industry) that tumours and unusual subcapsular cataracts of the eye can be caused by indiscriminate microwave exposure from radar and telecommunications equipment or leaky microwave ovens (Zaret, 1977). In England a prankster who shinned up a communications tower was blandly informed by the authorities that he had probably been rendered permanently sterile; they later admitted that this truth had been let out to discourage others. He might have been worse than sterile as far as possible future offspring might be concerned, because, as mentioned, Dr Jose Delgado in Madrid had found that exposure of hen's eggs to microwaves caused aborted or grossly malformed chicks just as did exposure to ELF fields (McAuliffe, 1985). We should remember, too, the microwave irradiation of the US Embassy in Moscow (see Chapter 10), as a result of which several diplomats developed leukaemia; two of the US Ambassadors serving during the period (1953–77) died of cancer and the third, Walter Stoessel, died in December 1986 of leukaemia, which was first discovered in 1975 when he was taken ill with nausea and bleeding from the eyes (Obituary, *The Times*, 12 December 1986).

Becker's postulation of synergistic effects concerned both microwaves and ELF irradiation in an area of New York State where the hilly terrain combined and concentrated these different radiations in clearly defined patterns, within which an unusually high incidence of cancer, especially blood cancers, was also revealed (Becker, 1977). It seems that we, too, discovered at least one person suffering from this combined effect – a farmer in Wiltshire whose land is crossed by HV lines and who wrote to us in 1978 describing his crippling headaches which vanished whenever he left home (in fact it was his doctor who had suggested that he should write to us). When we visited him, we found that his land was surrounded also by military microwave and radar installations. He subsequently developed cancer of the ear. An interesting connection may be made: an article (*Science News*, 1984) (Swicord and Davis, 1983) entitled 'DNA helix found to oscillate in resonance with microwaves' elicited a letter from a private nurse for cancer patients in California who was struck by how many of her patients lived near HV power-lines. As for ocular effects, at least one Fishpond and one Innsworth resident have been diagnosed by consultant ophthalmologists as having damaged retinas which show unusual signs, almost as if they have been burned. Another Fishpond resident has now developed a rare cancer of the eye so serious that the eye has had to be removed.

The possibilities of synergistic effects are countless. It has even been suggested that so-called lines of geopathic stress may contribute synergistically – and there is said to be a major ley-line running through Fishpond. Dr Michael Ash, who practises various forms of alternative medicine at his clinic in Cornwall, has measured electromagnetic activity from even minor earth faults; the faults underlying Fishpond, which he studied in 1979, display considerable activity which, of course, varies constantly. Innsworth, like Fishpond, is full of springs and streams – indeed, Innsworth's pylons now stand in permanently waterlogged land. In the light of what has been discussed in Chapters 6 and 7, the apparent ability of water to 'remember' frequencies to which it has been exposed may enhance the straightforward electromagnetic effects of environmental sources of highly coherent frequencies.

It is by now more than clear that this newly-emerging knowledge is not only vitally important, but also greatly under-researched or even suppressed. After the Innsworth Inquiry, the Health and Safety Executive (HSE) was approached by representatives from Japan (the CEGB had refused to talk to them); the HSE Inspector, who had by then visited Fishpond, referred them to us because, as he said, we had far more and far more up-to-date material on this subject than he had. Another group from Japan asked the Economist Intelligence Unit to prepare a report on the subject; they in turn referred to us for all our material.

We received other inquiries, too, from Australia, Canada, Scotland and Ireland, and in fact testified at a Public Inquiry in Haddington in south-east Scotland (the Torness Inquiry) in April 1982, on behalf of the farmers and villagers (Best, 1982). Dr David Melville, then at the University of Southampton (now a professor at the Lancashire Polytechnic in Preston), testified at this Inquiry on the results of his work on low-level pulsed magnetic fields, which affect the permeability of cell membranes (Braganza *et al.*, 1983); he also read out a statement by Professor Bernard Watson, who is researching brain effects from variously modulated electromagnetic fields at the Department of Medical Electronics at St Bartholomew's Hospital in London. Professor Watson quoted the work of Wever (1973) and others in warning against the disturbance of the body's circadian rhythms by ELF fields – the same effects as jet-lag, for instance, except that in the ELF environment these effects would be constant and therefore cumulative.

One of the many protesters at the Torness Inquiry was the Abbot of Nunraw who was deeply concerned about the effects of the proposed 400 kV lines on his enclosed order of monks and the monastery farm. By our greatest piece of good fortune since the Innsworth Inquiry, we now had Dr Cyril Smith working on the subject. I had seen him on a BBC Television programme – together with Dr Robert Becker and others – considering the question of the limits of ELF radiation applied externally for healing purposes. We wrote to him in 1979, but he was fully occupied at the time, although very interested; two years later, however, he asked for an account of our experiences in order to launch a graduate student on a research project. His work has since proved to be the most relevant and revealing of all. The night before the Abbot was to present his objections to the Inquiry, Dr Smith telephoned us some details of a letter he had just had accepted for publication, on the effects of low-level magnetic fields on the DNA of *Escherichia coli*, the most common bacteria within the digestive system. As the monastery farm would be over-wintering the cattle in barns directly below the proposed lines, where a silage pit would also be fermenting, and in view of the restricted sources of the diet of the Cistercian monks, this evidence was of paramount importance to the Abbot. The decision of the Reporter in charge of this Inquiry was the first really enlightened move on the part of any of the authorities in the UK – the HV lines were not to be erected near houses, schools or factories until further research proved them to be biologically harmless.

Meanwhile, further studies were showing up ELF effects and we gathered these in. It is precisely because they work at such a subtle level of biological information and instruction that ELF effects take so long to reveal themselves cumulatively; but within the last few years studies carried out in the United States, for example by Wertheimer and Leeper (1982), have shown an increase in cancer, especially leukaemia, among people whose early childhood had been spent close to HV lines. A report from Sweden in 1982 confirmed Wertheimer and Leeper's findings relating the incidence of tumours in children living near 200 kV lines to the strength of the magnetic fields (Tomenius, 1982).

Also in 1982, the *New England Journal of Medicine* (Milham, 1982) published a statistical study carried out by the State of Washington on workers subjected to ELF electromagnetic fields which showed a significantly higher than average incidence of acute myeloid leukaemia; the *Lancet* published similar findings in a study of workers in Los Angeles (Wright *et al.*, 1982). A third similar result, this time from the UK, was published in the *Lancet* (McDowall, 1983) with comment in the Editorial. And yet another UK study (Coleman *et al.*, 1983) found similar results in the incidence of leukaemia among men in ten electrical occupations in south-east England. Later in that year, Dr Ross Adey, a biophysicist at the Loma Linda Hospital in California who had formerly worked for the US Navy and whose work is in the forefront of research on ELF electromagnetic effects on the brain and the nervous system, particularly the binding of calcium to cell walls and the production of enzymes and hormones, presented a report to the Montana Department of National Resources and Conservation (Adey and Sheppard, 1983). When questioned by our correspondents from Ireland, whose electrical authority were misrepresenting (by omission) his conclusions, Adey, who is now an adviser to the White House on EMR, replied:

> From the available data, fields of 1 kV/m at power-line frequencies appear to be safe. However, I cannot emphasize too strongly that it is not now, nor may it ever be possible to determine that this or any other specific field level 'have no adverse effects'. The reasons relate to interactions between competing low-level environmental factors. This problem has been admirably addressed in the BIER III Report on effects of ionizing radiation. You may wish to consult a paper by the statistician Hoteling on this aspect of the BIER III Report which appeared in *Science* (I believe

around 1970). (Adey to Dr E.Hickey, Thomond College of Education, Limerick, 19 September 1985)

Such a time-lapse in obtaining accurate information illustrates all too poignantly the extreme difficulties which the ordinary public has experienced in trying to discover anything at all about this area of environmental pollution, which yet concerns them most closely.

A similar example concerns the biophysicist, Dr Louise Young, whose article in the *Sierra Club Bulletin* had given us our first hint that responsible scientists were seriously concerned. We held our original meeting with the CEGB in July 1976. What we did not know, and were not told (perhaps, shamefully, no one knew), was that in January of that year Louise Young had taken part extensively in a hearing held by the University of Mississippi on the management of rights of way under HV lines. Unfortunately, the same lack of information (it cannot always be called obfuscation, since these questions are so relatively new and profoundly radical) has dogged attempts to research into the other fields of radiation effects already mentioned. None the less, if country housewives and farmers can amass enough material on such a radically new subject to be consulted by people from many countries, including the Japanese government, surely it is time the official authorities informed themselves better than they have so far done – at the very least without insulting those possibly at risk with wilful irrelevancies or sins of omission.

Although the discovery of ELF electromagnetic bio-effects has been so extraordinarily exciting, both intellectually and now medically in the work of Dr Cyril Smith and Dr Jean Monro, the personal and social tragedies which might have been avoided had greater concern been shown sooner by authorities are irreversible: heart attacks, nervous disorders, epilepsies, suicides, deformed or stillborn children, lowered fertility – together with all the stigmas attached to so-called 'non-specific' symptoms such as headaches, sleeplessness, exhaustion and, of course, the additional anxiety of being trapped in a living or working environment which is increasingly felt to be hostile. Those who have campaigned on behalf of everyone else have had unwelcome publicity forced on them, as well as the more helpful kind which has elicited genuine interest and support. Of course, there have been some lighter moments, as when, at the Innsworth Inquiry, a very deaf farmer utterly silenced the barrister who was cross-examining him by describing in a booming voice how his cows preferred to gather around the pylons in his field instead, as he put it, of 'getting on with the job' – i.e. grazing which, although he did not know it, confirmed completely Dr David Smith's testimony on field enhancement and Dr Cyril Smith's ideas of electrical stimulation of endogenous opiates giving rise to what he humorously called 'junkie cows' (Smith and Aarholt, 1982).

It is, moreover, interesting to note that, as time has passed, our ideas, which were generally met with either a kind smile or a lifted eyebrow thirteen years ago, now tend to be received with, 'Well, it's sort of obvious, isn't it...'. The following remains true to this day: 'When a thing was new people said, "It is not true". Later, when its truth became obvious, people said, "Anyway, it is not important". And when its importance could not be denied, people said "Anyway, it is not new"' (Michel de Montaigne, 1533–92).

There is considerable truth and some solace in these thoughts; but against them must be placed the fact that it is, and always has been, ordinary people, electrical workers, the residents of Fishpond and many other places, who are dying off first, uninformed and often in great distress. I have drawn a diagram (Figure 8.1) to show what the residents of Fishpond have suffered over the years. I still receive letters or reports of suicides, heart trouble and cancers and other ailments from people like myself and my Fishpond neighbours, which could surely have been treated preventively and at the very least alleviated if the necessary research had been encouraged – and its conclusions accepted.

Yet, at long last it seems that the tide may possibly be turning in favour of the general public. The Christmas 1985 issue of 'Picture Week' (*Time-Life*, 1985) showed a startling photograph of fluorescent light tubes glowing brightly as they were being held under 345 kV lines that had been erected two years earlier by Houston Lighting and Power, and which cross the Klein Independent School District near Houston, Texas – 99 acres of land containing an elementary, an intermediate and a high school. The School District sued Houston Lighting and Power on the grounds of increased risk of cancer due to the HV lines, especially in children. Two things mark this case as a tremendous step forward. First, the jury took only two and a half hours of deliberation before awarding $25.1 million in damages against the power company – the first such award made against a power company anywhere; and second, one of the leading cancer specialists in the US, Dr Harvey Busch, chief oncologist at the Baylor School of Medicine in Texas, together with another cancer specialist, Dr Jerry Phillips, testified on behalf of the School District, supporting their claims. Houston Lighting and Power had produced as their chief witness only an electrical engineer. It is interesting, by way of comparison, that at the various Inquiries in England the CEGB, from the start, field only their own Medical Officer, Dr John Bonnell – a physician, but one who, resolutely refusing to accept the growing evidence, preferred to interpret my medical conditions in terms only of previous medical history and psychological factors, and

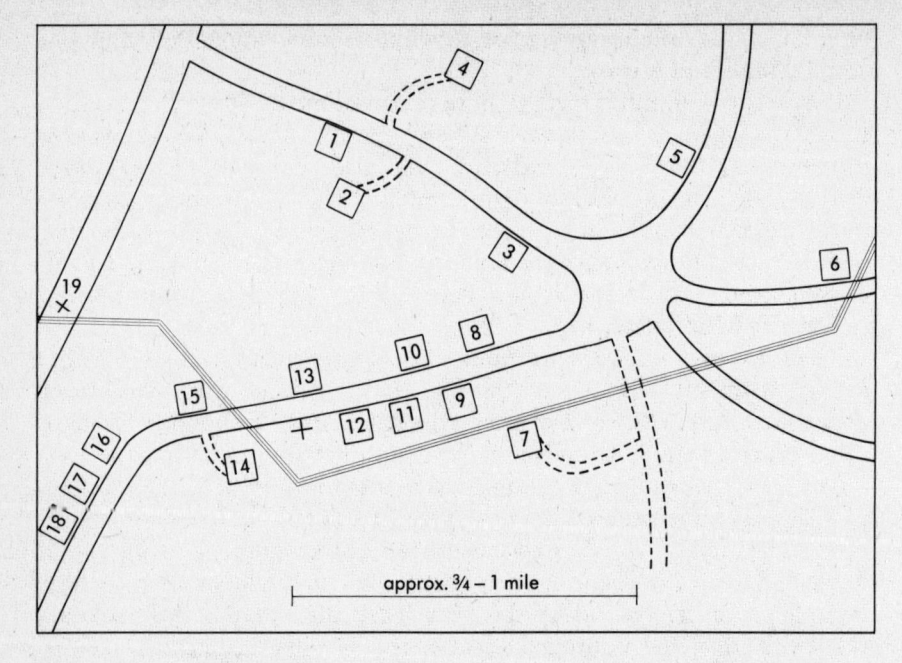

Fig. 8.1 Map of Fishpond.
Approximately 30 people in permanent residence: 23 reported 'non-specific' effects or presented clinical illness, or both, by 1987.

Effects by house (numbers equal houses on map):
1. Previous history of hypertension, retired early from merchant navy (captain of oil-tankers so large his wife said you could see them vibrating in waves from stem to stern); very sudden heart-attack death after working all weekend in part of garden of no. 7 directly under lines. Visitors reported sleeplessness and dizziness.
2. Petit-mal epilepsy in adolescent boy, now controlled by medication. Later, severe exhaustion illness in very lively mother.
3. Rare cancer of eye, eye removed. Bees swarm unusually angrily.
4. Very severe chronic heart condition, considerably relieved on leaving village.
5. Sleeplessness due to howling and throbbing of lines.
6. Holiday home, but vet advised owner not to leave donkey in field directly under lines. Night-light continues to glow after being unplugged.
7. Two separate cases of black-outs; one grand-mal epilepsy, food allergies, rashes, raised leucocyte count; sleeplessness, exhaustion, headaches, depression, muscular weakness.
8. Dizziness, some loss of muscle strength when outside.
9. One unexpected heart-attack death, apparently very difficult to diagnose, following a history only of one-sided headaches and persistent skin rashes; one case of recurrent severe heart palpitations; strong asthmatic reaction in daughter whenever visiting (although very fond of family and place).

10 Severely swollen limbs, with muscular distress and pain in joints; dizziness, sleeplessness.
11 Previous serious heart condition severely aggravated immediately on moving to village, death within a few months. Unusual irritability in very gentle wife after two or three years in village.
12 Original family: one cancer, progress improved on leaving village. Nervous tension needing medication, dizziness, severe eye-strain and drying-up of retinal fluid in one eye. Grandchild who visited frequently developed skin rashes when sleeping in pram under lines, later petit-mal epilepsy. Second family: former electrical engineer with history of heart trouble died suddenly of heart-attack shortly after returning from two months' holiday. Sleeplessness due to throbbing sensation throughout body.
13 One case of black-out, together with frequent dizziness and occasional total loss of muscle-power (i.e. collapse), even though inside. Severe headaches for all family. Very unusual and severe rash in small child, baffled the specialist (who even photographed it).
14 Cancer leading to hysterectomy; eye-strain, headaches.
15 No symptoms reported, but two new TV colour sets blew up in succession.
16 Dizziness, heart palpitations, headaches, near-clinical depression. Bees kept near lines became aggressive and stopped making honey until taken twenty miles away, at the advice of the Bee Inspector.
17 Holiday home, little used; but visiting friend fell off moped due to black-out under lines, broke ribs.
18 Two cataracts removed in middle age.
19 Well known dangerous accident spot (several fatal).

even wrote a letter to Mrs Stella Ross of Innsworth assuring her categorically that there were no harmful effects at all from the electromagnetic fields produced by HV lines. Dr Bonnell retired in September 1986.

The jury's decision in the Klein Independent School District case was appealed by Houston Lighting and Power in November 1986. No new evidence is allowed in the US appellate court; all the testimony originally offered must be re-considered by three judges unfamiliar with the case and the evidence. As this whole subject is radically new and has received little coverage, it is to be presumed that the original jury were unfamiliar with it, yet they took their decision with authoritative speed. Significantly, while the appeal was being heard the Texas Supreme Court refused to allow HL&P to energise the power line, reversing a previous court decision. In April 1987 HL&P applied for and was granted permission by the Texas Public Utilities Commission to re-route the lines at an approximate cost of $4.26 million (MWN, May/June 1987, p. 3). Such a victory will be music to many ears, besides providing a legal precedent for those engaged in, or thinking of engaging in, further battles over power-lines anywhere in the world. Although the punitive damages were overturned, the appeal judge upheld the original health hazard decision.

In May 1986, five months after the case was first decided, an editorial in *Science* took it as an example of the difficulties of deciding whether or not the bio-effects of ELF electromagnetic fields are indeed harmless, and whether the US government should have cut back its research support as it has done. The editor pointed out that research can never demonstrate that a risk does not exist. Is that why the authorities are cutting back on research funding – because it may never be possible to prove their point to all the people whose health and well-being should really be their first concern? From our own accumulated experience, now so hearteningly being backed up by increasingly widespread commitment on the part of the medical profession, we know that it is not simply a question of money for research, necessary as that is; it is a matter far greater and far graver than that, but with a tremendous potential for entirely new knowledge, and for the enlightened application of that knowledge.

* * *

Further accounts and details concerning the Innsworth Inquiry and the situation at Fishpond can also be found in Hildyard (1983) and Bacon (1986).

Fishpond and its 'problem' refuse to go away, despite the CEGB's disinclination to investigate the claims thoroughly. However, it is a little-known fact that five years after a Public Inquiry in the United Kingdom members of the public may apply to the relevant government department to have a case re-examined if significant new information has come to light that might strongly affect the original decision. Disconcertingly, it is up to the department in question to judge how substantial any such new information is (although this would seem to be a fruitful field in which to plant Parliamentary Questions). None the less, one or two cases have been successfully re-opened. Perhaps it is not yet over for Fishpond or Innsworth, even though many of the original inhabitants of Fishpond have died or moved away, while many of those remaining are still suffering, some severely. Certainly the world scientific situation has now fundamentally changed for any future such inquiry in the United Kingdom – or anywhere else for that matter.

Part 2 Towards an Explanation

The best way to escape a problem is to solve it.

Brendan Francis

Dr Cyril Smith takes up his account of Fishpond village, its residents and its pylons.

By 1980, the results of experiments on the growth of the bacterium *Escherichia coli* in the power frequency (50 Hz) magnetic field had been successful enough for their presentation in a preliminary form at a conference in Paris (Aarholt *et al.*, 1980) and, in October, for a paper to be submitted for publication in a scientific journal (Aarholt *et al.*, 1981). We now felt in a position of having something constructive to offer. Following a long telephone conversation with Hilary Bacon discussing the environmental effects being experienced at Fishpond, she wrote on 6 November 1980, kindly enclosing some of the reports which had been mentioned and the address of the general practitioner, Dr Stephen Perry, who had been investigating a possible connection between power frequency magnetic fields and suicides. I had a vested interest in one of these reports – the Report of the 1977 Working Group on Inequalities in Health. As an electrical engineer I came top of the class, having the highest death rate of men aged 15–64, 19.4 per 1000, but as a university teacher I came at the bottom of the low death rate class at only 2.87 per 1000, quite a Gilbertian situation in which to find oneself.

As I had a son at medical school in Bristol, it proved possible to visit Fishpond on my way from Manchester to collect him for the Christmas vacation. This was on Saturday 13 December, and a Saturday was a good day to catch all the villagers at home. Accordingly, I borrowed all the measuring apparatus that seemed relevant from the laboratory. I calibrated a meter in the high-voltage laboratory to measure the 50 Hz electric fields, and calibrated another meter to measure the 50 Hz magnetic fields. To look for other frequencies, I borrowed an oscilloscope which would run off the battery of my motor caravan which became a mobile laboratory for the occasion.

I planned a schedule of eight sets of measurements. The first step was to take a good look around and photograph the village of Fishpond and its power lines and to measure the heights of the cables with the camera's rangefinder. The ground plan of the village was, of course, available from Ordnance Survey maps (SY 370 982). I would then measure the frequency spectrum of the electric and magnetic fields in the vicinity, and the field strengths. Additional tests would include measuring the water and soil conductivity, taking some fingernail clippings for trace element analysis, and sampling the tap and well water for chemical and bacteriological testing. Finally, I planned to interview as many of the villagers as possible.

There was a bridleway running past Hilary Bacon's cottage at right angles to the power-lines which passed about 20 metres overhead. I could get the van along it and stop without inconveniencing anyone, and run out the cables to the apparatus without having the van close enough to disturb the field measurements. The electric field waveform was a good 50 Hz sinusoid. The values of the alternating electric field directly beneath the conductors went up to about 4 kV/m under one line and about 12 kV/m under the other. The fields had dropped to a few hundred volts per metre at distances of 100 m from the lines. No allowance was made for local screening or enhancement of the field by trees, hedges and earth banks because I was after the actual environmental values. It is quite likely that the two lines were energised at different voltages but, in any case, the values measured were typical of what one might expect under high voltage power-lines (Waibel, 1975; Banks et al., 1968). The quadruple, steel-cored, aluminium conductors would have been appropriate for a 3-phase, 400 kV supergrid lines with a capacity of 3600 MVA (Box and Symes, 1968). The full load current could rise to about 5000 A, although it might be allowed to rise further in cold weather because the increased cooling would reduce the thermal expansion sag at the lowest point of the catenary; this sets the limit to the current which may be passed. At the time the measurements were carried out, the magnetic field was about 10 milligauss beneath the lines, appropriate to a load current of about 100 A in the conductors. There were ELF variations amounting to ±20 per cent about this mean; this was presumably due to load fluctuations. Again, this is quite typical for locations under power-lines where magnetic fields may be up to 100 milligauss. More interesting was the finding that the magnetic field did not decrease as quickly as the electric field with increased distance from the lines. Inside Mrs Jean Wareham's farmhouse (100 metres from the power lines) the 50 Hz magnetic field was 1 milligauss even when the house electricity supply was turned off at the mains. This value is also typical of the fields produced by domestic house wiring and appliances. But, most importantly, it is more coherent in space. The field from a handheld appliance will at the hand be much greater than at the foot, whereas the field 100 metres away from the lines will be more uniform over the whole body. The mean of the results of Wertheimer and Leeper (1979) and Savitz (1987) suggests a three-fold enhancement of the cancer risk ratio at 1 milligauss (0.1 μT).

Dr David Smith, of the University College of North Wales, Bangor (personal communication), subsequently measured electric fields of 10 to 20 V/m inside Hilary Bacon's cottage, and 60 V/m to 4.8 kV/m in the garden. The magnetic field was 1 milligauss rising to 9 milligauss (extrapolated cancer risk ratio 23) in cold weather both inside and outside the cottage.

The waveform of the magnetic field was not so clean as that of the electric field. It carried about 20 per cent of the 300 Hz harmonic; this could have been due to the rectifiers for a direct current link connected to the power system. The frequency of 300 Hz is that which synthesises the homoepathic potency phosphorous 6X (Dr W. Ludwig, personal communication, 1987). The Boericke homoeopathic *Materia Medica* lists under phosphorus the following relevant symptoms for which it might be considered as a possible remedy, the corollary being that these symptoms would be triggered as 'homoeopathic proving symptoms' in healthy sensitive persons taking potencies of phosphorus or its equivalent electrical frequency:

> Phosphorus irritates, inflames and degenerates mucous membranes, irritates and inflames serous membranes, inflames spinal cord and nerves, causing paralysis, destroys bone, especially the lower jaw and tibia; disorganises blood causing fatty degeneration of blood vessels and every tissue and organ of the body and thus gives rise to haemorrhages, and haematogenous jaundice. Produces a picture of destructive metabolism.... Great susceptibility to external impressions, to light, sound, odours, touch, electrical changes, thunder-storms. Suddenness of symptoms, sudden prostration, faints, sweats, shooting pains, etc. ... Great lowering of spirits. Easily vexed. Fearfulness, as if something were creeping out of every corner. Clairvoyant state....

When the 50 Hz component of the field was filtered out, there remained trains of pulses at about 3 kHz. This note can sometimes be heard on a car radio when driving beneath power lines. The radio noise and corona loss from power lines has long been a matter for study and efforts have been made to reduce it (Banks *et al.*, 1968).

In 1980, the village of Fishpond was drinking the water from its own wells. I took samples of water in sterile bottles from the well and the tap in Hilary Bacon's cottage, and from the tap in Mrs Wareham's. These were subsequently plated out by Dr Aarholt back in my laboratory at Salford University. The sample from Mrs Wareham's house contained about 7000 bacteria per millilitre, but there is the possibility that the cells may have divided while in transit, thereby giving a high count. There were two types of bacteria: one was a motile bacterium, slow-growing at room temperature, with hardly any growth at 39°C; the other was a non-motile bacterium (size 0.8×1.5 μm) growing freely at room temperature, and again very slow-growing at 39°C. Neither were expected to be pathogenic.

Unusually, Hilary Bacon's water supply was found to be perfectly sterile; at least a few hundred cells per millilitre could be expected from any well water. The well water pH was in the range 6 to 8, that from the tap about pH 5. Dr Aarholt recalled that alternating magnetic fields had been experimented with for sterilising the water in space-craft, but that since these produce so much waste heat, distillation was preferred.

Mr Roger Hewitt, of Salford University's Geography Department looked up the geological maps of the area for me; they showed sands, shales and clays, nothing likely to give magnetic anomalies. Fishpond is situated upon an area of landslip and the water levels are distorted, although the importance of water to living systems was not well appreciated at that time. In a letter, Major Edward Golding, a retired geological engineer living near Dorchester, Dorset, confirmed and extended this view:

> Fishpond is a small village, scarcely more than a hamlet, in West Dorset. It is mentioned a number of times in the local Geological Manual because of its unusual geological make-up. The Manual lists three areas of 'landslips' in West Dorset and associates the origin of these 'landslips' with major coastal landslips that occurred in 1839. 'Landslip' areas are about six miles long and perhaps half-a-mile wide and are probably the result of earlier sub-erosion. When the sub-erosion has eaten sufficiently deeply under the higher ground, the whole mass slides into the hole. As it slides, it rides in any detritus already in the hollow and often finishes up with the strata tilted downwards towards the cliff face left standing after the landslip.
>
> Since the Greensand and the Lower Chalk were laid down in deep, and therefore, *still* waters, each contains a percentage of fine clays and in the case of Greensand is relatively impermeable until percolation has washed out finer particles and so made possible concentration of underground water flows, so re-starting the erosion process.
>
> At Fishpond [there is] 'an enormous slipped mass of Upper Greensand' with steep 'slip scarps' on three sides leaving a valley rather like a 'corrie' and with a 'back-slope' into the valley known as Fishpond Bottom. Moisture, therefore, tends to collect and be retained in the Greensand at the valley head. These conditions encouraged smallholdings and a road became desirable. The road will have, no doubt, helped the C.E.G.B to reach the decision to route its new transmission lines across the valley head. The steep-sided narrow valley keeps the wind away and the air, as well as the ground, is moist. (Golding, 1987)

The tendency for moisture to collect in Fishpond Bottom implies that whatever chemicals are applied to the land, these will finish up in the shallow well drinking water.

Mr Hewitt also kindly did a chemical analysis of the samples of water and soil brought from Fishpond; they gave sodium, potassium, calcium and magnesium as the main soluble components, with smaller amounts of phosphorus, copper, zinc, iron and lead. No unusual levels of minerals were present. At this time the importance of testing for organo-chlorides was not appreciated and the facilities now in Dallas, Texas, were not available anyway.

The Geography Department of Liverpool University kindly sent me copies of the Bouguer Gravity Anomaly and the Aeromagnetic Anomaly Survey maps covering the area around Fishpond. No anomalies were shown.

The fingernail clippings were analysed by Dr Nadir Ahmed using the Rutherford Backscattering technique. We had previously used this method with success on dental specimens (Ahmed and Smith, 1981). It showed the presence of oxygen, fluorine, sodium, magnesium, sulphur, calcium, copper and bromine, but nothing abnormal.

My interviews with the villagers had elicited the effects and symptoms already described by Hilary Bacon, and had convinced me that they were genuine. The problem was, why Fishpond? Depending on whom you ask and the criteria they use, there are probably between 15,000 and 80,000 persons in Great Britain living beneath high voltage power-lines. As there are 32,000 GPs in the UK, each should only see one or two such patients, an insufficient sample to detect a trend. Was there any additional factor besides the gossip of a close-knit community, which already resented having the power lines thrust upon it? None of the measurements that I had then done suggested that the fields were in any way atypical. Either, I was missing some contributory factor, or there was a mighty can of worms waiting to be opened.

Hilary Bacon pointed out to me that, at the Innsworth public enquiry, the Inspectors had asked why the CEGB had never done any health surveys on Fishpond in response to its complaints. The response was that it was not necessary to do so, because electrical workers were so obviously healthy. When asked if any health surveys had been done on electrical workers, the reply was, again, that it was not necessary because they were so obviously healthy! One might perhaps ask whether they are at work for almost 24 hours each day or, whether they sleep in the electromagnetic field conditions of their place of work, too? Taking account of the Report of the Working Group on Inequalities in Health, I clearly needed to do my own survey to be able to counter this. It reminded me of the story of the man who asked what the red light was doing at the top of a radio mast. Not satisfied with the answer that it was to prevent aircraft from flying into it, he asked what the mast was for: 'To keep the red lamp up, of course,' was the retort. Although this satisfied the man in the story, I was not going to be satisfied so easily.

It has become a common demonstration among environmental groups to stand beneath power lines in the dusk or dark, holding fluorescent lighting tubes aloft. The electric field is usually sufficiently strong for enough visible light emission to be photographed and give an impression of a candlelight procession. It clearly can be done without accident as many published photographs testify, but there is no point in putting Murphy's Law to the test. I have worked with high voltages and electrical insulation for long enough to have no confidence that the air around the pins at the top of such a hand-held fluorescent tube will always remain insulating enough to protect me from personally shorting 400 kV and shunting up to 5000 A to ground. However, I have calibrated a fluorescent tube under such conditions as simulated in the laboratory. With a fluorescent tube in an electric field of 2.8 kV/m there was enough light emission for photography in a darkroom; the current was 400 µA (r.m.s.), just below the threshold for most people's perception of a current; the electrical resistance of the fluorescent tube discharge was then 7 Megohms, somewhat more than dry skin. If the skin is very dry, it may have 1 megohm resistance, and the domestic 240 V will hardly reach the electric current perception threshold; if the skin happens to be moist, its resistance may drop to 1 kilohm, in which case the domestic 240 V supply will then pass a near-fatal $\frac{1}{4}$ Å through the body.

Back at Salford University, the basic research into electromagnetic field interactions continued. This has already been described in earlier chapters. By 1981, we were looking into the possibility of affecting a living system with a frequency and a magnetic field which combined to satisfy the proton magnetic resonance conditions. For example, at a geomagnetic field of 50 µT (0.5 Gauss), protons will interact strongly with a frequency of precisely 2130 Hz; the frequency can be supplied by an electric or a magnetic field. The protons (hydrogen atoms) in the water of living systems seemed to be sensitive to this condition (Jafary-Asl et al., 1982) and the necessary frequencies could conceivably be present as harmonics in a power distribution network. The situation combined both the high coherence of the 50 Hz and the uniformity of the geomagnetic field over the dimensions of the human body. It thus became necessary to know the precise values of the geomagnetic field in Fishpond, since the aerial survey could not resolve local variations, such as those due to the steel pylons and cables, for example. I visited Fishpond again on 6 June 1981 and measured the geomagnetic field with a laboratory magnetometer; the readings were between 45 and 48 µT. The aerial survey map had shown that the geomagnetic field over the Fishpond region was about -0.1 µT relative to the local reference field for the British Isles of 47.033 µT.

There are two ancient earthworks in Fishpond, Lambert's Castle and

Coney's Castle. The magnetic field readings taken at points just outside Lambert's Castle were 44 μT, against 42 μT inside the earthworks. There seemed to be some anomalous readings on the magnetometer going along the road through Coney's Castle but the instrument was not really sensitive enough for this purpose. These results did not seem to be particularly significant until subsequently, when the dowsing section for this book was being prepared (see Chapter 11).

However, in July 1981 something else happened. Overnight, and while many people in British universities had dispersed for a vacation, the government drastically cut the universities' funding. Salford University took a 40 per cent cut in resources. With most of a university's budget going on salaries, this meant that everyone over 50 years of age was strongly urged to take premature retirement, so as to pass the financial burden on to the pension funds. I was then 51, and, not wanting to be 'last on the scrap-heap', I had to give my mind to survival. I lost my interdisciplinary undergraduate course in Biomedical Electronics and with it a supply of students skilled in both biological and electronics experimentation. Interdisciplinary courses in British universities immediately became too demanding on the scarce resources remaining. About this time, I also had a verbal communication, discrete of course, asking me not to dispense material of assistance to the protesters from Fishpond. A letter to the presumed originator of that message produced for me written confirmation that it had in fact been sent, and conveyed the acceptance, with resignation, that I would continue to 'rock their boat' if I thought fit. At times like this, one is very glad of the remaining vestiges of 'academic tenure'. However, in view of the then current situation in universities, I was careful to make available on request only those results which had been referred and accepted for publication.

The Abbot and Community of Nunraw Abbey, in Scotland, must have been praying hard. At the time, I was unaware of the sequence of events, including their involvement in the Haddington Inquiry of April 1982, described above by Hilary Bacon.

Dr Stephen Perry very kindly let me have access to the 'raw data' on which his work on environmental power-frequency electromagnetic fields and suicides was based (Perry *et al.*, 1981). The work we had done with bacteria showed that the determining onset conditions were likely to be the most informative. I needed to get this information from the suicide data. At Salford University Dr Rose Baker did the necessary statistics for me and the threshold came out at about 140 microGauss (Smith and Baker, 1982). Because magnetic fields are quantised, it was immediately possible to conclude that whatever part of the body was being affected it must be at least 360 microns in size to accommodate a single quantum of magnetic flux at this threshold field. The other interesting feature of the results was that the 'rural' suicides' risk came out higher than that for 'urban' suicides. We could not suggest any reason for this. One would expect towns to be less healthy places in which to live than the country. Not until a conference in Dallas in 1985 did we realise that people living in the country were more at risk from being hypersensitised by exposure to pesticides and herbicides.

In 1981, the electrical utilities in the State of New York had been required to make $5 million available for a five-year research project into the effects of power-lines – the New York State Power Lines Project, which reported in July 1987. I submitted a pre-proposal for research funding from this source, but it was turned down. Without resources to do the work myself, I published one of the topics in the proposal (Smith and Aarholt, 1982), pointing out that the fields near power-lines could give body currents comparable to those used to give pain relief, which had in turn been associated with the stimulation of endogenous opiates; therefore, with long-term exposure, one must expect to find withdrawal symptoms. I concluded it with a reference to the Innsworth Inquiry 'cows'. Because that year there has already been reports at two conferences linking allergy with endogenous opiates, Dr Jean Monro contracted me to see whether I could help with her electrically sensitive allergy patients. The co-operation with Dr Jean Monro and, through her, with Dr Bill Rea in Dallas, Texas, developed from this rejected funding application. Research workers in the United States have since told me that I should be thankful I was unsuccessful in getting the funding, but for other reasons.

The health survey finally got going as a result of the help and publicity arising from a Channel 4 television programme, *4 What It's Worth*, made in Fishpond and in which I said my piece. My 'fan mail' over the years had also made it clear that the power-lines problem was not confined just to Fishpond.

My attention was called to the General Health Questionnaire published by Professor David Goldberg (1972). This has the great advantage for such research that each of the 140 questions has already been analysed in respect of scores to be expected from normal, mildly ill, and severely ill subjects. Thus the answers to even a single questionnaire could be so classified. Since I planned to use the questions for an objective assessment of the general problem as well as each correspondent's state of health following long-term exposure to electromagnetic fields rather than for the detection of psychiatric illness, I had no grounds on which to base the simplifying reduction in the number of questions which Goldberg proposes for psychiatric purposes. This could now be done with the information generated in the first trial.

The GHQ questions are collected into seven generalised groupings which are not subscales of the test, but which cover:

A General health and central nervous system.
B Cardiovascular, neuromuscular and gastrointestinal.
C Sleep and wakefulness.
D Observable behaviour – personal behaviour.
E Observable behaviour – relations with others.
F Subjective feelings – inadequacy, tension, temper, etc.
G Subjective feelings, mainly depression and anxiety.

In the event, I was able to get 41 persons who lived close to power lines to answer the 140 questions; of these 8 were residents of Fishpond and their scores were representative of the general results described below. The General Health Questionnaire (GHQ) Scores came out into two non-overlapping groups as shown in Table 8.1. The high score group

Table 8.1 Groups by GHQ score

GHQ score	Numbers in score range
0–10	6
11–20	5
21–30	4
31–40	4
41–50	2
51–60	0
61–70	7
71–80	6
81–90	3
91–100	3
101–110	1

averaged 77.9 ± 11.8, the low score group averaged 21.1 ± 14.1. Other details of the two groups given in Table 8.2 show that chance had favoured me with a pair of reasonably balanced sets. There was no selection – this is just what arrived in the mail and I had to do the best I could with it. The GHQ scores, as percentages, for the above seven sections and the low and high score groups respectively, are compared in Table 8.3 with the GHQ results given by Goldberg. On this basis it is seen that the high score group correspond in general to the severely ill, while the Low Score Group come between normal and mildly ill.

Table 8.2 Averages against GHQ score groups

	High score group	Low score group
Total	20	21
Male	8	8
Female	12	13
Ages	42.0 ± 14.4	43.4 ± 15.7 years
Years at address	12.2 ± 9.4	10.6 ± 6.0 years
Hours/day in fields	19.8 ± 5.5	18.2 ± 5.0 hours
Direction sleep		
E/W	8	9
N/S	8	12
Distance from lines		
< 160 metres	(60 ± 102)	(75 ± 84) yards
Direction of lines		
E/W	10	12
N/S	2	5
Scores on GHQ	77.9 ± 11.8	21.1 ± 14.1

The Low score group come out as normal in respect of G – depression, while the high score group come out as only mildly ill. The high score group exceed the scores of the severely ill in respect of Groups A, B, C and E. Given the resources, more information could have been gleaned from the existing completed questionnaires and a larger-scale survey could have been initiated. However, before stirring too thoroughly, one had to consider whether, in the then *Zeitgeist*, resources would merely be directed to keeping the lid on this particular 'can of worms'; today with the 'greening' of politics, the situation may have changed.

Goldberg (1972) points out that as one proceeds through his Questionnaire, the items become more overtly psychiatric. Since the low score group tends toward normal scores in all but the first three sections of the questionnaire and the high score group is only mildly ill in respect of depression and anxiety (G), it would seem that power-line illnesses are not 'all in the mind' but rather, that some organic condition is present. Dr Jean Monro has commented that sections A, B and C would also be scored high by allergic subjects. Medical histories are not available for those completing the Questionnaire.

It would now be possible to select those questions which were given high scores by persons living under power lines and complaining of illness, and to produce a shorter form of the Questionnaire. As an attempt to make further progress researching into the electromagnetic field effects, I looked at the questions scored highly and ranked those which the

Table 8.3 GHQ sections

	Power-line subjects low-score group (%)	Power-line subjects high-score group (%)	GHQ results normal (%)	GHQ results mild (%)	GHQ results severe (%)
A General health and CNS	13	47	3	23	41
B Cardiovascular, neuromuscular and gastrointestinal	7	39	4	19	32
C Sleep and wakefulness	13	68	5	33	58
D Observable behaviour – personal behaviour	7	50	5	31	52
E Observable behaviour – relations with others	8	50	6	32	47
F Subjective feelings – inadequacy, tension, temper, etc.	5	52	5	37	58
G Subjective feelings – mainly depression and anxiety	½	37	5	40	64

Sections A, B, C would also be scored high by allergic subjects.

high score group had scored higher than the severely ill, and those which the low score group had scored higher than the mildly ill. Then, because of Hahnemann's Law of Similars in homoeopathy, it seemed reasonable to find out what caused these high-score symptoms in healthy persons by looking up a homoeopathic pharmacopoea. The first place to look was under 'Electricitas' and 'Magnetis' – potencies made from tinctures exposed to electric currents or magnetic fields. Table 8.4 compares the high-scoring questions and the homoeopathic listings; the similarity is quite remarkable, although it should not be unexpected.

Examination of a homoeopathic *Materia Medica* (Boericke, 1927) shows that the above symptoms are not unique, and that they can also be elicited by a number of environmental and nutritional substances, at least when homoeopathically potentised. The possibility that electromagnetic fields can enhance, or potentise, the effects of such substances should be considered. The Chinese homoeopaths have been reported to be able to potentise remedies by burying them in the ground for

Table 8.4

High-scoring questions	Homoeopathic characteristic
Blushing easily	Face-colour, bright red (E)
Noises in ears	Fullness in ears, ringing in head (X)
'Pins and needles' in hands and feet	Pains in arms and legs – tingling extending to foot (E)
Worried about heart	Anxiety. Pain from heart (E)
Palpitations	Palpitations especially before storm (E)
Diarrhoea	Diarrhoea (E)
Bad headaches	Violent headaches (E)
Aches and pains	Aches and pains (E & M)
Exhaustion, weariness	Generally depressed and weary (E)
Sleep does not refresh	Sleep disorder (E & M)
Worry about health	Anxiety (E)

E = Electricitas; M = Magnetis; X = X-ray.

a period. It may be significant that this would have the effect of screening them from all electromagnetic radiation except that in the ELF part of the spectrum, which includes the Schumann band. Table 8.5 lists some homoeopathic remedies and their symptoms which are often encountered in electromagnetically triggered allergic responses. It is based on the Questionnaire scores and on the case histories of more than 60 electrically sensitive allergy patients.

This was the 'Fishpond Story' up to the time of writing this book. With the above as background information, I was able to ask Hilary Bacon some more questions when we met to discuss this chapter. She and one of her sons again completed the same Questionnaire, three and a half years after they had first completed it in 1983; I have not disclosed the scoring method I used, and their first intimation of the scores they actually obtained on either occasion was when they read the draft of this section. In the intervening period they both left Fishpond. In 1984, Hilary Bacon moved to the San Francisco area of California (USA) and into a 60 Hz environment. In 1983, she scored 97, putting her at the upper end of the high score group and definitely in the seriously ill category. In January 1987, she scored only 1 – very 'normal'. She told me that it took her a whole year after leaving Fishpond to regain positive good health. Her younger son, whom she describes as 'not an allergic person', scored 7 in 1983, and 8 in 1987 – 'normal' each time.

Table 8.5

Homoeopathic remedy	Symptoms from 'provings'
Amyl nitrite	Anxiety, redness of face
Coca	Noises in ear, headache, palpitation
Coffee	Headache, sleep disorder, noise sensitivity, palpitation
Digitalis	Palpitation, anxiety about future, breathing, dullness of sense, noises in head, etc. (All questionnaires came from areas of the UK where the foxglove grows wild.)
Ferrum Met.	Face flushes, headache, breathing difficult, palpitation, noise unbearable
Phos. Ac.	Mental debility, noise in ears
Sulphur	Oversensitivity to odours and sounds, thinking difficult, sick headache, sleep disorder, relationship to magnetis
Tabacum	Muscular prostration, band round head, vision through veil, heart palpitation, angina, insomnia
Thea	Mental exhaustion, headache, hearing, sleep disorder, palpitation
Zincum Met.	General and mental 'fag', headache, noise sensitivity, blurred vision, chest constricted, back pain, convulsions

Synergistic effects of electrical and chemical pollution

I asked Hilary Bacon whether she had ever been exposed to any chemicals which could hypersensitise her to electromagnetic fields. I learned that when she left Oxford University, she was in Eugene, Oregon, (c.f. p. 228) from 1958–60. She spent some of that time with an uncle and aunt on a former fruit farm. There was then a State programme of pest control. While she was there the whole farm was sprayed three times a year by men wearing complete protective clothing; she could not have avoided some of the drift spray and eating contaminated fruit. The Oregon programme was subsequently discontinued on environmental grounds. Throughout the USA as a whole the problem still remains. In 1950, 200,000 lb of pesticide was used; the figure for 1986 was

4,000,000,000 lb yet in the intervening period the percentage loss of crops to pests doubled (Seba, 1987, 1988).

Immediately Hilary Bacon moved into the cottage in Fishpond, in 1973, she set about painting it throughout and at once suffered loss of voice; possibly an allergic response triggered by the paint fumes and involving a regulatory system already damaged by the Oregon pesticides. In the presence of the fields from Fishpond's overhead power lines, such an allergic response would be very likely to have its triggering stimulus transfer to the electromagnetic fields. This mechanism commonly occurs in hayfever sufferers. The year's initial reaction is triggered by pollen, but after the pollen season has finished, the reaction transfers and continues to be triggered by mould spores from wet grass and then in the autumn from the dead leaves. Respite is obtained only when the frosts come and kill everything.

I then learned that the hill farms around the village of Fishpond do not have any crops that require to be sprayed. The region is mostly pasture. However, they do get good crops of stinging nettles, and these get sprayed with herbicide. There was still ample evidence of this when I visited Fishpond and the surrounding district in May 1987. The local authorities in the area did not spray the roadside verges even in their more affluent days, but they did scatter pellets of weedkiller, so I am informed. Bearing in mind that the village is on a hillside and that it was then on well water, there is at least a possibility that these sprays and herbicides could have been the pathway for hypersensitisation of the other residents. Weedkillers used to contain dioxin as a contaminant and some would readily decompose to give this chemical, as discussed in Dallas (1985). Texas is very fertile agriculturally; the farms get three crops a year. Because of the enormous scale of distances, the crop spraying is done from fixed-wing aircraft, and there may be three aerial crop sprayings each year. Not only does Texas have to cope with problems of allergic reactions triggered chemically, it has to consider the synergistic effects of chemicals and petrochemicals with electromagnetic fields. In Houston, Texas, the successful $25 million action against a utility for siting powerlines over a school has already been discussed by Hilary Bacon (see p. 147). A farm in Texas situated on wet land in a sprayed area, between two power lines and at the intersection of microwave beams, had strong magnetic fields around the house wiring. There were also ground currents outside. The environment was so bad that electromagnetic de-sensitisation, effective in Dallas, could not help a patient from this environment.

At a panel session during a Symposium on the Health Effects of Electric and Magnetic Fields held in Toronto in September, 1986, a questioner asked the panel to suppose that they had a family with two young children and were buying a house. Would they take a house next to a transmission

Electromagnetic environmental pollution

line which was $25,000 cheaper than an identical one elsewhere? The replies were (*Microwave News*, September/October 1986, p. 9):

> 'Yes, no question about it, I'd buy the home along the right-of-way.'
> 'No. If I was bald and 65 years old, I might.' ($25,000 was not enough money to take the risk.)
> 'If it bothers you don't buy the house.'
> 'No.' (Not because of adverse health effects but because of corona noise and the loss of aesthetics due to the power line.)
> 'Yes, I would buy the house next to the transmission line and pocket the difference.' (Would not live right under a 500 kV line, but would do so along the right-of-way.) (None presently required in UK.)

Dr Cyril Smith's comments on the above would have been as follows. Only buy the house, if:

1 There is no family history of allergies on either side for three generations (e.g. eczema, asthma, hayfever, migraine, food intolerance).
2 The family doctor can recognise an environmentally triggered illness if it presents, and knows how to treat it, and is aware of homoeopathic effects.
3 The family can afford the loss, if after a year or so there is an enforced sale on health grounds, assuming that the housing market may have moved against such properties.
4 The family is not into eating 'junk' (high additive-containing) foods and has not been, and will not be exposed to chemicals, especially as pesticides, herbicides, fungicides.
5 The house does not contain recently 'treated' timber, or formaldehyde vapour emitting insulation, decoration or furnishings.
6 No environmental sources of coherent electromagnetic fields affecting the house appreciably exceed 15 nT (150 microGauss) in magnetic field strength (based on my interpretation of Perry's data (Smith and Baker, 1982), that of Wertheimer and Leeper (1979) and of Savitz (1987)).
7 The occupants acquire no exposures to ionising radiation, including the naturally occurring radioactive gas radon (prevalent in certain geological locations) followed by the equivalent of incubation in an alternating magnetic field (based on my interpretation of Tumanyan and Samolienko (1983) concerning possible synergistic effects of ionising and non-ionising radiation.

The controversy over the health risks of living near power lines is having an impact on property values in at least two states of the USA

(*Microwave News*, September/October 1987, p. 7), and could begin to do so in Britain and elsewhere. In the light of the growing evidence, it is time to establish rights of way in the UK along existing pylon routes and a moratorium on any further erection of pylons within 200 metres of dwelling-places or the building of houses within 200 metres of existing pylons, as a growing number of US States have now done (see Chapter 9).

Hilary Bacon's move in 1984 was a very good move for her health and in view of what continues to emerge in this saga. She is fortunate in having had that option. Those less fortunate need to be enabled with knowledge and resources to create an electromagnetically safe-haven, at least for sleep, and for electromagnetically improving the workplace. There is a precedent in respect of the provisions for the sound insulation of houses near airports and motorways. Nothing can happen quickly at the other end. Heavy electrical plant and distribution systems and other major sources of electromagnetic pollution have a decade or more of lead time between conception and implementation and are expected to last at least 25–40 years. Thus, most of the existing systems will take us well into the 21st century. Our vast investment in all the electrical and electronics systems of present day convenience compares with our investment in motor vehicles and roads. There has never been any suggestion of abolishing these because of road traffic accidents; rather, there is a policy of safety and a system of insurance with compensation for the victims of accidents which is perhaps the way forward for victims of environmental electromagnetic pollution.

CHAPTER 9

Chronic electromagnetic field exposure, health risks and safety regulations

There should be a major research effort on means of power delivery and use that would reduce magnetic field exposure.

First recommendation of the Final Report of the New York State Power Line Project, 1st July 1987

The 'fan-mail' following newspaper and television reports of Hilary Bacon's campaign and Cyril Smith's work on the effects of coherent electromagnetic fields on living systems has brought them many letters giving accounts of personal illnesses and tragedies involving their writers. The following accounts, all taken from published material, including newspaper reports and evidence presented at Public Inquiries, are quite consistent with the tenor of these letters.

Since the Innsworth Inquiry in 1978 and the Haddington Inquiry in 1982, other groups in the UK have protested over proposed power-lines with varying degrees of success. In the Republic of Ireland, objectors have met with what they felt to be a very unsympathetic Electricity Supply Board (ESB) in their fight to stop proposed 400 kV transmission lines between Moneypoint, in County Clare, and Dublin from being erected on their land, especially near their homes. In 1982, a group of landowners led by Dr Ted Hickey, a lecturer in Horticultural Science at the Thomond College of Education in Limerick, protested to the ESB that the proposed line constituted a health hazard and should be re-routed (N.Smith, 1982). In Dr Hickey's case, a pylon was to be sited just 50 m from his house in Cloonfadda, outside Killaloe. Other protesters included two medical doctors, Dr Frieda Keane and Dr Paschal Carmody. The latter recounted the case history of a patient who consulted him in 1978 with a multiplicity of complaints that did not fit into any pattern, including eight consecutive miscarriages, before which she had had four healthy children (Walsh, 1985). Medical investigations produced neither evidence nor conclusions and by 1983, she weighed only 6 st 4 lbs (40 kg). When Dr Carmody asked her if there was anything in her environment that could be causing her problems, she told him that there was a transformer at the end of her house that had been put in about eight years before, which coincided with the start of her troubles. After representations were made to the ESB, the transformer was removed. Walsh (1985) reported that, 'Shortly afterwards she gained weight, to 10 st 7 lb [67 kg], and her depression lifted. She became a happy person and is now in the seventh month of a pregnancy which has been totally uneventful.' But despite much protest and mounting publicity, Dr Hickey and his supporters failed to prevent the ESB from erecting a pylon near his house in 1986, forcing him and his wife to sell their house and move. None the less, Dr Hickey is continuing his opposition and is presently studying the effects of electromagnetic fields on plants.

However, other protesters and groups have taken up Dr Hickey's fight. A number of them, including residents' associations, the Irish Bord Fáilte (Irish Tourist Board) and An Táisce (Irish National Trust) objected, in September 1986, to the ESB's plans to erect a 220 kV double-circuit line between Carrickmines, Co. Dublin, and Arklow, Co. Wicklow, through some of the most beautiful areas of County Wicklow, including the Glen of the Downs, the Sugar Loaf and Enniskerry (Brennock, 1986). However, in a decision on 6 January 1987, An Bord Pleanála (Irish Planning Appeal Authority) turned down the appeals and granted permission, with a few minor conditions, to the ESB. The terms of the permission do specify that pylons shall not be erected closer to dwelling houses than 30 m (or, if already closer than 30 m, must not be moved any closer), though the reason given is, 'In the interests of clarity and residential amenity.' From the data reproduced in the WHO (1984) Publication (Chapter 3), at 30 m there will be electric fields of the order of 0.5 kilovolt per metre and magnetic fields of the order of microTesla (10,000 microGauss). This is large in respect of what may be deduced about the onset of effects from the work of Perry, Wertheimer and Leeper, Savitz, and Tomenius as discussed below.

In rejecting possible health hazards from the proposed lines, Dr Joseph Cunningham, the ESB Medical Officer, referred to two World Health Organisation publications (WHO, 1982, 1984) as concluding that, 'electric and magnetic fields caused by transmission systems up to voltages of 420 kV do not constitute a danger to human health' (*Irish Times*, 6 September 1986). Such a blanket statement clearly omits proper consideration of the question of residential proximity to such lines, as well as whether the occupants might be babies, children, pregnant women, the old, the infirm, or those suffering from certain illnesses or receiving special medical treatments. Because of the duality between coherent oscillations and chemical structure, synergistic effects may occur at any frequency. Microwaves, for example, have been found to potentiate the action of a number of drugs, including the tranquillizer Librium (*Microwave News*, 1981, February), and a team at the Johns Hopkins University headed by Dr Sam Koslov have observed the tell-tale Alzheimer's pattern of neurofibrillary tangles in a monkey chronically exposed to microwaves (*Microwave News*, 1986, September/October). In fact, Mr John Royds, probably one of the few Irish farmers to hold a physics degree, has accused the ESB of distorting their evidence, pointing out that the above statement is in fact taken from the 1982 WHO Report and that their 1984 one is far more cautious (McDonald, 1987). The 1984 WHO publication deals specifically with Environmental Health Criteria for Extremely Low Frequency (ELF) Fields and in its conclusions and recommendations it states that:

> It is not possible from present knowledge to make a definite statement about the safety or hazard associated with long-term exposure to sinusoidal electric fields in the range of 1–10 kV/m. In the absence of specific evidence of particular risk or disease syndromes associated with such exposure, and in view of experimental findings on the biological effects of exposure, it is recommended that efforts be made to limit exposure, particularly for members of the general population, to levels as low as can be reasonably achieved. (WHO, 1984, p. 18)

This places the risks from ELF fields in the same category as road traffic accidents (which currently run at epidemic proportions!); an acceptable risk is one which society will accept.

Despite the apparent status of the published material, the discussion and interpretation of the material presented in the two WHO publications is slanted toward the view that there are no effects to worry about or that, where they occur, they are entirely due to thermal factors. The reason is not hard to discern. Since these documents were prepared, considerable theoretical and experimental advances have taken place, making them unreliable and in need of updating.

This is underlined by the more emphatic statements in the latest 1987 WHO Report (not actually available till May 1988), produced in conjunction with the International Radiation Protection Association (IRPA), on static and time-varying magnetic fields (WHO, 1987): 'There is an urgent need for well designed experimental studies on the carcinogenic effects of ELF electromagnetic field exposure', and 'the possibility of some perturbing effects occurring following long-term exposure cannot be excluded.' It should be noted that even these and other statements in the report are dated, the final draft having been reviewed in July 1986, just before the results of Savitz's research were reported in November 1986 and then published in the Final Report of the New York State Power Lines Project in July 1987 (discussed below), which is not included.

All this seems to have had little effect on the Irish authorities responsible for allowing the new Arklow–Carrickmines 220 kV line to be built. To galvanise public opinion, Mr John Royds, together with Mr Valentine Byrne, in September 1987 formed SPARKS ('Stop Powerlines Across Residences, Kindergartens, and Schools') and have petitioned the Irish Minister for Energy for a moratorium on energising the line until an independent scientific commission has been set up and has fully assessed the significance of the latest research on the health hazard question, an assessment to which the ESB has agreed. Unfortunately, a report prepared by the Department of Energy (McManus, 1988) is extremely biased and selective in the evidence it presents. But as a result of it, the Minister of Energy has seen fit to energise the line, despite further protests

It is beyond the scope of this chapter to attempt a comprehensive assessment of all the recent evidence – biochemical, epidemiological and animal studies – that support the view that powerline EM fields can be hazardous to human health. Many such studies have been assessed elsewhere and the reader is referred to such sources as Becker and Seldon (1986), Marino and Ray (1986), Dutta and Millis (1986), Polk and Postow (1986), the PhD thesis by Florig (1986) and, especially for the campaigner, the excellent Australian source document by Macmillan (1986), mentioned below. Recent books by Marino (1988) and Fröhlich (1988) are also recommended. The aim in this chapter is to give a broad overview of the more recent developments in the debate, focussing chiefly on specific epidemiological studies, possible mechanisms of interaction and the establishment of feasible guidelines for protecting the public, based on the latest understanding of the health risks involved.

Dutta and Millis's book contains 'An Overview of the Electropollution Literature', with 150 abstracts culled from the BENER (Biological Effects of Non-ionising Electromagnetic Radiation) Digest. Covering 13 different aspects of the problem, it is a good introduction for the interested but uninitiated scientist. That by Polk and Postow contains some fine treatments by authorities in various areas of bioelectromagnetics, although some of the reviews of the biological studies, including the cancer/ELF connection, are dated or fail to present a full picture of the research by omitting important data.

One book that cannot be recommended, despite its seemingly authoritative title, is that by Cartensen (1987). Approaching the subject as an engineer, Cartensen betrays not only his considerable bias but also his inability to get to grips with some of the essential issues. As Dr Abraham

Liboff points out in his review *Microwave News*, 1987, July/August, p. 11), much of the most critically important work is 'summarily dismissed in tables bearing the presumptuous legends "negated" or "unconfirmed"'. Cartensen constantly attempts to explain away non-thermal effects as ill-perceived, and tends to see all the work done on calcium efflux effects as flawed. He has great difficulty in accepting the concept of 'biological window' as an explanation of different frequency effects and the non-linearity of response of biological systems, and shows himself at his most biased and blinkered when he comments that the 'failure of biological effects to be dependent on the magnitude of exposure is one of the traits which characterize "pathological" science' (p. 158). Clearly, such views do not assist the rapprochement between those able to accept the implications of the growing body of evidence and those who remain fixed in viewing the data in the context of an increasingly outmoded paradigm. That such reactionary views tend to favour the position of certain vested interests is now generally appreciated by those involved in the debate.

The best source of information concerning current developments in this area is the bi-monthly US journal, *Microwave News* (see Postscript for details). This was launched in 1981 by New York publisher and editor Dr Louis Slesin as a result of the burgeoning controversy and research concerning non-ionising radiation. It provides excellent and not too technical coverage of world-wide, but especially American, research and we are indebted to it for much of what follows. Slesin also publishes the equally useful *VDT News*.

A landmark pronouncement was made early in 1986 by the American Advisory Committee on the Non-Thermal Effects of Non-Ionizing Radiation who reported (NRC, 1986) to the United States National Academy of Sciences' National Research Council (NAS–NRC) that, 'Abundant fragmentary evidence has been presented in support of possible biological effects from non-ionizing radiation, at both transmission and microwave frequencies. These effects often appear to be unaccompanied by macroscopic thermal changes' (*Microwave News*, 1986, May/June). In the light of the NAS–NRC Report, it is hard to see how power utilities will be able to rely any longer on outdated work dismissing non-thermal effects, which was, in many cases, funded to demonstrate that the sponsors were blameless.

The point at which a biological effect becomes a hazard is open to debate, but this is often terminated with the remark that, of course, more research is needed. It only remains for funding for the necessary research to be withheld, usually for quite plausible reasons such as the need not being proven and the money not being available, for the status quo to be allowed to persist. In the USA, two major NIR bioeffects research programmes have been shut down recently: the EPA's in September 1987 and that of the National Institute of Environmental Health Services (NIEHS) in July 1987, although the Department of Energy has allocated $3 million in research funds for their 1988/9 financial year.

Such cutbacks in research funding are all the more remarkable in the light of a further landmark in power-line ELF research – the conclusion of the five-year, $5 million American research project, the New York State Power Lines Project, in mid-1987. As mentioned in Chapter 8, the Project was set up as a result of a Public Service Commission Inquiry in 1978, which ordered New York power utilities to fund the research. The Final Report on 16 funded studies was published on 1 July 1987 (Ahlbom et al., 1987), and received worldwide publicity. One study in particular, by Savitz (1987) at the University of North Carolina, attracted considerable attention as it attempted to replicate the findings of Wertheimer and Leeper's 1979 study suggesting that children living in homes with elevated electromagnetic field levels due to power lines near the house are at increased risk of childhood cancer. Savitz improved on their case-control study design and was able to evaluate various aspects, such as differences between high-power and low-power conditions. Using direct point-in-time measurements within the home and the coding of wires and other transmission facilities, he was able to show that magnetic field measurements correlated with the wire codes. He also confirmed via a questionnaire that a variety of possible confounders, such as socioeconomic status, smoking and X-rays, did not appreciably change the results. These indicated that the chronic, low-power-condition magnetic fields (appliances turned off) as well as wire codes were associated with cancer risk that was most pronounced for leukaemia. The shorter duration, high-power-condition magnetic fields (appliances on) did not show an association. The Final Report concluded that if one accepts a causal link between power-line magnetic fields and cancer, the percentage of childhood cases attributable to such fields would be 10–15 per cent. The Report discusses Savitz's result in relation to previous findings and accepts that it 'adds to the credibility of the hypothesis'.

Of the other projects reported, the Panel acknowledged that they indicated 'a variety of effects' not previously appreciated and that 'Several areas of concern for public health have been identified.' The results of one study in particular, by Dr Kurt Salzinger (1987) at the Polytechnic University in Brooklyn, NY, were singled out as 'dramatic'. He found that adult rats previously exposed to 60 Hz electric and magnetic fields in the womb and for the first few days of their lives responded to behavioural conditioning significantly more slowly than unexposed controls. Salzinger is attempting to follow up his findings but, like other NYS researchers, has found it difficult to raise funding since the NYSPLP ended (*Microwave News*, 1987, July/August). Such apparent lack of support is in direct contrast to the panel's final recommendations in their Report, which stated:

1. There should be a major research effort on means of power delivery and use that would reduce magnetic field exposures.
2. Further study should be made of the interactive effects of the Earth's geomagnetic field and 60 Hz fields.
3. The determination of the existence of thresholds for biologic effects of magnetic flux densities should be pursued.
4. The experiments on field effects on learning ability should be replicated.
5. The possible association between cancer (especially leukaemias) and magnetic fields must be further investigated. Several avenues of study should be pursued.
   (a) There should be further epidemiologic study of residential exposure, conducted at more than one site with careful measurement of exposure.
   (b) Attempts should be made to correlate cytogenetic and diagnostic subgroups of cancers with exposures.
   (c) Further investigation of occupational exposure and cancer incidence should be conducted with improved documentation of actual exposures.
   (d) Animal models should be developed and laboratory investigations designed to explore possible mechanisms of field-induced carcinogenesis. If an effect is documented, then the dose-response relationship should be investigated.
6. Further research on the biologic effects of electromagnetic fields is very important. It should be administered by an agency, preferably federal, which is credible by virtue of being clearly independent of partisan influence.' (Ahlbom *et al.*, 1987, pp. 134–5)

The last recommendation is especially significant in view of the involvement in funding in North America and the UK of the respective power utilities and military establishments (the latter is further discussed in Chapter 10).

As a result of the NYSPLP, the American House Subcommittee on Water and Power Resources held a hearing on the health risks associated with exposure to power line EMFs on 6 October 1987, in Washington, DC. Among the witnesses heard by the Committee were Dr Robert Becker, Dr Jerry Phillips of the Cancer Therapy and Research Foundation, San Antonio, Texas, Dr David Savitz, Dr Ross Adey, Dr Richard Phillips from the EPA, Dr Leonard Sagan, of the Electric Power Research Institute (EPRI), and Dr Philip Cole, of the University of Alabama.

Extended excerpts of the testimonies of Becker, Jerry Phillips and Savitz are reproduced in the September/October 1987 issue of *Microwave News*, while the recommendations made by Ross Adey appear in the following issue. Democrat Congressman George Miller of California canvassed each of the witnesses with a number of probing questions; their responses are included in the transcript of the Hearing which is now available. As a result of the Subcommittee Hearing and the NYSPLP, the health hazards of power line EMFs have become a major public health and environmental issue in the USA, and will become so in the UK, Europe and other countries as scientists and the public become more informed of the mounting evidence.

Recently more research has been focussed on the mechanism of operation of EM bio-effects. Besides the work of Fröhlich, Smith and others mentioned in earlier chapters, recent work by Ross Adey at the VA Medical Center in Loma Linda, California, and Byus and Pieper at the University of California at Riverside, throws light on a possible mechanism (Byus *et al.*, 1987, 1988). These researchers found that low energy EMR, producing fields comparable to those from power lines, increases the activity of the enzyme ornithine decarboxylase in human, rat and mouse cancer cells grown in culture. This enzyme produces putresene, a polyamine that accelerates the growth and proliferation of both normal and cancerous cells. Contrary to beliefs that the electric field across the cell membrane would insulate the cell interior from external fields, Adey found that threads of protein protruding from the cell walls can sense weak electric fields and transmit them to the inside of the cell. He also observed that radiofrequency fields only influence cells if they are modulated at frequencies below 100 Hz. This implies that the high frequency carrier must be even more coherent and again emphasises the importance of Fröhlich's work. Adey's conclusions agree with those of Dr Jerry Phillips (discussed below), in San Antonio, Texas, which implicate the magnetic field as the more biologically active component and indicate that it may act as a cancer promoter rather than an initiator.

Work by Wertheimer and Leeper (1979, 1982), Perry *et al.* (1981), Tomenius (1986) and recently Savitz (1987, 1988) may allow the specification of that value of magnetic field at which an enhanced risk of illness commences. If their data is extrapolated back to zero enhancement of effects, the projection does not pass through zero field, but gives a value of field below which the illness statistics are the same for persons not so exposed. However, since we all live in a polluted world environment (the only clean air is now that coming off a glacier), if the general baseline of environmental pollution levels were to be reduced, it might be found that the statistical effects of pollution would appear worse, because all the controls would have become healthier; a point also made by Wertheimer. If we compare the acutely ill with the chronically ill, where shall we find health?

The above recent reports by Savitz and Tomenius have confirmed the earlier work by Wertheimer and Leeper linking all forms of childhood cancer, especially leukaemia, with environmental ELF magnetic fields at the homes, but not the fields associated with domestic appliances. Tomenius originally reported his finding of a correlation between childhood cancer and 50 Hz magnetic fields from ELF sources, particularly power-lines, in Stockholm in 1982. Savitz, from the University of North Carolina, produced further confirmation that implicated the North American 60 Hz power frequency fields, using Wertheimer and Leeper's technique of estimating the fields from an electrical-wiring index. For some 'high exposure' groups, the cancer risk was more than five times higher than that for the 'controls'. Wertheimer and Leeper's wiring coding index (see *Microwave News*, 1986, July/August, p. 9) has been independently assessed as a reliable indicator of residential magnetic fields by Dr Bill Kaune at Battelle Northwest Laboratories, in Richland, Washington State (*Microwave News*, 1986, July/August p. 4).

Although domestic appliance fields may be stronger locally than other environmental sources, they have a strong localised gradient of the field so that the whole body is not in a uniform (spatially coherent) ELF field. Furthermore, domestic appliances, but not TVs and computer terminals, are usually only in use for relatively short periods of time compared to those geophysical and environmental fields which are present throughout the sleep period, or in the work-place. It may be significant that, whereas during the day the body's constant movement through the various fields creates time and space variations and reduces their coherence, at night the body is relatively stationary for 7–8 hours in whatever environmental fields are present. If so, EMF measurements in the bedroom may be the most important factor in determining the chronic residential health risk and differences in the functioning of the body's defence systems while asleep are then likely to be of crucial importance.

Most people have not yet realised that living systems function in a non-linear manner; a consequence is that electromagnetic field effects cannot be predicted, estimated or extrapolated on the basis of simple proportionality of time or field strength exposure.

In other countries, pressure from residents' groups or labour unions has forced new legislation or increased research by the authorities. In the State of Victoria, Australia, a proposed 8 km length of 220 kV (50 Hz) line between Richmond and Brunswick has caused concern and public opposition, particularly because the line would cross the grounds of a public school. As described by Hilary Bacon in Chapter 8, in November 1985 a court in Texas handed down a US$ 25,100,000 judgment against the Houston Lighting and Power Co. for 'reckless disregard' of children's health in siting a 345 kV power-line over school property (*Microwave News*, 1985, November/December). In November 1987, the Texas Court of Appeals upheld the jury's previous decision that there was 'clear and convincing evidence' of health hazards associated with exposure to power-line EMFs (*Microwave News*, 1987, November/December, p. 1). However, Judge Paul Pressler overturned the $25 million award for punitive damages against Houston Power and Light for building a power line across school property without getting proper permission, on the legal grounds that it was not guilty of trespass and therefore could not be held liable for punitive damages. Both sides filed for a re-hearing before the Texas Supreme Court, but this has been turned down.

The fight against the power-line in Victoria, Australia, has been led by the Collingwood Community Health Center, whose highly informative 240-page community resource document produced by Ian Macmillan (1986) is of great practical value to any group opposing power-line proposals. Besides presenting the growing evidence for various health effects, the document criticises the review by American consultant Dr H.B. Graves, submitted in March 1986 on behalf of the Victoria Health Department, as being strongly biased and for not citing 62 important papers relevant to the issue. At least another 60 have become available since the Graves' report was issued. Macmillan's report includes testimonies from three leading American researchers, including ex-patriot Dr Ross Adey, now an advisor to the White House on EMR, who all rejected the Graves' report as biased. Yet, despite the Victoria residents' association flying in Dr Jerry Phillips from San Antonio, Texas, to rebut the Victoria Government's testimony, approval for the line was given in August, 1986. Commenting on Dr Phillips's research (Phillips *et al.*, 1986a, 1986b), which has shown that human tumour cells proliferate more easily and are more immune from attack when exposed to power-line fields, the Victoria State Minister for Health, David White, said that experiments on cell tissue are of 'limited value only' in resolving questions about the health effects of electromagnetic radiation (*Microwave News*, 1986, September/October).

Interestingly, in 1985, Australia instituted one of the strictest safety standards for public and occupational exposures to radiofrequency and microwave radiation outside the Soviet Union and Eastern Europe (Standards Assoc. Australia, 1985). Based on the 'as low as reasonably achievable' (ALARA) principle, the architects of the Standard recommended 'that the levels of all electromagnetic fields to which people are non-occupationally exposed should be kept *as low as possible*' (italics in original). Health Minister David White appears to have disregarded this principle, as well as the work mentioned above. As it happened, in late

March 1988, under much public pressure, the State postponed the Brunswick–Richmond line, pending a review panel's report.

Coincidently, the *7th International Congress of the International Radiation Protection Association* (IRPA) was held in Sydney from 10 to 17 April 1988. For the first time, ionising and non-ionising radiation were addressed together in many of the sessions. A week earlier, a workshop on *Non-Ionising Radiation Biological Effects, Protection and Standards* was held in Melbourne. The IRPA's International Non-Ionising Radiation Committee agreed on draft guidelines proposed in May 1987, on exposure limits for power frequency electric and magnetic fields as follows: the general public should not be exposed to rms unperturbed electric fields greater than $10 kV/m$ or continuous exposure above $5 kV/m$. Magnetic field exposure should be limited to less than $0.2 mT$ ($200 \mu T$). Occupational exposure to electric fields should not exceed $30 kV/m$, with continuous exposure limited to $10 kV/m$. Continuous exposure to magnetic fields should not exceed $5 mT$ (*Microwave News*, March/April 1988). Many will still argue that these figures are too high, especially when field enhancement around a person entering an unperturbed electric field can raise the field strength considerably, particularly around the head. The IRPA says the guidelines will be subject to 'periodic revision'. Given the rate of development of research, this should be at least every 18 months.

In New Zealand, power-line disputes have not attracted much attention. However, a Wellington team led by Pearce (Pearce et al., 1985) carried out a case-control study of 546 male leukaemia patients and showed that the excess of leukaemias 'was entirely due to significant excesses for electronic equipment assemblers and radio and television repairers.' However, since electrical engineers, technicians and fitters, by contrast, showed no such excess, the idea that metal fumes and substances used in electrical components or assemblies (such as the formerly used poly-chlorinated biphenyls) were responsible in whole or in part was proposed – as it has been to explain other inconvenient statistical results. As already discussed, electromagnetic radiation may potentiate the action of chemical stressors. However, in a study reported in the same issue of the *Lancet*, Milham, who had previously reported an increased mortality due to leukaemia in men whose death-certificate occupation suggested exposure to electromagnetic fields (Milham, 1982), found a similar increased risk in American amateur radio operators ('Hams') (Milham, 1985). The significant excess was confined to myeloid and unspecified leukaemias. But, unlike Pearce, Milham noted that both those with and those without occupational exposure had a proportional ratio considerbly above that expected, which thus supported the hypothesis that electromagnetic fields themselves are carcinogenic. Pearce et al.

(1988) have since reported corrected data showing a significant increased risk for 'electricians', in place of 'electronic equipment assemblers'.

In Canada, Drs Michel Plante, of Hydro-Quebec, and Gilles Theriault, of McGill University, are carrying out a large-scale epidemiological study of workers exposed to power-line fields, in the hope of providing a 'definitive answer' to the question of cancer risk. The study was requested by the Quebec Government after a public hearing in 1983 (*Microwave News*, 1986, May/June, p. 2). To gauge individual exposure levels, Hydro-Quebec engineers have developed a new pocket-sized 'electromagnetic dosimeter' which can measure both the 60 Hz electric and magnetic fields every minute for 18 days over a wide dynamic range, starting at 0.5 V/m and 3 nT and extending to 16,000 times these minimum values. High frequency fields in the range 5 to 20 MHz are also monitored. The data can be unloaded into a microcomputer for analysis (*Microwave News*, 1986, September/October). A handy instrument, the 'Kombi-Test' is marketed by Bioset in the UK and by Bio-Physik Mesmann in the USA.

Other Canadian/US research is focussing on ocular effects from pulsed microwave radiation. Dr John Trevithick, at the University of Western Ontario, in Canada, working with the Walter Reed Army Institute of Research (WRAIR) in Washington, DC, has found that pulsed 918 MHz microwaves damaged the eye lens cell membranes in rats nearly five times more than continuous wave radiation at the same average power level (*Microwave News*, 1986, September/October, p. 5). He and his colleagues (1985) had earlier studied the relationship between exposure and dose rate of pulsed microwaves to induce cataracts *in vitro*. Funded by the US Army Medical R & D Command, Trevithick is now collaborating with WRAIR in a further three-year study exposing the corneas of anaesthetised rabbits to 35 gHz (8.6 millimeter) waves. Trevithick's findings are notable in the light of the new, strict Australian exposure standard for RF and MW radiation mentioned above, among whose key features is a recommendation of eye examinations for non-ionising radiation workers before and after employment and at least every five years, if not more frequently.

Cyril Smith (Smith *et al.*, 1985) has studied cataractogenesis in bovine eyes *in vitro* and been able to show that highly coherent radiation, including weak microwave radiation, can exert a cataractogenic effect on such lenses, particulary if the residual if the residual modulation on the microwaves satisfied magnetic resonance conditions in the ambient magnetic field. His results are in agreement with the theoretical predictions of Professor Fröhlich concerning the effects of coherent excitations in biological systems.

In the USA Dr Milton Zaret, in Scarsdale, New York, is probably the world's leading researcher of ocular effects, especially cataracts, in

RF- and MW-exposed personnel. He first identified a posterior, subcapsular cataract as a signature of such irradiation in 1964 while carrying out a study of radar maintenance men for the US Air Force (Zaret *et al.*, 1963; Zaret, 1964). Although controversial, independent studies of other microwave and radar technicians have corroborated his finding (Bouchat and Marsol, 1967; Carpenter and Donaldson, 1970; Sadcikova, 1974; Hollows and Douglas, 1984). From further research (Zaret, 1969; Zaret, 1973), including cases of air traffic controllers (Zaret and Snyder, 1977; Zaret, 1979) and journalists using VDUs (Zaret, 1980, 1984), Zaret has described a specific 'microwave cataract' which originates in the elastic membrane or capsule that surrounds the lens, as opposed to the other types of cataract (hereditary, metabolic and senile) which originate in the lens. According to Zaret, exposure to either thermal or non-thermal radiation can cause microwave cataracts, which can remain latent for months or years.

Fears of ocular and other effects from irradiation by radar and similar installations have caused concern in a number of residents' groups in the USA. Vernon Township, in New Jersey, is the site of three satellite stations with more than 15 uplink antennae and numerous point-to-point transmitters. Residents have complained of excessive exposure since a cluster of Down's Syndrome (DS) cases were identified between 1975 and 1981 and confirmed by the Centers for Disease Control in 1985. Previously, Sigler and his co-workers (1965) found that mothers of DS babies were likely to work in the medical field and to have been exposed to X-rays, while fathers were significantly more likely to have had radar exposure, either as a technician or operator. However, EPA measurements have apparently indicated 'significantly lower levels' of EMFs – typically 226 picowatts/cm^2 – than those to which most Americans are exposed (*Microwave News*, 1986, July/August, p. 8). But this result (EPA, 1986a) was based on only 25 measurements and has been condemned by a leading authority, Dr Robert Becker, as 'completely inadequate' (*Microwave News*, 1986, July/August, p. 8). A power density of 2,810 pW/cm^2 in the 11 GHz band measured at a school near the American satellite facility is due, Becker believes, to a side-lobe from a low-power relay station which Becker assumes must indicate the presence of further side-lobes from all higher power earth-to-satellite stations, which the EPA has failed to identify. Becker recently updated his analysis to show that from 1975 to 1987 there had been a 500 per cent increase in the number of DS and other genetic defects (*Microwave News*, 1988, March/April).

In another example of environmental exposure Becker and Marino cite, in their book *Electromagnetism and Life* (1982, p. 179), a report (Tell and O'Brien, 1977) that Mount Wilson, in California, which is host to

27 radio and TV antennae radiating approximately 10 MW, produces 120–840 $\mu W/cm^2$ power densities inside Mount Vernon post office.

A recent EPA national exposure survey (1986b), however, found that in 15 major US cities over 99 per cent of the residents were exposed to less than 1 $\mu W/cm^2$ at AM, FM and TV frequencies. (The current and much criticised ANSI recommended safety standard, adopted in 1982 and due for revision in 1987, is 10 mW/cm^2 but many think that this should be reduced by a factor of 10.) In high-rise buildings near FM and/or TV antennae, the levels can be much higher. For example, power densities on the roof of the Sears Tower in Chicago measured 230 $\mu W/cm^2$ (*Microwave News*, 1986, November/December, p. 4). Measures in downtown Honolulu in 1984 were the highest ever recorded in a US urban area and have resulted in the prohibition of new broadcast towers in residential or business districts. All new FM and TV transmitters must be sited at least 2,500 feet from the nearest dwelling; AM broadcast towers must not be nearer than 500 feet.

The EPA report notes that the strength in the main beams of some tracking radars at airports or military bases can be up to 100 $\mu W/cm^2$ at nearly five kilometres from the antennae of some large-diameter systems. High-power radars in general contribute little to urban electromagnetic pollution because their beams are usually directed away from centres of population. However, near airports and military bases the electromagnetic environment increases and is further reinforced by airborne radars.

Besides the possibility of cataracts, an elevated risk of cancer has also been associated with residence close to radar installations. Lester and Moore (1982a) studied the geographic incidence of cancer in Wichita, Kansas, relative to the local Mid-Continent Airport and McConnell Air Base. Both cancer morbidity and mortality between 1975 and 1979 were assessed and mapped against line-of-sight projections of radars from each base. Cancer morbidity was found to be significantly related to the degree of radar exposure. It was also found that the highest cancer incidence tended to occur on leading terrain crests in the path of radar transmissions, with the lowest occurring in the valleys, shielded from the radar beams. They cite one residential building with 100 occupants, situated so that the upper levels were directly exposed to both beams, whose cancer morbidity rate was over six times greater than that for a sample of six nursing homes in the city.

In a second study Lester and Moore (1982b) analysed the cancer mortality rates from 1950 to 1969 in areas surrounding 92 US Air Force bases containing radar. Using as controls the nearest county within the State having the most similar population size but lacking an Air Force base, they found that counties with an Air Force base had a significantly higher incidence of cancer mortality for the period in question. The authors conceded that other factors besides EMFs may account for this finding. They cited a study (Meecham and Shaw, 1979) which found a 20 per cent higher mortality for residents living 2–3 miles from the touchdown point of Los Angeles International Airport when compared with a similar neighbourhood 8–9 miles from the landing-strip, and which the authors attributed to noise. However, both the latter results and those of Lester and Moore may equally well be due to microwave radar irradiation, noise, or a combination of both or other factors. Although their results were criticised as due to incorrectly assembled data (Polson and Merritt, 1985), Lester and Moore (1985) showed that this was not the case and that re-analysis confirmed their original association. A further threat for those irradiated is that the various scanning systems for the radar beams will produce ELF modulation of the microwaves.

Such repeated indications have prompted many scientists to call for a reduction in the present American National Standards Institute (ANSI) RF/MW exposure safety standard of $10\,\mathrm{mW/cm^2}$ to $1\,\mathrm{mW/cm^2}$ at its most stringent for frequencies from 30–300 MHz. Adopted in 1982, it is in fact due for revision every five years, i.e. in 1987. It is based on limiting the whole-body average specific absorption rate (SAR) to 0.4 watts per kilogram of body weight for both public and occupational exposure. In July, 1986, the American EPA proposed four options for the revised standard, on which it invited public comment: maximum SARs of 0.04, 0.08 or the present 0.4 W/Kg. These correspond to power densities of 100, 200 or 1000 $\mu\mathrm{W/cm^2}$, respectively. The fourth option is to pass no binding official regulation (*Microwave News*, 1986, July/August, p. 2).

The EPA has been considering public reaction and was due to issue a final guidance in December 1987. The three key questions that the EPA has to resolve before making its final choice are: 'What safety margin should it adopt to protect the public?' 'How should it take account of non-thermal effects?' and, 'How should it accommodate the risk of RF/MW-induced carcinogenesis?' But, as *Microwave News* editor Dr Louis Slesin observed in the July/August 1986 issue, it is more likely that, due to on-going battles between its own Office of Management and Budget since 1984, it will be forced to issue a new proposal, with a further request for public comments, when it finally selects one of the four options. If this happens, the final guidance could be delayed until 1989 or beyond. In fact it is likely to be even later since, in August, 1987, the EPA postponed, yet again, its final guidance date to July, 1989. As Slesin notes, having begun work on the guidance in the late 1970s, the EPA was on the point of proposing option 1 (100 $\mu\mathrm{W/cm^2}$) in 1984 but was forced to back down under pressure from its own policy office. At the time of writing, the EPA has just announced that it is postponing its decision indefinitely (*Microwave News*, September/October, 1988).

Just before the EPA released its four proposed options, the National Council on Radiation Protection (NCRP) published its long-awaited report on RF and MW radiation (NCRP, 1986). It recommended, as expected, a 200 $\mu W/cm^2$ standard in the 30-30 MHz band for the general population, which covers the 300 kHz to 100 GHz frequency range. This represents a fifth of that advocated for occupational exposures, the latter being the same as that adopted by the ANSI in 1982 (*Microwave News*, 1986, May/June, p. 3). The decision to set the public exposure limit by reducing the occupational limit by a factor of five rather than the more commonly used factor of 10, was based on the NCRP's assessment of the total number of hours in the average working week to that in the whole week being approximately 0.2. For the public the proposed limits are averaged over a 30-minute period, whereas occupational exposures are averaged over six minutes.

The NCRP report also recommends extra precaution for the public regarding the hazards of modulated fields. SUch concern is based on such work as that of Dr Ross Adey on the effects of specific frequencies on calcium efflux from the brain (Bawin and Adey, 1976; Adey 1980; Adey *et al.*, 1982). His findings have been confirmed by Dr Carl Blackman, at the EPA's non-ionising research laboratory, which, however, has recently closed down (Blackman *et al.*, 1977; 1980; 1985).

One of the results of the concern among those chronically exposed to radar was the formation, in 1976, of the Radar Victims Network (RVN). This was founded by Joe Towne, who served from 1957 to 1966 as a radar technician at McClellan Air Force Base in Sacramento, California, with a small group of mainly ex-Forces personnel in Framlingham, Massachusetts (*Microwave News*, 1986, January/February, p. 2). Towne developed cataracts, heart trouble and many other problems, and after much legal wrangling the Veterans Administration awarded him a 100 per cent disability. In 1969 he sued a number of companies that designed and built the EC-121 Constellations on which he had worked, and eventually accepted a $55,000 settlement. He carried out an informal survey of other EC-121 radar technicians living near McClellan Base and found that a high percentage had developed cataracts at an early age. This prompted him to warn people of the dangers of microwaves and to help others to sue and to obtain treatment. At its peak the RVN had more than 150 members but at Towne's death in April 1985 – he remained in a coma from his last stroke the previous January until his death – this had dropped considerably, with many having died and others being too sick to be actively involved. No other such organisation is known to exist, as yet, in any other country.

Since the formation of the Radar Victims Network in 1976, the public's growing concern has been fuelled by increasing reports of links between power-line EMFs and raised cancer risk, leading to further protest/pressure groups across the USA and in countries such as Canada, Britain, Scotland, the Republic of Ireland, France and Australia. These groups have tended to focus on the links with residential exposure, and Savitz's recent 1987 confirmation of Wertheimer and Leeper's 1979 childhood leukaemia findings (already discussed above) has certainly raised the temperature of the debate and attracted wide press coverage and demands for action. In response the American Electric Power Research Institute (EPRI) met in January 1987 to consider research priorities. Among its seven area proposals, the panel of experts stated regarding childhood leukaemia: 'The strongest evidence points at leukaemia as the major outcome of interest, but there is also evidence that brain cancer, and perhaps, other cancer sites are similarly at risk' (*Microwave News*, 1987, March/April, p. 9.). The panel recommended two types of study.

> The first is a more careful look at residential exposures with 24-hour measurements of EMFs and estimates of exposure based on appliance use. Likewise, estimates of exposure from schools, daycare centres, playgrounds, etc. should enter the exposure assessment effort.... Following this, ... a large 'megachild' study covering a significant part of the US should be considered. (*Microwave News*, 1987, March/April, p. 9)

The duration and cost of the first study was estimated at about three years and between $750,000 and $1 million.

The EPRI also called for studies of occupational exposure. The growing body of evidence in that area was recently summarised by Savitz and Calle (1987) who combined data sets from eleven different occupational surveys (many of them mentioned by Hilary Bacon in Chapter 8) and found that telegraph, radio and radar operators had 2.6 times the risk of acute myeloid leukaemia (AML), as well as a two-fold increased risk of acute leukaemia, compared with other workers. Power and phone linemen also had a greater risk of developing AML, while aluminium workers and power station operators showed a greater likelihood of getting acute leukaemia. The authors accepted that other occupational factors might have contributed to the results, but also suggested that the inclusion of many unexposed individuals may have diluted what could be a much higher risk.

A recent report from Sweden, however, is less conclusive. Tornquist (1986) found that Swedish power linemen had a slightly increased risk of leukaemia and brain tumours but that power station operators had normal cancer rates. Also, none of the workers showed an elevated risk of any particular type of leukaemia, although, unexpectedly, both groups did have a greater risk of kidney and urinary cancers. It is worth noting that both groups were exposed to chemicals on the job, raising the possibility of synergistic interaction.

By contrast, Stern (1986) and his colleagues at the National Institute for Occupational Safety and Health (NIOSH), while looking for any connection between leukaemia and exposure of naval shipyard workers to ionising radiation or solvents, instead detected a six-fold and three-fold increased risk of lymphatic leukaemia and all leukaemias, respectively. Welders had nearly four times the expected rate of myeloid leukaemia. The trend of similar studies was emphasised by Dr Tom Tenforde, of the Lawrence Berkeley Laboratory in California, when, in February 1986 at a 'Panel Session on Biological Effects of Power Frequency Electric and Magnetic Fields' in New York City he noted that, at that time, 15 out of 17 studies showed 'some apparent correlation between cancer and EMFs' (*Microwave News*, 1986, March/April, p. 4). The first number now exceeds 20, and includes a recent study by Milham (1988) who found a significant increased mortality from acute myeloid leukaemia and multiple myeloma in 2,485 US radio hams, reinforcing his earlier finding (Milham, 1985).

In the UK the NCRP's equivalent body, the National Radiological Protection Board (NRPB), has also recently issued similar proposed standards for frequencies below 300 GHz, including in the ELF power-line range (NRPB, 1986). It proposes one set of standards for workers and two different sets (short- and long-term) for the public. At 50 Hz the guidelines for workers are linked to 2-hour exposures per day: 30 kV/m and 1.88 mT for electric and magnetic fields, respectively. For the public, the proposals are: 12 kV/m and 0.76 mT (up to 5 hours a day) and 2.6 kV/m and 0.174 mT (continuous). Based on the same 0.4 W/kg SAR as the present ANSI standard, the NRPB proposes for the public, in the 30-300 MHz range, a power density of 400 μW/cm^2 over five hours or, between 10–300 MHz, 80 μW/cm^2 for continous residential exposure. At 1.5 GHz the limits increase to 2 mW/cm^2 (5 hour) or 400 μW/cm^2 (continuous). For workers the limits, for 30–300 MHz and 500 MHz to 300 GHz, are 1 mW/cm^2 and 5 mW/cm^2, respectively.

The proposals, however, have come under criticism from both UK (Dr Brian Maddock of the CEGB) and US specialists as 'too complicated'. Dr Czerski, of the US Center for Devices and Radiological Health at the Food and Drug Administration (FDA) in Rockville, Maryland, has also criticised the scientific groundwork for the limits, saying, 'They have sacrificed basic physical and biological accuracy for some rather doubtful mathematical elegance' (*Microwave News*, 1986, September/October, p. 7). The NRPB is presently reviewing invited comments on their proposals, which include those from the senior author. Originally, it planned to issue its final standard in early 1987; that has now been postponed to the spring of 1989. It is likely that it will seek to achieve agreement with the IRPA's latest recommendations (see p. 175).

The prospective publication of the EPA and NRPB reports comes in the wake of the publication of yet a third report – this time on static and time-varying ELF magnetic fields by the WHO and the International Radiological Protection Association (IRPA) (WHO, 1987). The report took 10 years to complete and the committee of experts from 13 countries has concluded, as mentioned elsewhere, that there is an 'urgent need' for research to resolve the suspected link between very weak ELF fields and cancer (WHO/IRPA, 1987, p. 114). The report states that induced current densities of less than $10\,mA/m^2$ have not been shown to produce any 'significant biological effects' and that such a level, at 50/60 Hz, is induced by a field of approximately 5 mT (50 Gauss). 'The suspected carcinogenic effects of ELF magnetic fields occur at $0.1–1\,\mu T$ at more than a 1000 times lower' (WHO/IRPA, 1987, p. 116). This figure of $0.1\,\mu T$ is somewhat nearer to extrapolations of an onset threshold based on the work of Savitz and Wertheimer and Leeper, together with the authors' assessment of a threshold based on Dr Perry's research into suicides, as discussed earlier.

However, rather than wait for the ANSI or EPA to come to decisions or research agreement, a number of American states have introduced their own laws. Among them, Massachusetts adopted in December 1985 the most stringent regulations in the US designed to protect workers from RF/MW radiation, having been the first state, in 1983, to set an exposure standard for the general public – at a level five times more stringent than ANSI's (*Microwave News*, 1983, September, p. 5). Radio, TV and radar stations with an input power of more than 100 W, RF sealers and heaters, industrial microwave ovens, and diathermy and hyperthermia equipment are among those sources covered, although all facilities maintained by the federal government are exempt from the rules! Among other requirements of the standard are the appointment of an 'RF Safety Officer' by each employer using radiation equipment, and annual survey checks by all employers, including the checking of all new equipment, with records being kept for 30 years.

In Florida, the Department of Environmental Regulation (DER) has set up a six-member advisory panel to establish 'reasonable' standards to protect the public from powerline fields (*Microwave News*, 1986, September/October, p. 14). At an April 1988 meeting the DER proposed EMF standards at the edges of rights of way (ROW) of 1.5 kV/m for the electric field and 50 mG for the magnetic field under maximum loadings (see Table 9.1 for comparison with other states). In the summer of 1985 the DER recommended a 190-feet ROW for the ultimately rejected 500 kV line from Lake Tarpon to the town of Kathleen, and the siting of power-lines has since been at a standstill until the rule-making process is completed (*Microwave News*, 1987, March/April, p. 7).

Table 9.1 Maximum electric field levels (kV/m) for high-voltage transmission lines in seven US states

State	In ROW*	Edge ROW	Comments
Minnesota	8	–	
Montana	7	1	In ROW at road crossings
New Jersey	–	3	
New York	7	1.6	Interim magnetic field of 100 mG at edge of ROW suggested
North Dakota	9	–	
Oregon	9	–	State law
Florida	–	1.5	50 mG magnetic field for average load, 100 mG magnetic field for maximum load at edge ROW suggested

* ROW = right of way.
Based on information in NYSPLP Report, July, 1987, by Ahlbom *et al.* (1987).

In New York a Bill before the State legislature would require no new above-ground 23 kV or greater power line to be built within 50 feet of a residential building, no new residential building to be built within 50 feet of a 23 kV or greater power line, and no new power line or residential building to be built such that a power line magnetic field of 2.5 mG is present anywhere in the building (*Microwave News*, 1988, May/June). And in California, which has approved $2 million for ELF EMF research, the Department of Education has proposed possibly the first guidelines on siting power lines near schools, as a result of the recent Klein School District lawsuit in Houston, Texas. Its interim policy calls for minimum distance between the edge of a school's property and the edge of a right-of-way (ROW): 100 feet from a 100–110 kV ROW, 150 feet from a 220–230 kV ROW, and 250 feet from a 345 kV ROW. At present the UK has no such ROWs around overhead power-lines.

It remains to be seen what impact such decisions have on other states – as well as other countries such as Britain – and especially on new power-line projects, for example the two proposed 500 kV lines for the California–Oregon Transmission Project and California's Los Banos-Gates Transmission Project, both of whose draft environmental impact reports (EIR) have dismissed any health risks from ELF electric and magnetic fields (*Microwave News*, 1987, January/February, p. 7). Any decision on these and other projects might best wait until the completion, around spring 1989, of a two-year study by Dr John Peters, at the University of Southern California, to replicate the findings of Wertheimer and Leeper, Tomenius, and Savitz. Funded by the EPRI, Peters is investigating the link between all types of childhood leukaemia and power-line fields, using data with information on both parents' occupational and chemical exposure (*Microwave News*, 1986, November/December, p. 12). A number of studies (Hicks *et al.*, 1984; Spitz and Johnson, 1986) have found a marked link between the occupation of the father, in particular, in electrical and electronics jobs and an elevated risk of cancer in children.

Besides power-lines, recent research is indicating possible hazards from other electrical sources. In a study first presented to the New York Academy of Sciences in 1984, Wertheimer and Leeper (1986) reported that pregnancies among couples using electric blankets are more likely to end in miscarriage than those among couples who do not heat their beds electrically. Their results also showed a trend toward slower foetal development among babies born to parents using electric blankets or water beds, both of which generate ELF electric and magnetic fields. The researchers observed a clustering of spontaneous abortions from September to June among electric blanket users, and for those relying on either electric blankets or water beds the miscarriage rate was significantly higher during the September–June period. No such seasonal pattern was observed among non-users. Although the results could be attributed to either EMF exposure or possibly excessive bed-heating, Wertheimer and Leeper favour the former, based on related suggestive evidence (*Microwave News*, 1986, May/June, p. 6). Recently, Wertheimer and Leeper (1989) have reported a further link between miscarriages from EMFs from ceiling cable heating in homes.

A study by Dr Bary Wilson, based on previous results (Wilson, 1988) indicates that sleeping with an electric blanket may affect a woman's menstrual cycle, an effect that Wilson believes is mediated by the pineal gland (*Microwave News*, July/August, 1988). In a conference report that has yet to be published, Wilson described 'dramatic' changes in the cycles of 33 women whose urine and melatonin metabolite samples he analysed. The EPRI is now funding a pilot study by Dr Michael Bracken at the Yale School of Medicine on the prevalence of electric blanket use in a group of 4000 pregnant women to determine the feasibility of studying the growth and development of children exposed to EMFs *in utero*. Meanwhile, Stevens (1987a) has hypothesised how alterations in melatonin rhythm by EMFs and light – among other factors – may provide a framework for understanding mechanisms of action of hormone-related cancers, especially breast cancer, which he is now attempting to study in relation to electric power use.

Research in Britain on EMFs has been more sporadic and less co-ordinated. Some has already been mentioned, such as the results of Staffordshire GP Dr Stephen Perry linking residential exposure to power-line frequency magnetic fields to suicide incidence (Perry et al., 1981). Although dismissed by the then Chief Medical Officer of the CEGB, Dr. John Bonnell, as lacking 'any biological hypothesis' and for 'incorrect use of epidemiological techniques' (Bonnell, 1982; Bonnell et al., 1983), Smith and Baker (1982) calculated the onset level of magnetic field at which the effects began to occur from Dr Perry's raw data. The onset level (14 nT) corresponds closely with that calculated by Wertheimer and Leeper (1987) in a new re-analysis of their data on childhood leukaemia and EMF exposure. For overhead 400 kV powerlines operating at full load, such a field would occur at 250 metres either side of the lines. This observation should be a major consideration in establishing a minimum corridor along power-line routes in the UK within which no human dwelling should be permitted, as has become law in certain states in the USA. How to control exposure to underground power-line frequencies presents a more difficult and, as yet, unresolved problem. Perry and Pearl (1988) have recently produced further evidence linking power-line fields in high-rise buildings with depression and other illness (see p. 190).

As a result of the Innsworth Inquiry in 1978, the CEGB were required to carry out annual research on the possible health effects of EMFs to which the public and workers are exposed. To date the only survey of Fishpond residents has been carried out by Hilary Bacon, Dr David Smith, at the University of Bangor, Wales, and Dr Cyril Smith (see Chapter 8), while residents near the erected Innsworth line, some of whom have suffered illnesses worthy of investigation (Ross, 1987), have not been monitored. Published CEGB reports have been confined to the effects on implanted pacemakers (Butrous et al., 1982) and a study, carried out with the help of two Oxford psychologists, D. and M. Broadbent, that concluded that the health problems of a sample of CEGB workers were due to other aspects of their jobs, such as working overtime or alone or changing shifts several times, rather than to any measured or estimated exposure (Broadbent et al., 1985).

By contrast, in 1983, two years before, three independent UK reports had linked EMFs with increased risk of leukaemia. McDowell (1983), at the Office of Population, Censuses and Surveys in London, in a case-control study, found raised leukaemia, particularly acute myeloid leukaemia, in those whose occupation registered on their death certificates in 1973 indicated electrical occupations, the highest being for telecommunications engineers. Coleman and colleagues (1983), now with the International Agency for Research on Cancer in Lyon, France, produced similar results analysing the occupation of patients registered with malignant disease in south-east England. Finally, Swerdlow (1983), at the University of Glasgow, studied adult eye cancer rates around Britain and Wales between 1962 and 1977 and found a significantly higher incidence in electrical and electronics workers. None of these studies, nor that of Tomenius reported in 1982 (published in 1986), were mentioned in the Broadbent study. Indeed, in a review paper, also published in 1985, Norris, Bonnell and their colleagues at the CEGB not only dismiss any 'deleterious effects on health that might arise from living or working near electric power equipment', also without mentioning the four above studies, but baldly state: 'It is not unreasonable to suppose that further work ... will equally show nothing. However, perhaps partly pushed by the need to calm fear engendered by the press but partly with a sense of public duty, it is likely that the electric utilities and others will continue to press the search' (Norris et al., 1985, p. 141). This statement contains so many misrepresentations it could be dismissed as laughable were it not for the power and authority that its authors and funding body wield – the review having being 'published by permission of the Central Electricity Generating Board'. First, on the basis of all the studies published to that time, it was wholly unreasonable to suppose or hope that further studies 'will show nothing' – and indeed this has been borne out by subsequent research. Second, the prompting 'to calm fear engendered by the Press' rings somewhat hollow alongside the CEGB's constant dismissal of embarrassing evidence. Best's 1984 *Guardian* article on the electrical sensitivity of one of Dr Monro's patients to the fields from power-lines (Best, 1984) is not mentioned (in fact, no press reports are specifically referred to); however, neither Best nor the *Guardian* received any letter from the CEGB afterwards detailing errors or disagreements. Indeed, the open invitation to Dr Bonnell and others from Dr Monro to visit her clinic and observe the electrical hypersensitivity claimed by some of her patients (some of whom are now on film) has never been taken up. If there is any fear that needs calming it might more plausibly be that the CEGB's chiefs suffer, or at least suffered until the retirement of Dr Bonnell in 1986, from scientific tunnel-vision of the worst kind.

Finally, their 'sense of duty' that apparently motivates them to 'continue to press the search' seems to have deserted them as far as, for example, investigating the repeated claims by the residents of Fishpond of numerous illnesses due to the power-lines over their village – now finally detailed by Hilary Bacon and Cyril Smith (see above). As for 'continuing to press the search', it was not until 1979, with the decision of the Innsworth inquiry requiring them to carry out research, that the CEGB really started to do any in this area – witness the total lack of published research (as opposed to literature assessment) by them until 1985, despite the first reports of health effects in Russian workers appearing as early as 1966.

However, with the decision of the New York Inquiry into the proposed powerline between Albany and Canada which, in 1978, required New York utilities to provide $5 million for research into power-line effects – the New York State Power Lines Project – it is not surprising that the CEGB should begin to feel it was time to start doing some research of its own. However, waiting until required by a Public Inquiry and until prompted by the need to combat the increasing reports of health effects hardly merits the phase 'pressing the search'. Compared to the actual research carried out by individuals and utilities in North America, the CEGB's research effort had, up until 1987, been minute.

A year after the above statements by Norris and his colleagues, a team from the Medical Research Council's Epidemiology Unit at Southampton, including no less a person than Dr Donald Acheson, now the Government's Chief Medical Officer, reported a study of cancer in young and middle-aged people (Coggon *et al.*, 1986) in which they observed acute myeloid leukaemia in five men who had worked in electrical trades, a finding they describe as 'striking'.

A further study assisted by the CEGB was reported in December 1985, at an International Conference on Electric and Magnetic Fields in Medicine and Biology in London, organised by the Institution of Electrical Engineers. The leader of the team, Dr A. Myers (1985), of the University of Leeds, reported preliminary findings of a study of childhood cancer related to residence near overhead power-lines. The authors concluded that there was 'no apparent relationship' but admitted various shortcomings of the study, including an estimate of up to 15 per cent of the total data set of diagnosed children missing. Also, no field work supports the contention that the population Myers considers exposed, really was exposed to ELF magnetic fields. The study's calculations are based on at least two probable errors. First, they assume no current return in either the earth wire or in various ground-return paths, and, second, they assume that the effect of nearby buried cables, household ring-mains, etc. will not matter. Thus, their calculated fields at the children's homes bear little, if any, relationship to reality, especially for homes farther away from the lines. In addition, they used a current-flow estimate based on maximum current flow in years after almost half the children had already been diagnosed. Thus, no firm conclusions can be drawn from the results, although a fuller report, promised since 1985 but still not published, may allow a more complete assessment. Nonetheless, some interesting measurements were reported; the major contribution to domestic EMF exposure was confirmed to result from underground or overhead power-lines and, for a sample of 40 properties, the magnetic fields ranged between .01–3.2 mG (1 nT–0.33 µT) and .002–16.8 mG (0.2 nT–1.68µT), respectively. In high-rise flats the average magnetic field on the ground floor was

2.0 mG (200 nT) (peak: 4 mG or 400 nT) as against .15 mG (15 nT) for the top floor, a difference of some 13-fold. These figures are in line with those measured by Dr Perry in his suicide study, mentioned above, in which he found, among other things, a higher suicide rate for those living on the ground floor of flats. The view that the magnetic field is the more hazardous component of EMFs is supported by the fact that, whereas electric fields from three-phase cables tend to be balanced, the associated magnetic fields can easily be unbalanced and surprisingly high depending on the loading of the line at any given time, as Olsen (1985) has shown. There will also be other frequency components in the magnetic field arising from load fluctuations. In general, the fields generated by electrical appliances fall off in proportion to the inverse of the cube of the distance from the source; balanced power-line electric and magnetic fields fall off in proportion to the inverse of the distance squared, whereas similar unbalanced fields only dissipate in proportion to the inverse of the distance. Such a difference (for example, between 3, 9 and 27 feet) emphasises the importance of the balancing of the currents in the lines and cables passing dwellings. Present evidence seems to suggest that perhaps as much as 80 per cent of domestic exposure is due to external overhead and underground power lines, the rest being due to domestic appliances. A TV, for example, generates a field of 2.5–50 μT at 3 cm, .04–2 μT at 30 cm, and less than .01–.15 μT at 1 m; comparable figures for a safely functioning microwave oven are 75–100μT, 4–8μT and .25–.6 μT, respectively (WHO, 1987).

The CEGB has been engaged on two further studies since 1985, according to Dr Robin Cox, who took over as its Chief Medical Officer in October 1986. The results of two epidemiological surveys of both adult and childhood leukaemia are awaited with great interest. They are being carried out by a team headed by Dr R.A. Cartwright at the Cookridge Hospital in Leeds and follow on from the report by Myers and Cartwright mentioned above. The results for the adult study were due to be published in late 1987 but have been delayed, while the childhood study should have been completed in early 1988.

Noting the recent results worldwide, Dr Cox said, in early 1987, 'I accept that there is growing evidence that there is an association between electromagnetic field exposure and cancer risk' (Cox, 1987). Such constructive attitude by Dr Cox contrasts markedly with the entrenched attitude of his predecessor, Dr John Bonnell, who has always maintained that there are no health effects associated with power-line frequencies, a view he put in writing to Mrs Stella Ross, an Innsworth resident, after the Innsworth Inquiry, and one which, by early 1989, flew in the face of over 20 studies indicating the opposite:

'... I am writing to repeat my firm assurance that the overhead power lines owned and operated by the CEGB at Innsworth and elsewhere will not cause ill effects to your health or that of others living near the lines ...' (Bonnell, 1979).

Of the more recent studies in Britain, Dr Stephen Perry (1988), assisted by Pearl, published further research on people living in multi-storey blocks (having nine or more storeys) in Wolverhampton, showing a significantly higher number of people suffering from certain types of heart disease and from depression had been living near the main electrical supply cable. Magnetic field strengths measured in all 43 blocks with a single rising cable showed very significantly higher readings ($p<.0002$) in the apartments 'near' the cable, averaging 3.15 mG (highest: 3.77 mG) against 1.61 mG (lowest: 1.48 mG) in the 'distant' apartments (1 mG = 100 nT). They also contradicted the CEGB finding (Myers *et al.*, 1985) that field strengths are highest on the lowest floors of multi-storey buildings, an observation that the researchers attributed to the balanced 3-phase supply to the lower floors. Significantly more 'myocardial infarction, hypertension, ischaemic heart disease and depression' was observed in the 'near' group but, strangely, significantly less 'personality defect, anxiety, agitation, young confused' traits. One intriguing finding was that, if only those blocks with underfloor or storage electric heating were considered, the proportion of cases of 'depression' living in flats categorised as 'near' the rising cable rose to 82 per cent, although this was the only category of illness to show such a change. Perry and Pearl's study received favourable comment in the *British Medical Journal* (Dixon, 1988). Perry is carrying out further studies of depression and heart attack.

Another study looking at the incidence of depression and also chronic headache was reported by GP Dr David Dowson (1988) and his colleagues in Southampton. Using a questionnaire to study patients living within various distances of overhead lines and a control group living three miles away, their analysis revealed that 15 in the former group versus one in the latter reported recurrent headaches, the highest number (10) living at 80–100 metres from a 132 kV line. A further significant finding was of nine patients in the study group reporting depression (seven lived within 40 m of the lines), as against one in the control group. A larger follow-up study is in progress.

In the USA a number of challenging studies have been published recently. Looking at the risks associated with medical exposure, Dr Jacob Paz *et al.* (1988) and a team at New York Medical College simulated a normal operation and found that surgeons using electrosurgical units (ESUs) were being exposed to very high levels of RF radiation, especially their eyes and foreheads which registered electric and magnetic fields as high as 9,000,000 V/m and 3.5 A/m respectively, far above the ANSI standard of 4000 V/m and 0.0025 A/m between 30 and 300 MHz. An ESU, used to cut and seal tissues during operations, might be used up to 100 times depending on the particular operation being performed.

In another occupational study following up his 1985 research, Dr Samuel Milham (1988), at the Department of Social and Health Services in Olympia, Washington, found that a sample of 2,485 amateur radio operators ('hams') in California and Washington States showed a significant excess of deaths due to acute myeloid leukaemia (AML), multiple myeloma and possibly certain types of malignant lymphoma. Milham, who was the first to report a link between occupational exposure to EMFs and cancer (Milham, 1982), observed that the death certificates of 31 per cent of Washington State radio ham licensees listed occupations with EMF exposure. (Similar information was not available for the Californian deaths.)

One criticism of occupational studies has been that very little information on actual levels of exposure of electrical workers has been available. But Dr Joseph Bowman (1988) and his colleagues at the University of California's School of Medicine, in Los Angeles, have now measured such fields and found that they are 'significantly above the levels encountered in residences and most offices.' Among those exposed to the highest magnetic fields were: electricians working with industrial power supplies; underground and overhead power-lines workers; welders; and transmission station and distribution substation operators. Exposures varied considerably; most were between 10 and 50 mG, although some exceeded 100 mG. Residential exposure, by comparison, was usually below 1 mG. The researchers noted that high exposure can also occur in other occupations not usually considered under the category 'electrical worker', e.g. battery-driven fork-lift truck drivers. One implication of Bowman's findings is that future studies of residential or occupational exposure need to evaluate the contribution from each source of exposure to the illness under study. On the evidence to date, one would expect an electrical worker living on the cable side of a high-rise apartment block to be at much greater risk than a non-exposed worker living in a detached house in the country. Bowman is now carrying out a more detailed study of occupational exposure funded by the EPRI.

Most recently, Speers (1988) and her co-workers at the Centers for Disease Control in Atlanta, Georgia, found a 13-fold increased risk of brain tumour in electrical utility workers against the expected rate for unexposed workers. Brain cancer risk in other occupations grew linearly with the probability of EMF exposure on the job. Her findings corroborate those of Lin *et al*. (1985) who also reported an excess of brain tumours in electrical workers.

Turning to residential exposure, Drs Wertheimer and Leeper (1987), at the University of Colorado, have carried out an extended analysis of cancer incidence among adults living near high current power-lines in and around Denver, Colorado. Certain cancer subtypes, particularly nervous system cancers, were associated with two measures of exposure to alternating 60 Hz magnetic fields (AMFs). Both those exposed occupationally and residentially showed similarities in the subtypes they contracted. Second, by dividing cancers into those which peak in incidence before old age and decline late in life (Type A, e.g. nervous system cancers) and those which continue to increase in incidence throughout life (Type B, e.g. adult leukaemia), the incidence-age patterns observed in exposed and non-exposed groups suggested that prolonged EMF exposure may act as a cancer promoter (as opposed to an initiator).

The researchers also noted that in their previous 1982 adult study, certain patterns were observed that supported the idea that cancer promotion underlies the connection between high current configurations (HCCs) and cancer. The effect of HCC exposure seemed to be reversible, that is, the cancer incidence was no longer high in those who had lived at an HCC house if they had left that home for 3 years or more. (Savitz's study deals almost entirely with addresses occupied within three years preceding diagnosis.) Also, a latency period of seven years or less was usually seen between first occupation of an HCC home and cancer manifesting, which is a shorter latency than has usually been seen for most carcinogens (Wertheimer and Leeper, 1987, p. 43).

In a memorandum in the January/February 1988 issue of *Microwave News*, Wertheimer and Leeper discuss the above possible pitfalls in the interpretation of ELF research findings as explanations which could explain results where increased cancer may not be observed with increased MF exposure. They emphasise that not to include them in evaluating studies could lead to false negative conclusions. They suggest, for example, that little increase in cancer should be expected among children exposed prenatally to the most extreme sources of magnetic field exposure. They confirm this observation in their own data and in that of Fulton (1980) (whose negative results they re-analysed and reached a positive outcome (1980)), Myers (1985), Tomenius (1986) and Savitz (1987). In each case moderate exposures were associated with increased cancer after birth, but extreme exposures, prenatally, were not. Wertheimer and Leeper hypothesise that this pattern occurs because magnetic fields 'can have an adverse effect on tissue development which, if it is severe and occurs in the first trimester of pregnancy, may often lead to prenatal abortion rather than postnatal cancer.' Clearly, such a hypothesis needs to be considered in evaluating the results of other and future childhood cancer studies, including some recent contradictory findings on leukaemia clusters and ionising radiation in the UK.

Another negative result that Wertheimer and Leeper (1988a) have re-analysed is the study, funded by the NYSPLP, by Dr Richard Stevens (1987), at the Battelle Pacific Northwest Laboratories in Richland, Washington, on the incidence of acute non-lymphocytic leukaemia (ANLL) in a sample of Washington State adults exposed to ELF electric and magnetic fields residentially. No significant increased risk among those exposed to the greatest EMFs was found by Stevens, although in his report he admits the study has certain shortcomings. Using Stevens's data, Wertheimer and Leeper were able to take account of the chronic use of electrically heated beds – electric blankets, waterbed heaters and electric mattress pads – whose use they had previously linked to an increased risk of miscarriage (Wertheimer and Leeper, 1986). Taking these and other refinements into account, the researchers found that in those exposed to EMFs from either power lines or electrically heated beds the risk of leukaemia increased 50–90 per cent, and if exposed to both, by 110–260 per cent. The single or synergistic contribution of electrically heated beds to leukemia risk and their link with increased miscarriage has prompted Leeper (1988) to outline some cost-efficient methods to waterbed heater manufacturers for reducing the generation of magnetic fields by 95 per cent or more.

Savitz (1988), also, has reanalysed and added to his data reported in the 1987 NYSPLP Report, and strengthened his original link between childhood cancer and power-line magnetic fields by removing some earlier ambiguities. He also checked and rejected other possible confounders, such as air pollution from traffic, and determined that the association is now similar for both estimated and measured magnetic fields. Originally, he only found a weak association between measured magnetic fields and cancer when he used a 2 mG cut-off for classifying the 60 Hz exposed group; when he changed this to 3 mG, the risk became 'notably larger'.

Mainly as a result of the NYSPLP Report and the associated publicity, the CEGB (1988a) in Britain announced in March 1988 a £500,000 research programme to study EMF bioeffects. No specific details are yet available but the study programme will include:

* Electricity supply industry staff volunteers wearing small exposure meters to measure their personal exposure to magnetic fields at home and at work.
* Assessing magnetic fields in homes without the need for access by using new vehicle-mounted sensing equipment.
* A proposed study by an independent epidemiological group of all new diagnosed childhood cancer cases in England and Wales which will enable the child's past exposure to be much better estimated. Similar estimates will be made for other children not suffering from cancer.
* Funding an independent programme of basic research on the key biolo-

gical interactions to access their significance, if any, for human health. (CEGB, 1988)

The CEGB made much of the amount of money to be spent; in fact it exceeds what they had spent on the area in the previous 10 years, and against an annual environmental budget of approximately £25 million represents 2 per cent. By comparison, the American EPRI spent $6.1 million alone on ELF EMF research from 1985 to 1987, and budgeted $4.7 million in 1988 and $6.0 million in both 1989 and 1990 (*Microwave News*, 1988, March/April).

Just prior to their announcement, the CEGB also produced pamplets and brochures, made available to their own personnel and the public, explaining why they were extending their research in this area. As might be expected, the publications (CEGB, 1988a) play down any possible hazards and are somewhat economical with details when referring to the accumulated research and range of opinion on this subject.

Despite intending to pursue such new projects since the publication of the NYSPLP in July 1987, the CEGB, with the obvious intent of defusing criticism, delayed the announcement of their plans till just four days before a critical BBC TV *Panorama* programme 'Electricity – A Shock in Store?' on 21 March 1988, which assessed some of the recent evidence relating to the power-line–cancer connection. But despite the CEGB's carefully timed publicity, the programme provoked considerable public reaction, so much so that the Secretary of State for Energy, Mr Cecil Parkinson, felt obliged to tell the Houses of Parliament: 'I believe the *Panorama* programme was essentially a scare-mongering programme.' ... 'There has to date been only one authority for this thesis ...' (Pienaar, 1988). His views were not shared, however, by the *British Medical Journal*'s reviewer, Dr Neville Goodman (1988), who described the programme as 'well balanced'.

But, besides being factually incorrect as to 'one' authority for the claim, Parkinson's remarks should be viewed in the context of his appointed task of bringing the Government's planned privatisation of the CEGB to fruition, an enterprise he clearly perceives is threatened by any acceptance of the mounting evidence of the hazard posed by power-line EMFs. Certainly, the successful and pending legal actions in the United States raise the likelihood of renewed public objections against new power-line route proposals in the UK, as well as possible claims for damages against the CEGB and other regional electricity suppliers, especially now that such litigation can be pursued on the basis of the recently introduced 'class actions' in such cases. In the USA, besides the Klein School/HP&L case in Houston, Texas, referred to earlier, a suit against the New York Power Authority by landowners in the state claiming that the proposed

345 kV Marcy-South power-line will create a 'cancerphobia' corridor which will destroy the value of their property, came to court in September 1988. The plaintiffs want the NYPA to establish a right-of-way of 2400 feet around the line, thus limiting the magnetic field exposures to a maximum of 0.5 mG (50 nT). As pointed out earlier, the UK does not recognise the need for any such ROWs around power-lines related to possible health hazards from EMFs. Further cases are pending in other states.

Regarding the question of objections to power-line proposals, it should be noted that the Select Committee on Energy (1988) published a First Report on recent changes to the 1981 inquiry proceedings Rules concerning electricity generating stations and overhead lines. The new Rules were introduced on 14 December 1987, two days before the House rose for the Christmas recess and just three days before the first public intimation by the Government that a public inquiry would be held into the CEGB's proposals to build a pressurised water reactor at Hinkley Point C in Somerset. The new Rules came into force on 14 January 1988, and on 22 January, just eight days later, Mr Michael Spicer, Parliamentary Under-Secretary at the Department of Energy, announced that an inquiry would be held into the diversion of transmission line entries at Hinkley Point C. The new Rules thus apply to this enquiry.

Another report that was presented to Parliament in December 1987, with relatively little attention, by the then Secretary of State for Social Services, Mr Norman Fowler, was by the Industrial Injuries Advisory Council (IIAC) on the question of whether the terms of prescription for occupational diseases induced by NIR should be amended to include a wider range of conditions (IIAC, 1987). The Report, which followed a previous one on ionising radiation in 1984, concluded that there was no need to change the schedule of presently prescribed industrial diseases. Under MW and RF effects the Council deemed evidence that low intensity MW and RF is associated with cataract development and other eye damage as 'not conclusive', and stated: 'In general, any risk of injury appears to be confined to exposures at levels greater than 10 milliwatts per square centimetre of body surface' (p. 4), a statement likely to be contested by many researchers in this area. (The significance of 10 mW/cm^2 is revealed in Chapter 10.) Under electric and magnetic fields, the Report states (p. 5): 'In our view there is insufficient evidence linking exposure to electric and magnetic fields with any harmful effects on humans.' No indication is given of exactly what evidence was assessed by the Council but such a view will be met with derision by most independent researchers and seriously calls into question the objectivity of the Council or their Research Working Group. What is listed, however, are those individuals and organisations who gave evidence, among them the CEGB, NRPB and MoD. The timing of the submission of the Report to Norman Fowler

(March 1987) is noteworthy in view of the imminent publication of the NYSPLP Report on 1 July 1987, which the Council must have been aware of and which the CEGB certainly were. Since the Report was not actually submitted to Parliament until December 1987, it seems odd that its completion and final assessment could not have been delayed until the very important NYSPLP Report – whose conclusions carry far more weight and totally negate the above Council statement – had been received, particularly since the Council's Report had already taken some two years to produce. It is to be hoped that the NYSPLP Report (a copy of which now resides in the House of Commons library) and other more recent evidence will serve to modify the views of the Council's Research Working Party, which is apparently keeping the various areas under review. Certainly, as they stand, the Council's views on MW/RF effects and ELF EMFs are at considerable variance with a wide body of opinion, particularly in the USA where most of the research has been done.

That such new evidence requires constant reassessment of potential hazards is underlined in the Council's view on VDUs (p. 5): 'In our view there is no evidence to support the prescription of any condition due to electromagnetic radiation emanating from VDUs.' This echoes a similar but more recent statement by the IRPA in February 1988. By contrast a WHO panel in January 1987 endorsed a report by two Canadian health officials (Marriott and Stuchly, 1986) that VDT operators (as they are referred to in North America) should not work within one metre of the rear or sides of nearby terminals unless the machines have been tested and confirmed to emit only low levels of non-ionising radiation (*Microwave News*, 1987, January/February). The panel also recommended that 'it is good practice to avoid unnecessary exposure to non-ionising radiation from adjacent VDTs'.

Most recently, a study by Goldhaber, Polen and Hiatt (1988) at the health organisation Kaiser-Permanente, in Oakland, California, found that women who used VDTs more than 20 hours a week had more than twice as many miscarriages as women doing other types of office work. Their survey of 1,583 pregnant women showed that the risk of both early (less than 12 weeks) and late (12 weeks or more) miscarriage increased approximately 80 per cent for all women who worked on VDTs for more than 20 hours a week, compared to those doing similar work without VDTs. A 100 per cent increase in miscarriage was found when VDT operators were compared to non-working women. The results also found a 40 per cent increase in birth defects for both moderate (5-20 hours/week) and heavy (over 20 hours/week) use, but the number was too small to support a statistically significant link at any level of exposure.

The Kaiser study is important because, with all the controversy over possible alternative explanations for observed correlations, it is the first to consider seriously low frequency EMFs, which are at their highest at the sides and rear of sets – not at the front – and which thus means that the number of hours at a terminal may not be a reliable index of exposure. In fact it will tend to under-estimate an operator's exposure, depending on office seating and co-workers' use of machines, so that if there is a risk to pregnancy outcome from VDT EMFs, the risk is likely to be greater than suggested in the study. Dr Irving Selikoff, editor-in-chief of the *American Journal of Industrial Medicine* and a world-renowned specialist in occupational health, told *VDT News* (1988, July/August) that the findings add 'substantial authority' to concerns about VDT-related reproductive hazards. And in the *AJIM*'s July issue editorial, Dr Baruch Modan, referring also to two other recent papers, states that EMR from computer screens should now be considered an environmental health hazard until proven otherwise. Needless to say, the UK's Health and Safety Executive officially considers it harmless, although it is funding research at the London School of Hygiene and Tropical Medicine on VDUs by Drs Beral and Roman, which is due in 1989. Meanwhile, the London Hazards Centre (1987a, 1987b) has produced a useful handbook on VDU hazards, with a wealth of references, as well as one on the possible hazards from standard – as opposed to full spectrum – fluorescent lighting. Taking a strong line, the EEC wants to make members pass laws covering VDUs by no later than January 1991 (*New Scientist*, 9 June 1988). It plans to lay down minimum health and safety requirements to force employers to modify workstations if any risks to workers are discovered. Eye tests will have to be provided for workers before they start working on VDUs, and subsequently if necessary, although it has not been decided yet whether shielding of screens will be required.

Against such new evidence and opinion the IIAC's comment above stands in immediate need of revision, and the speed with which EMF bioeffects research is progressing emphasises the need for an annual review of the potential hazard from all sources, not just VDUs.

Future studies by the CEGB and other independent organisations and researchers will doubtless help to elucidate the contribution of EMFs to cancer and other diseases, as well as their mechanism of effect. According to their corporate plan for research until 1991, the NRPB (1987) plans to continue to study ocular hazards, including cataract formation, from intense infra-red radiation since such understanding 'may have relevance to the possibility of this hazard from exposure to microwave radiation'. The Board also intends to monitor and, where appropriate, study reports that non-ionising radiation can induce subtle effects in tissues, as well as supporting a study of the effects of magnetic fields on metabolic reactions at Oxford University and one on intense static and time-varying magnetic field effects on cardiac function at Cambridge University.

COMARE (the Committee on the Medical Aspects of Radiation in the Environment) was set up at the end of 1985 by the Government 'to assess and advise Government on the health effects of natural and man-made radiation in the environment and to assess the adequacy of the available data and the need for further research'. Its 18 members were chosen by Dr Donald Acheson, the Chief Medical Officer, with Government departments represented by assessors. COMARE has not published many research projects to date. A recent one that it did carry out (COMARE, 1986) came to the controversial conclusion that the amount of (ionising) radiation emitted around the Sellafield reprocessing plant was too low to have caused clusters of child leukaemia near the site. A more recent study (COMARE, 1988), however, found a significant increase in leukaemia in young people near the Dounreay nuclear reprocessing plant in Scotland. It is difficult to know what, if any, research COMARE is conducting or advocating into non-ionising radiation since COMARE will not divulge what exactly it is doing in order to avoid, according to a DHSS spokesman, 'pressure' from others, including the general public.

At the University of Birmingham, Dr Alice Stewart is carrying out research relating the incidence of childhood cancer in parts of Britain to geographic variations in radiation exposure. The main aim is to separate the effects of medical and background radiation and to estimate the contribution of each (Prentice, 1986). Although the survey only covers ionising radiation, its comprehensive geographical mapping will allow a much more accurate assessment of the relative risks and contribution of non-ionising radiation to childhood cancer.

Cancer in childhood affects only about one in 650 children up to 15 years of age but leads to about 400 children dying each year in the UK. In Britain the largest and longest-running study of childhood cancer is the Oxford Survey – begun in 1953 and since 1974 located in Birmingham – which comprises the medical and family details of 15,000 children who have died from cancer since 1953, together with the same number of healthy controls. Using such data Stewart and her colleagues at Oxford were the first to identify the association between diagnostic medical X-ray exposure of pregnant women and subsequent cancer in their children (Stewart *et al.*, 1956). Since the general population receives an annual dose of background radiation about five times as great as that from X-rays, a high proportion of childhood cancers could be due to background gamma radiation. The NRPB has recently surveyed levels of such radiation and has readings for every 10 square kilometres of the national grid. Stewart's initial results should be ready in 1989, her research being funded by the EEC's radiation protection programme. However, according to the EEC Commission in London, there are no

EEC-funded projects to study non-ionising radiation exposure at present, nor any joint EEC proposals on exposure guidelines.

One British, non-Government body that is planning research into EMF bioeffects is the London-based Institution of Environmental Health Officers. Representing some 7000 officers who advise local health authorities, the Institution recently published a report on the extent of the radon hazard in Britain, from which it considered 50–70,000 people to be at risk, approximately two and a half times the number suggested by a previous NRPB report (Wrixon et al., 1988). The NRPB (1989) has since produced a report estimating that over 2500 people in the UK die each year from lung cancer caused by radon.

The possibility of synergistic effects between electromagnetic fields and ionising radiation should not be ignored. The senior writer wrote to the Black Commission of Inquiry into the ionising radiation at the Sellafield Nuclear Materials Re-processing Plant, Cumbria, pointing out that the synergistic effects of ionising radiation and the overhead power lines from the nearby electrical power generating stations needed consideration. Both separately had then already been associated with leukaemia. Hawkins and D'Auria (1987) recently suggested synergistic interaction as a possible explanation for similar reported clusters of leukaemia around other nuclear sites (Cook-Mozaffari et al., 1987). A Russian paper (Tumanyan and Samoilenko, 1983) reports that the effects of an alternating magnetic field and ionising radiation delivered separately or in combination on micro-organisms of differing radiation resistance were studied. While the alternating magnetic field had no pronounced bacteriocidal action, a synergistic increase in the sterilising effect of ionising radiation was demonstrated after incubation of irradiated bacteria in alternating magnetic fields. These workers have subsequently reported on the use of combined radiation and heating methods for the sterilisation of proteolytic enzymes (Samoilenko et al., 1984). Reports of synergistic interactions between ionising radiation and microwave radiation are cited by Fröhlich (1980). It is likely that these effects involve free-radical reactions.

An area which has resulted in co-operation between US and UK researchers is the allergy work of the senior author, at the University of Salford, with Dr Jean Monro, previously full-time at the Allergy and Environmental Medicine Unit at the Lister Hospital, London – where she remains medical director – but now based at the new private Allergy and Environmental Medicine Hospital at what was formerly Breakspear College, in Abbots Langley, Hertfordshire. This has been converted into a hospital suitable for highly allergic patients. As described in Chapter 6, they have shown that weak EMFs can cause allergic reactions, including fatigue, hyperactivity, migraine and convulsions (Choy et al., 1987; Smith and Jafary-Asl, 1986; Smith, 1984). Dr Monro has described her work in her recent book (Mansfield and Monro, 1987). They have examined many individuals with multiple allergies who react to various types of electrical equipment, including power-lines, electric typewriters, VDUs, hair dryers, microwave ovens and fluorescent lights. Smith, Monro and Choy emphasise that the frequency is the all-important parameter in electrically sensitive patients and that the signal strength is of secondary importance once a critical strength – which may be as low as $1\,\text{mV/m}$ for electric fields and well below the $50\,\mu\text{T}$ geomagnetic field strength for magnetic fields – has been reached (Choy et al., 1987). The most sensitive patient Smith and Monro have tested was a woman allergic to EMFs from less than $1\,\text{Hz}$ up to $2\,\text{GHz}$ and to a wide range of chemicals, who went into convulsions when taken to within 200 metres of a power-line while allergically reactive (Best, 1984).

Similar results have been obtained by Dr William Rea, at the Environmental Health Center in Dallas, Texas, who is collaborating with the British researchers. They have tested over 100 patients to a wide range of frequencies and presented their findings at the 5th Annual International Symposium on Man and his Environment in Health and Disease in Dallas in February, 1987 (Rea, 1987). Partly as a result of this co-operation, Dr Rea has recently accepted a post at a British university, as will be described.

As discussed in Chapter 6, Smith and Monro believe that electrical reactions are the basis of most allergies and that EMFs and chemical allergens are electrically related; in other words, that an allergy triggered by one can be neutralised by the other, and vice versa. If the distribution of people's responses to EMFs is similar to those for chemical and nutritional allergies, Smith calculates that one person in a thousand is appreciably allergically affected by EMFs – amounting in Britain to approximately 55,000 people functioning substantially below par.

One family which has suffered, both medically and financially, from hypersensitivities is the Rudd family living on Corfe Farm near Bridport in Dorset. Mr and Mrs Rudd and their three children have suffered varying degrees of multiple allergy for 10 years and possibly longer. In 1981 Mrs Rudd was referred for allergy treatment (her face constantly swelled up) on the NHS but had to wait 11 months before anyone could see her. Despite the treatment, no improvement occurred (NHS treatment only tests for nutritional not chemical allergies). Finally, in 1983, she obtained the help of Dr Monro who, within a few months, was able to bring her allergies and, in due course, those of the rest of her family under control. (Fortunately, certain private medical insurers in the UK are now beginning to recognise Dr Monro's work.) The Rudds' experience was made even more burdensome when their eldest son was diagnosed, in 1983, as having developed the devastatingly debilitating (and controversial) condition known as myalgic encephalomyelitis (ME), also known as post-viral fatigue syndrome.

ME attacks the muscles and nervous system, leaving the victim constantly tired, weak and, in many cases, unable to work. Various outbreaks of the disease have been noted in different countries since ME was first recognised in 1934 in Los Angeles. In 1939 the first outbreak occurred in the UK where there are now estimated to be some 100,000 sufferers. Predisposition to the illness is thought to be linked to previous infection with certain viruses, such as Coxsachie B, and in the Rudds' case the son had 18 months earlier been infected by the Epstein-Barr virus. Recent research has produced evidence of previous viral infection among sufferers (Yousef *et al.*, 1988). Failure to recover fully from such an infection is thought to make the immune system vunerable to ME, which is suspected to be triggered, if not exacerbated, by environmental stressors, particularly pesticides. Psychological factors also appear to be involved.

No NHS treatment for ME offers much relief but Dr Monro was immediately asked to treat the son and managed to bring the worst symptoms under control. For two and a half years the Rudds battled with the West Dorset Health Authority (WDHA) over whether it would pay the crippling cost of their son's continuing treatment by Dr Monro. Finally, with the help of their MP and a sympathetic Manager of the WDHA, they were informed, in June 1986, that the WDHA would pay, but that such payment was not to be retrospective. Despite the recognition of the benefits of Dr Monro's treatment, the Authority would not pay for the other members of the Rudd family to be treated for their allergies, fearing, according to Mrs Rudd, an avalanche of requests from patients for reimbursement or treatment by Dr Monro. Nonetheless, since then a further eight health authorities have agreed to pay for Dr Monro's treatment of ME sufferers. Tragically, the Rudd's eldest son took his own life in June 1988 after suffering further setbacks triggered by an emotional crisis.

However, cases such as the Rudds have been taken up at Parliamentary level. In March 1986 an all-Party group met at the Houses of Parliament to discuss ways of promoting Dr Monro's work, with the ultimate aim of getting it generally recognised and available on the NHS. A major development took place in March 1988 when Dr Monro, with the help of backing, bought Breakspear College, at Abbots Langley, Hertfordshire, and opened the Allergy and Environmental Medicine Hospital, one of the few facilities of its kind in the world and Europe's first purpose-built environmental hospital. Containing 33 beds, the hospital within the old building was built with and uses only environmentally safe products and furnishings, selected for their allergy-free properties. The air is filtered and an electromagnetically screened room is available.

Dr Monro is Medical Director of the hospital and is assisted by a number of staff. Dr Frank Binks, formerly Consultant Physician in Medicine at the Edgware General Hospital, is Consultant Advisor to the hospital, while Dr Philip Barlow, formerly senior lecturer in Aston University's Environmental Health Department, is Consultant in Environmental Health. There are presently four physicians, some of whom are engaged in research (e.g. Mirakian *et al.*, 1986), as well as other visiting staff from Europe and America undertaking specific research projects.

In 1986 a charity, The Environmental Medicine Foundation, to which Dr Monro is a medical advisor, began fund-raising for £1 million to establish a Chair of Environmental Medicine at a British university which has included a Sponsored Carriage Drive, organised by Sir John and Lady Colfox (Chairman of the Foundation) in May, 1987, starting at their home and ending at Chideock Manor in Dorset, the then home of the Duke and Duchess of York. However, in April 1988 the Foundation was able to announce it had reached agreement with the University of Surrey in Guildford to endow the first British university Chair of Environmental Medicine, based at the Robens Institute, to start in September 1988 under the Professorship of the eminent American authority Dr William Rea, from Dallas, Texas, mentioned above. The Chair is based in the Department of Epidemiology and Public Health, under Dr Ballarajan who, together with Dr Rea, intends to research a number of areas of environmentally induced illness, including EMF bioeffects. The Environmental Medicine Foundation also publishes *EMF Newsletter*.

In fact, the Prime Minister herself, Mrs Thatcher, has shown an interest in the new allergy treatments of Dr Monro and others. In a letter replying to Mrs Elizabeth Scott, of North Finchley, London, Mrs Thatcher, referring to Dr Monro's treatment, expressed her hope 'that the treatment you have been receiving will continue to be of benefit.' She continued: 'If a hospital consultant felt that no suitable NHS facilities were available, he could ask the Health Authority to finance treatment for an NHS patient at a suitable private facility.' Referring to treatment based on the principles of 'clinical ecology', the Prime Minister added encouragingly: 'If this form of treatment is to expand in the NHS, those doctors who believe in the methods involved will have to convince more of their colleagues that they work perhaps through properly validated research or trials' (Thatcher, 1986). At the time of writing, Dr Monro is engaged on just such research and an Early Day Motion supporting the Foundation's work has now been signed by more than 150 MPs. A film of her work and treatment can be hired from the Environmental Medicine Foundation.

As for other individual investigations of EMF effects, Professor Bernard Watson, in the Department of Medical Electronics at St Bartholomew's Hospital, London, has been able to prevent tumours implanted with an electronic probe from growing (Bellamy *et al.*, 1979). His success parallels the pioneering work on cancer treatment of Dr Björn Nordenström (1984) at the Karolinska Institute in Stockholm. According to Watson, Nordenström has now succeeded in shrinking the size of some 40 lung tumours by passing an electric current into them. In 1983 Nordenstrom published (himself) a book entitled *Biologically Closed Electric Circuits* (1983) in which he presented the evidence from 30 years research for a revolutionary ideal – an additional circulatory system (McAuliffe, 1985). In a foreword to the book, Professor Watson stated: 'The new concept of energy conversion in tissue over biologically closed electric circuits (BCEC) ... offers a unified theory even for such diverse phenomena as acupuncture and the effects of electromagnetic fields on man and increases our understanding of the mechanism of tumour growth.' It is to be hoped that Nordenström's work and ideas will receive much wider currency from now on, perhaps as a result of Professor Watson's associated work.

Watson has also investigated bone healing using pulsed, low frequency magnetic fields, as well as showing that they can reduce the growth of bacteria (Lunt and Watson, 1982). With Dixey, a former PhD student, his team was able to show that pulsed magnetic fields, with the characteristics of those used for bone healing, produced a release of nor-adrenaline from a cultured cell, which implied an effect on the cell membrane (Dixey and Rein, 1982). In a recent report of the work carried out in his department, Professor Watson states that a recent study on the immunological changes brought about by exposing human lymphocytes to pulsed magnetic fields 'indicates that we should be aware of the dangers of environmental electromagnetic fields caused by 50 Hz power transmissions. We intend to pursue this work to establish the therapeutic use and also the dangers involved' (Watson, 1986).

Another person who has been interested in the effects of EMFs on cell membranes is Professor David Melville, formerly at the University of Southampton and now at Preston Polytechnic. Melville has shown that it is possible that homogeneous magnetic fields as low as 0.2 mT may cause significant changes within the membrane which, in turn, may trigger changes in cellular biochemical processes (Braganza *et al.*, 1984).

Dr Leslie Hawkins, who appeared as an expert witness at the Innsworth Inquiry, is now with the Southern Counties Occupational Health Service (SCOHS) linked to the Robens Institute at the University of Surrey in Guildford. He is continuing his work on the effects of air ionisation, particularly regarding the Sick Building Syndrome (SBS), a syndrome including fatigue, headaches, lack of concentration and associated symptoms observed in office workers under certain conditions and now officially recognised by the WHO (Sykes, 1988). SCOHS has the facilities to measure environmental EMFs and can advise on current UK exposure guidelines.

The pervasive influence of chronic exposure to low-level, non-ionising radiation and associated EMFs may contribute to a number of diseases whose aetiology is still obscure. In a book offering a new theory of the cause and possible cure of multiple sclerosis (MS), Dr June Clarke (1983), based in Sheffield, outlines her main thesis that the damage seen in MS is due to degeneration of the insulating coverings of the nerves, the myelin sheath, brought on by various factors including microwave exposure, particularly radar frequencies in the 10 cm waveband which bypass the skin's heat receptors. Clarke suggests that those least able to dissipate excess heat are likely to be most vulnerable, i.e. people adapted to living in cold climates and women of child-bearing age, a fact borne out by the unique worldwide distribution of MS. Symptoms of radar over-exposure are remarkably similar to the major symptoms of MS. An epidemiological survey of MS sufferers seems warranted to test Dr Clarke's provocative theory.

It is not only scientists in the Western world that are becoming increasingly aware and concerned about long-term exposure to EMFs. The Russians, who have been researching them since long before the Second World War (see Chapter 10), are stepping up their research on the biological effects of EMFs, according to two US scientists, Dr Bill Guy, of the University of Washington, and Dr Don Justensen, of Kansas City's VA Hospital, who visited various laboratories in the Soviet Union in October 1985 (*Microwave News*, 1985, November/December, p. 1). The scientists report that the Russians work in large, interdisciplinary teams, with no skimping on equipment. Both admitted envy at what they saw and compared the obviously flourishing Soviet bioelectromagnetics programme with the faltering American one. Justesen predicted that, based on their progress, the Soviets would soon begin exporting medical devices such as magnetoencephalographs.

Regarding exposure standards, the Russians introduced a new occupational standard in January 1986, limiting workers' exposure to 25 $\mu W/cm^2$ for an 8-hour day over the frequency range 300 MHz–300 GHz. The standard is based on the total amount of energy absorbed and permits exposures for shorter time periods, e.g. 100 $\mu W/cm^2$ for 2 hours. As for the general public, the Soviet Union relaxed its exposure standard in 1984 from 5 $\mu W/cm^2$ to 10 $\mu W/cm^2$ above 300 MHz. By contrast, the American National Standard Institution presently only voluntarily requires a limit for worker and public exposures of 1–5 mW/cm^2 (1000–5000 $\mu W/cm^2$) above 300 MHz, while the US Occupational Safety and Health Administration's standard is 10 mW/cm^2 (10,000 $\mu W/cm^2$).

The new Soviet standard for ELF electric fields from power-lines (Soviet distribution operates at 50 Hz) is 5 kV/m for a full, 8-hour day, though it does not cover switchyard workers. The similar magnetic field standard is 50mG.

The Chinese, perhaps conscious of being responsible for the health of one-quarter of the world's population, are also carrying out research into EMFs. The first Chinese Scientific Conference on Bioelectromagnetics took place in 1984, while the second was held in Hangzhou in October 1986, according to a report by Dr Chiang Huai at Zhejiang Medical University in Hangzhou (*Microwave News*, 1986, November/December, p. 6). Four major areas were covered: theoretical dosimetry, biological effects of EMFs, public and occupational protection, and biological and medical applications of EMFs. One report discussed the substantial progress being made toward the use of microwaves for birth control, in both animal studies and in pilot clinical trials. (In both the UK and Israel there has been work on the electrical detection of estrus in ewes.) Another report detailed work on synergistic effects of microwave and ionising radiation. Concern was also expressed in some sessions about the connection between cancer and EMFs, an area in which some participants are now working. Their results are likely to be presented at the next conference, scheduled for spring 1989, possibly in Xian.

Any discussion of the possible health effects of EMFs must eventually lead to a consideration of safety standards for both public and occupational exposure. The level that any committee will recommend is liable to be a compromise between that at which health effects are observed in the most sensitive person and that level deemed reasonably achievable by the power companies and associated industries within a reasonable time-scale. Even if one is able effectively to inforce a law that covers 99 per cent of the population, there always remains a fairly large number of people (1 per cent of the UK adult population is about 250,000 people) for whom a solution must be found. Part of the solution, of course, is to test all those who live within a certain distance of overhead and underground cables, or whose homes (and gardens) are found to be exposed to a certain minimum EMF. Monitoring such people would not only help to identify any problems or highly sensitive people, but would also provide very useful on-going epidemiological data. Certainly, it might also raise questions of loss of property values and compensation for medical expenses and possible removal costs; whether such investigation and expense is deemed cost-effective in the long term or unnecessary will, in part, depend on the prevailing social climate. But beyond such measures it is important to make doctors and other medical personnel aware of the symptoms of acute and chronic exposure to EMFs – and environmental pollutants in general because of synergistic effects – so that such conditions are recognised and referred immediately for (required) specialist treatment. Whether the CEGB in Britain, or other utilities abroad, should be required to fund such treatment is a matter for debate.

Ten years ago, at the time of the Innsworth Inquiry in Britain and the Public Service Commission hearing in New York, the respective power companies argued their case on three main grounds: there was insufficient evidence for the health effects of power-line EMFs; there was insufficient evidence for the non-thermal effects of EMFs; and, there was no plausible model for how such alleged bioeffects could occur. Ten years later, in 1989, there is a growing number of independent and replicated studies, now exceeding 30, linking residential and occupational exposure to EMFs to a variety of diseases, especially leukaemia. (for a comprehensive review covering frequencies from ELF to RF/MW, including 300 references, see Brown and Chattopadhyay (1988).) In July, 1986, the National Academy of Sciences' National Research Council finally officially accepted the reality of non-thermal EMF bioeffects, thus ending a 25-year debate. Finally, although not complete, there now exists empirically supported, plausible models of how weak but coherent EMFs in the power-line ELF range can interact with and affect biological systems. As described in earlier chapters, strong evidence now supports an understanding based on coherent EMFs producing frequency-specific effects via resonant amplification properties across cellular membranes.

There is now sufficient evidence and theoretical understanding of the effects produced to call for a moratorium on the erection of overhead power cables near any human dwelling, especially schools. By implication, no future buildings should be built near overhead power-lines. The placing of present and future underground cables should also be carefully evaluated, as well as those serving high-rise buildings for which lead or aluminium insulation should be considered around the 'dry riser'. Britain should follow the example of an increasing number of American states and introduce a minimum corridor around overhead power-lines. That distance should, according to the evidence available, be at least 150 metres either side of 400 kV lines to take account of varying load characteristics, although this may be conservative, and require a health warning to be added to descriptions of properties near power-lines; the law in certain US states, which admittedly have up to 765 kV lines as opposed to only 400 kV in the UK, requires 350 metres. The relevant British authorities should be aware, in light of the present and growing evidence for health effects and the recent successful and pending lawsuits in the USA over the health hazards of power line EMFs, that any further delay in implementing enforceable legislation on this issue may prompt litigation on the part of individuals, community/pressure groups, labour unions or even commercial concerns, whose outcome – now that 'class actions' are to be allowed in Britain – are likely to be very different from that of Public Inquiries ten years ago. The possibility that the Ministry of Defence may need to be consulted on the question of enforceable legislation only adds a further, sinister dimension to the issue, which requires a separate chapter to elucidate.

In conclusion, the recommendations of Dr Ross Adey, an Advisor to the White House on EMR, in his testimony before the House Subcommittee on Water and Power Resources on 6 October 1987, are especially relevant for future research and the adoption of enforceable standards in the UK and, ultimately, the EEC. Under the heading 'Steps Towards Implementation of Health Safety Standards', he stated:

1 There is a growing and even urgent need for early establishment of national safety standards that would govern exposures to non-ionising EM fields in the workplace, in the home and in the general environment.
2 These standards would be regarded as interim at the time of promulgation, since current epidemiological knowledge and experimental evidence remain incomplete in precisely defining mechanisms of EM interaction with body tissues and in evaluating the exact role of these EM fields in human disease. Although incomplete, current knowledge may be considered adequate for establishment of interim standards.
3 Interim standards should cover exposures to environmental fields from ELF frequencies (below 300 Hz) to millimeter waves at 300 GHz. For radio and microwaves, an early requirement involves consideration of pulse- or amplitude-modulation of the carrier wave, since these low frequency characteristics of the field largely determine modes of tissue interactions at athermal field levels.
4 Beyond establishment of interim standards, a major new effort will be necessary in reviewing current research developments and incorporating new knowledge into more refined and more comprehensive standards.
5 There is a need for an interagency coordinating group with cognizance over the whole spectrum of the national research and regulatory effort. In the last, [in the USA] the Electromagnetic Radiation Management Advisory Council (ERMAC) offered much-needed foci for research planning and dissemination of information. This need is now especially acute, in times of small budgets and restricted funding. Lack of communication between federal agencies and other funding bodies hampers research and enhances risks of duplication of effort. (*Microwave News*, 1987, November/December, p. 10).

Adey's last point is in line with Recommendation 6 of the NYSPLP's Panel who called for an *independent* agency to be set up to administer and oversee research on electromagnetic bioeffects. Such an agency or committee should be constituted for similar work in the UK, especially in view of the growing problems surrounding university research funding. Following Ross Adey's recommendation, its first urgent priority should be the establishment of national safety standards for exposure to non-ionising electromagnetic fields in the home, workplace and the general environment. Unfortunately, the NRPB's final *Guidance to Restrictions on Exposure to Time-varying Electromagnetic Fields and the 1988 Recommendations of the 1988 Non-Ionising Radiation Committee*, published just as this book went to press, does not go far enough.

CHAPTER 10

Beware: military at work

All the armies of the world are not as powerful as an idea whose time has come.

Victor Hugo (1802–85)

It is, perhaps, one of the black ironies of scientific research that a significant proportion of the beneficial information it yields is discovered, almost incidentally, from research into the possibly harmful applications of the subject under study. Even Michaelangelo was not above defending Florence by his skill in the design of fortifications, and Leonardo da Vinci, one-time ducal engineer of Milan, petitioned for the appointment referring to his military designs – adding that he was a passingly good artist. The history of research into electromagnetic field effects is no exception. The nature and progress of research in this area has been and continues to be strongly influenced by military interest and involvement. Considerable evidence has been amassed, much of it presented by Brodeur (1977), that the US military, in particular, has deceived committees, delayed safety standards, denigrated opponents and damaged the health of its own personnel and citizens in its urge to protect its interests and to develop microwave and other NIR weapon systems.

As evidence, both experimental and anecdotal, steadily accumulated after the Second World War and pointed to certain harmful effects on humans of exposure to specific levels of electromagnetic radiation, it is not surprising that the military began to take more than a passing interest in its use and potential. Indeed, through their classified research both Eastern and Western military establishments may well know a lot more about the harmful potential of MW radiation than one might prefer.

The USSR has researched the area at least since the Second World War and, through their long-term irradiation of a specific group of American personnel, eventually caused the USA to take the possibility seriously. The result was one of the few occasions on which the US military – or any military establishment for that matter – has been forced to discuss such matters in public. It also spawned some of the first research in the West to examine just such possibilities and is therefore worth assessing in some detail. It should be noted, in the light of the new Official Secrets Act in Britain, that material in this chapter has been collated solely from information available in the public domain through the world's free press even though this may no longer be a sufficient defense under the new Act.

Microwave irradiation of the US Embassy in Moscow

The general public – particularly in America – got their first real idea of the potential military applications of electromagnetic fields in 1976, when the United States claimed that their Embassy in Moscow was being irradiated with microwave beams by the Russians. (There had been a brief newspaper report about it in 1972 but with few consequences.) The Russians denied the charge but measurements in and around the building indicated that irradiation was indeed occurring. However, what was perhaps equally if not more disturbing was the eventual disclosure that the irradiation had been happening since 1953 and that the US State Department and five previous governments had known about it since it started. This, together with the private and public concern as to what effects the exposed personnel might have suffered, prompted a Congressional inquiry and report (US Congress Senate, 1979). It is also comprehensively covered, with detailed descriptions of other military research on microwaves, in the highly recommended book, *The Zapping of America. Microwaves, their Deadly Risk and the Cover-up*, by prize-winning *New Yorker* magazine journalist Paul Brodeur (1977).

The congressional report showed that, rather than inform their embassy staff or take any preventative action, the US military authorities apparently allowed the former to act as guinea pigs to observe what effects they might suffer. It was only in 1976, when the US finally decided to install defensive screens to protect its personnel, that the staff discovered what had been happening, a situation roundly condemned in the official report:

> The State Department, thus, used the analogy of individual physicians withholding medical information from patients when, in their judgment, the well-being of the patient was better protected by so doing. But this substitution of a doctor/patient relationship for an employer/employee

relationship is not defensible, regardless of the outcome of the studies. The employees should have been promptly informed of the situation. (US Senate, 1979)

The report details a number of surveys and studies that were carried out on the staff both before and after the irradiation was made known to them. Without admitting liability, the State Department eventually tried to appease the embassy staff by re-grading Moscow posts as carrying an extra health risk and gave all staff a 20 per cent salary rise. None the less, a number of the staff have tried to sue the US Government and cases are still being filed today.

To understand in part how this cover-up developed requires following the evolution of research in this area over the period in question. In 1953 little was known or suspected (in the West at least) of the biological or psychological effects of exposure to MW radiation. Few, if any, of the Russian studies that had been done had been translated, and reports of what they were doing were generally mistrusted. Thus, after it had been established that the Moscow signal was too weak and irregular to be used for jamming or activating eavesdropping devices in the Embassy, little notice was taken of it until the early 1960s when equipment was made available to measure, mainly, its intensity, frequency and duration (US Senate, 1979). In 1963 continuous recording was started. From August 1963 to May 1975 the frequency ranged from 2.56 to 4.1 GHz and the intensity remained at about 5 $\mu W/cm^2$ at the strongest point of the beam. Two additional beams appeared, one in January 1973 and the other in August 1975, and continued almost daily, boosting the intensity at times to 18 $\mu W/cm^2$. When the protective screening was installed in February 1976 the intensity dropped to about 2 $\mu W/cm^2$, at which level it remained until all radiation ceased abruptly in January 1979 – to reappear only briefly in 1983. However, very recently, in March 1988, irradiation has again been reported, this time primarily in the 9–11 GHz range, producing power levels of 0.1 $\mu W/cm^2$ outside the building and 0.01 $\mu W/cm^2$ inside. A US State Department statement acknowledged that the signals were usually on for a couple of hours a day but refused to comment on the possible reasons for the irradiation (*Microwave News*, 1988, March/April).

By the mid-1960s growing concern by a number of medical scientists over possible biological effects of microwaves prompted the Medical Services Office of the State Department to carry out the first of a number of studies involving the Moscow personnel. An internal retrospective survey of the medical records of 139 staff and 268 dependants assigned to the Moscow Embassy yielded inconclusive results. It was followed by a project carried out by George Washington University School of

Medicine, led by Dr Cecil Jacobson, under the official title 'Cytogenic Evaluation of Mutagenic Exposure' (i.e. evaluation of the effect on cell structure of exposure to an agent capable of causing changes in genetic material). However, within the State Department it was referred to as the 'Moscow Viral Study' to avoid concern among personnel. It involved comparing blood samples from 71 employees before, during and after exposure to radiation at the Moscow Embassy with 13 personnel before assignment to the Embassy, who acted as controls. The results were also deemed inconclusive since although 43 per cent of the exposed subjects 'should be classified as either having actually experienced high risk of mutagenic exposure or were highly suspect, thereof', 38 per cent of the control subjects also fell into the same high risk category (US Senate, 1979). It was also considered difficult to quantify the contribution of other factors, such as caffeine intake.

Project Pandora

Thus, in 1965 a classified project, Project Pandora, was initiated through funding at the Walter Reed Army Institute of Research, to 'investigate possible behavioural and bioeffects (primarily the former) on primates when the latter were irradiated with microwave signals simulating the exposure of Embassy employees in Moscow' (US Senate, 1979). In fact the intensity of the signal was set at 4–5 mW/cm^2 compared to the Moscow one, whose average intensity varied between 2 and 18 μW/cm^2. Again, however, results were inconclusive and a record of what was done is 'scattered and incomplete'. No comprehensive report was ever prepared and parts of the record were destroyed in September 1973, about two years after the project was terminated.

However, this has not prevented Dr Samuel Koslow, a leading government scientist who investigated the Moscow radiation, from commenting in a recent interview: 'The Moscow signal was definitely not used to modify health or behavior. ... No one knows for certain what it was used for. But we have pretty good suspicions, which I'm not at liberty to discuss. They have nothing, however, to do with biology or psychology.' (McAuliffe, 1985).

His views contrast markedly with those of Dr Milton Zaret, an ophthalmologist in Scarsdale, New York, who was asked by the CIA in 1965 to review Soviet medical literature on microwaves to try to discover what the Russians were attempting to do. He concluded: 'Whatever other reasons the Russians may have had, they believed the beam would modify the behavior of the personnel' (Schiefelbein, 1979). Since then Zaret has carried out extensive research on the effects of microwave exposure on the formation of cataracts in the eye and has concluded that microwaves cause a special type of cataract that develops in the rear part of the capsule surrounding the lens. He has found such cataracts in at least 50 definitive cases, mainly comprising airline pilots and air traffic controllers (who are constantly exposed to radar), as well as microwave workers (Zaret and Snyder, 1977). Others have confirmed his observation, to the point that this type of cataract can now be interpreted to indicate sustained microwave exposure by the subject (see Chapter 9).

Project 'Big Boy'

In 1968 a designated Pandora Science Advisory Committee (SAC) was established to guide the project and it quickly decided that experimentation with human subjects was essential due to the limitations of animal studies to inform about human behaviour. Thus was born Project 'Big Boy'. This involved crewmen from the USS *Saratoga* who were divided into three groups: those exposed to the highest levels of radar on the ship, those exposed to low levels and those with no expected exposure. Dockside and seagoing tests were carried out but no significant psychological or physiological findings were obtained. As a result yet a further study was proposed in May 1969 – this time of eight humans to be exposed to a synthetic 'Moscow' signal but with special protective measures to safeguard the subjects involving independent medical and psychiatric monitoring. However the study was never carried out because after much discussion and review of previous inconclusive results the SAC decided in early 1970 not to carry out any further studies. Project Pandora was officially terminated on 20 March 1970. Thus, despite a number of studies since 1965 the SAC felt only able to conclude that, basically, no conclusions could really be drawn from any of the animal studies and that future studies needed to rely upon human subjects, 'even though grave questions as to the ethical acceptablity of such studies were still unanswered' – an absurd Catch 22 situation.

Moscow Embassy personnel studies

No further studies were carried out until February 1976 when protective screens were erected at the embassy and the irradiation suddenly received wide publicity. At that point a Study of Lymphocytes was started by Dr Thomas Stossel of the Massachusetts General Hospital. Earlier blood counts from Moscow personnel had indicated a higher than average lymphocyte count and the study set out to determine whether this finding could be attributed to the irradiation. The main causes of elevated lymphocyte counts are either as an acute reaction to infection or invasion by a foreign body, or as an indication of a neo-plastic condition, one sub-category of which is termed acute lymphatic leukaemia in which rapid accumulation of lymphocytes in the bone marrow occurs and is generally fatal if untreated.

Some 350 Moscow personnel, two-thirds of them male, constituted the study group, with a group of approximately 1,000 foreign service personnel resident in the US acting as controls. Although mean lymphocyte counts among Moscow personnel were approximately 41 per cent above those of the control group, this high count was present equally among those personnel who had arrived before February 1976 (when the screens reduced the radiation to very low levels) and those who arrived afterwards. The counts were also equally high regardless of where the person worked in the Embassy and showed a sharp and sustained drop-off after August 1977, for unknown reasons. In other words, the elevated counts were found to be reversible to the control group's levels both for those remaining in Moscow after August 1977 and for those leaving before then. Concluding that the elevated counts could not be due to the irradiation, the investigators were left to speculate that they might have been due to a parasite associated with the Giardia infection, an outbreak of which had occurred among tourists returning from Leningrad in 1976, although no Giardia epidemic had been reported neither in Moscow or among Moscow Embassy personnel. Whether the raised lymphocyte levels were due to the radiation or not and notwithstanding that they dropped off sharply after August 1977, it is perhaps worth noting that both Moscow Ambassadors Charles Bohlen and Llewellyn Thompson died of cancer and that Ambassador Walter Stoessel – on whose office the beam was centred – was, in 1976, suffering from a blood disease, nausea and bleeding in the eyes, and has since died from leukaemia (*Times*, 1986).

The final, and possibly most extensive epidemiological study of ex-Moscow Embassy personnel was initiated, at the request of the State Department under public pressure, in June 1976 by Dr Abraham Lilienfeld of Johns Hopkins University's School of Hygiene and Public Health. Known as the Johns' Hopkins Foreign Service Health Status Study, it assessed the mortality and morbidity of all Moscow Embassy personnel and dependants from 1953 to 1976 and matched them with a control group of US personnel who had been stationed in other East European embassies, none of which had reported microwave irradiation.

The analysis of the medical records of some 3,100 Moscow personnel and 2,336 dependants, 1,468 of them children, yielded some provocative findings. Although overall mortality favoured the Moscow group, females in the latter showed a higher than average death-rate from malignant neoplasms, though this was not statistically significant. However, Moscow males showed a definite significantly raised rate of protozoal intestinal diseases, benign neoplasms, and diseases of the nerves and peripheral ganglia. Moscow females had a significantly higher rate of protozoal intestinal diseases also, as well as complications of pregnancy and childbirth. As a group, Moscow personnel suffered significantly more eye problems, psoriasis and other assorted skin conditions (mostly cysts, dermatitis and eczema), as well as depression, irritability, loss of appetite and difficulty in concentrating. Within the Moscow group the incidence of other than skin cancer was higher in the exposed group, despite the amount of smoking being similar. And in the children four diseases – mumps, anaemic blood diseases, heart disease and respiratory infections – occurred in significantly higher numbers. In view of the variety of findings mentioned above and the greater knowledge of MW effects that the Russians undoubtedly possessed at that time, it is very difficult to understand how Dr Koslow could be so emphatic in his insistence that the irradiation was not intended to harm the Embassy occupants, when it so clearly did.

However, this official position becomes more understandable when one realises that the Moscow Embassy affair brought into sharp focus one very important question: what was a safe level of exposure to microwave radiation for both the public and military personnel?

When radar was first introduced in the Second World War there was little discussion of safety guidelines or possible health effects on the servicemen exposed to it, perhaps understandably when Nazi domination of the world was the uppermost fear in everyone's minds. After the war, however, in the early 1950s, disturbing reports of cataracts in animals and technicians exposed to relatively low levels of microwaves prompted the military and burgeoning commercial interests to search for an acceptable exposure standard, in particular one that avoided the numerous problems of trying to extrapolate one for humans based purely on animal studies. A solution was provided by one Professor Herman P. Schwan.

Schwan entered the United States in 1947, under 'Project Paperclip' (see below), where he accepted a post at the University of Pensylvania, remaining there ever since, largely funded by the Department of Defense (Becker and Selden, 1985). Schwan assumed that the only effect radio and microwaves could have on living tissue was one of heating – when absorbed in sufficient amount. He used metal balls and flasks of salt water as a model of the human body's ability to dissipate heat to help estimate a danger level of exposure. Finding that significant heating of such a model only occurred at 100 mW or more, he incorporated a safety factor of 10 and, in 1953, proposed a safety limit of 10 mW/cm^2 for human exposure (Schiefelbein, 1979). With little real debate or further experimentation, industry and the military had, by 1957/8, accepted the level as an informal guideline. Dr Solomon Michaelson, a veterinarian at the University of Rochester – also chiefly funded by the DoD – induced gross burns in test animals at much higher intensities and thus said he had confirmed that the $10\,\text{mW/cm}^2$ limit should be safe (Schiefelbein, 1979). However, no one tested for non-thermal effects, which were thought not to occur. In 1965 the Army and Air Force formally adopted the $10\,\text{mW/cm}^2$ limit and one year later the ANSI also adopted it as an occupational exposure guideline (though not for the general public). The ANSI decision is remarkable since, according to Becker, even Schwan has consistently maintained that his dosage limit is safe for probably no more than an hour. But Becker has accurately exposed the sinister reasons behind the endurance of the Schwan standard:

> There were persuasive economic reasons why the 10,000-microwatt [$= 10\,\text{mW/cm}^2$] standard was and still is defended at all costs. Lowering it would have curtailed the expansion of military EMR use and cut into the profits of the corporations that supplied the hardware. A reduced standard now would constitute an admission that the old one was unsafe, leading to liability for damage claims from ex-GIs and industrial workers. One of the strongest monetary reasons was given in a 1975 classified summary of the DoD's TriService Electromagnetic Radiation Bioeffects Research Plan: 'These [lower] standards will significantly restrict the military use of EMR in a peacetime environment and require the procurement of substantial real estate around ground-based EMR emitters to provide buffer zones.' The needed real estate was estimated to be 498,000 acres. The price of this much land would surely run well into the billions of dollars. (Becker and Selden, 1985, p. 305)

It now becomes clear why Dr Koslov, and indeed the whole US Government, cannot admit that the Moscow Signal caused health effects to its exposed personnel: to do so would be to admit that the US $10\,\text{mW/cm}^2$ standard was, and remains, inadequate, thus unleashing a flood of damage claims. (In fact a number of former Embassy personnel have successfully sued the US Government and received out-of-court settlements.) Because the peak exposure only ever supposedly reached $18\,\mu\text{W/cm}^2$, the US Government has never had any formal grounds on which to object to the irradiation as a health hazard. Requests to the Russians during the whole episode were mainly fairly low-key and perfunctory, probably because the US DoD realised that if the Soviets were to reveal their research on health effects at exposure levels well below the $10\,\text{mW/cm}^2$ level, they would acutely embarrass the US scientifically, expose the scandal of the $10\,\text{mW/cm}^2$ standard, open the way for massive negligence and damage suits, and jeopardise the entire American EMR weapons programme. They also faced the problem of explaining away why the Soviet equivalent microwave exposure standard at

that time was set at a thousand times below the US limit: at 10 $\mu W/cm^2$!
Caught between public pressure and secret collusion, the only way out
was the denial of a hazard, based on the dubious interpretation of some
questionable epidemiological studies. Although some 2,500 documents
about the Moscow irradiation have been released under America's Freedom of Information Act, all have been edited as to the probable reasons
for the signal.

However, on-going research may provide more evidence to support
the above view, besides further embarrassing the US DoD. Dr Stanislaw
Szmigielski, internationally known for his work on RF/MW radiation
effects on the immune system, and his colleagues at the Centre for Radiobiology and Radioprotection in Warsaw, Poland, have produced preliminary results supporting a link between cancer and exposure to RF and
MW radiation among military personnel (*Microwave News*, 1987,
January/February). The results are from a five-year prospective, epidemiological study, started in 1985, of new cancer cases among Polish
military personnel and will involve detailed analysis of past service history, including the duration and intensity of RF/MW exposure. The
initial results support an earlier retrospective study by Szmigielski, published in 1985, which showed that exposed military personnel, over a
period from 1971–80, were three times more likely than unexposed servicemen to develop cancer, especially tumours of organs involved in
blood formation and lymphatic tissue which were nearly seven times
higher than among unexposed personnel. The earlier study was published in Polish but the first English summary has appeared in a chapter
by Szmigielski in the recent *Modern Bioelectricity* (Marino, 1988) (to
which the senior author has also contributed). After making probably
the most complete review of the link between RF/MW radiation exposure and cancer, Szmigielski draws the following conclusions from his
1985 study:

- The risk of developing clinically detectable neoplastic disease was about 3 times higher for personnel exposed occupationally to RW/MW radiations. The highest risk appeared for malignancies originating from the hemato-lymphatic systems (morbidity about 7 times higher). Other more frequent neoplasms were located in the alimentary tract and in skin (including melanomas).
- The highest risk factor of cancer morbidity related to occupational exposure to RF/MW appeared for subjects at the age of 40–49 who had a 5–15 year period of exposure.
- Morbidity rates of neoplasms in those exposed occupationally to RF/MW showed strong correlation with the period of exposure.
- Neoplasms of the same localisation and/or type developed earlier (by about 10 years) in personnel exposed occupationally to RF/MW than

in those not working in the RF/MW environment. (*Microwave News*, 1987, January/February.)

Referring to immunological effects, the Polish researchers feel that research to date suggests that the immune system exhibits a 'biphasic' reaction to RF/MW radiation, with initial exposure stimulating the whole system, followed by a gradual suppression of the whole immunity with increasing exposure and/or power densities (Marino, 1988).

Thus, although the exact levels of irradiation are not clear, Szmigielski's 1985 results, together with his recent preliminary findings, certainly reinforce the proposition that the intentional low-level irradiation of America's Moscow Embassy between 1953–76 (and beyond) was carried out, at least partly, to harm the health of those exposed.

Certain other research during that period, some of it for the military, seems to point in the same general direction and, at the very least, must have raised suspicions. One such piece of research was carried out by Dr Dietrich Beischer.

Project Sanguine/Seafarer

Since 1958 the US Navy has wanted to construct an ELF radio network to be able to communicate with its nuclear submarines such that they would be able to remain hundreds of feet below the surface rather than near it as required by their present systems, thus rendering themselves vulnerable to enemy detection. The concept was known as Project Sanguine – later renamed Project Seafarer – and by 1976 had already cost some $100 million (Brodeur, 1977).

Basically, the intention was to bury some 6,000 miles of antenna cable below the ground near Clam Lake in northern Wisconsin in a grid-like pattern to cover approximately 22,500 square miles – about 41 per cent of the state. The area was apparently chosen mainly because the underlying rock does not conduct electricity well, a factor that would enhance the efficiency of the antennae. The transmitters were also to be buried, making the complex fairly impervious to attack.

However, as well as local opposition, the Navy ran into problems with the results produced by one of their leading scientists who was asked to investigate the possible hazards to humans involved, Dr Dietrich Beischer. Beischer arrived in the USA after the Second World War, along with some 1,400 other German scientists under a deal known as 'Project Paperclip', whereby they had to agree to work for the US military establishment. (Others include von Braun, designer of the V2 rocket and eventual architect of America's space programme.) In 1973 Beischer and his colleagues at the Naval Aerospace Medical Institute at Pensacola, Florida, published research results which found that nine out of ten Navy volunteers who had been exposed to an alternating magnetic field of 45 Hz and 100 μT had shown a rapid build-up of serum triglycerides, an accepted warning of potential heart problems (Beischer et al., 1977, p. 252). According to Brodeur (1977), another study of eleven men exposed to ELF showed a significant decline in their ability to perform simple addition and both results were kept secret by the Navy for two years.

In the meantime a report reviewing biomedical and ecological effects of ELF radiation by the Department of the Navy in December 1973 stressed the need to investigate matters further: 'Detailed animal experiments on triglyceride levels should be undertaken simultaneously with a continuation of the human experimentation.' But public fears about exposure of people and animals to electromagnetic radiation and that the proposed system would make any area that accepted it a potential enemy target, besides depressing property values, forced the Navy to scale down the proposed system, which it then renamed Project Seafarer. The latter would cover only 3,000 to 4,000 square miles, with antenna cables buried 3 to 6 feet below the surface and fed by less transmitters which would be housed on the surface. Other sites were also eventually considered, such as the Upper Peninsula of Michigan, and an Army base in New Mexico (Boffery, 1976).

However, although research continued Dr Beischer's funded work in the area ceased. His findings were never adequately followed up and he himself retired early – and became mysteriously difficult to contact. Dr Robert Becker, an orthopaedic surgeon and pioneer in the field of regeneration and its relationship to living things, was on the committee set up in 1973 by the Navy to review 15 years of research on ELF radiation, which included Beischer's results. In his very important book, *The Body Electric* (which recounts his own research and battles with various committees and authorities), Becker recalls the extraordinary circumstances surrounding his last communication with Dietrich Beischer:

> In 1977 the Erie Magnetics Company of Buffalo, New York, sponsored a small private conference, and Beischer and I both planned to attend. Just before the meeting I got a call from him. With no preamble or explanation, he blurted out: 'I'm at a pay phone. I can't talk long. They are watching me. I can't come to the meeting or ever communicate with you again. I'm sorry. You've been a good friend. Goodbye.' Soon afterwards I called his office at Pensacola and was told, 'I'm sorry, there is no one here by that name,' just as in the movies. A guy who had done important

research there for decades just disappeared. (Becker and Selden, 1985, p.325)

Not only did Beischer disappear but so also did reference to his work – at least by the military. Whereas the 1973 ELF research for the Navy acknowledges his findings on serum triglycerides, by 1980 a review covering from 1968 to that year conveniently omits any reference to any of his 19 years' of research for the Navy (Grissett, 1980), despite the fact that its author, Dr James Grissett, then still working at Pensacola Naval Base, had been one of Beischer's co-authors on his 1973 paper (see reference).

However, in 1984 Beischer was tracked down – by a British Channel 4 TV crew making an illuminating series of documentaries, entitled *The Good, the Bad, and the Indefensible*, about the positive and negative effects of EMFs (Central TV, 1984). The series, co-funded by WGBH-Buffalo, New York, was shown in Britain in August/September 1984 but, possibly due to the sensitive nature of the third episode – on the US military involvement – was apparently never shown in America.

When visited at his home, Beischer agreed to talk and be filmed provided no sound was recorded. The interviewer, David Jones, reported his comments in the third episode, 'Opening Pandora's Box':

> He refused to disown his discovery that low level magnetic fields could adversely affect the heart. He also revealed that a secret survey of the workers at the Wisconsin transmitter had produced similar results. But these had been classified and never released. As for his sudden retirement, that had been for personal reasons, and any other suggestion was a gross defamation of his former employers.

Despite such findings by Beischer and others, and the opposition of groups in Michigan and Wisconsin backed by Congressmen, together with controversy over the research presented in Environmental Impact Statements (EIS) (mainly funded by the Navy), Project ELF, as it is now called, has been pushed through and is nearly ready to become operational. Transmitter antenna sites are virtually completed and the production of submarine receivers is under way (*Microwave News*, 1987, May/June). Opponents had hoped to stall such construction until a more advanced system, the Satellite Laser Communications (SLC) system, using a blue/green laser, had been developed, but the US Navy recently stopped further development by refusing to fund the SLC system to the tune of $100 million over the next couple of years which, according to officials at the Defense Advanced Research Projects Agency (DARPA), will kill the project, (*Microwave News*, 1987, May/June). The Agency has previously also considered such ideas as using natural 'resonances' of the ionosphere (see Chapter 1 on Tesla's ideas), or subatomic particles – neutrinos – as a communication channel, but none matched the potential of the laser system, which would be able to transmit data at a higher rate than ELF.

Ever-watchful of what their American colleagues are doing, the British MoD announced in March 1985 that it was planning a £300 million ELF system, using some 30 miles of pylons along sections of the Scottish Highlands, to contact its nuclear submarines (Brown, 1985). A number of prospective sites were being considered, aided by Sussex University's Armament and Disarmament Information Unit who helped to identify high resistive rock in the area. In a further press report (Hughes, 1985), it was disclosed that the test rig alone would involve 12 miles of cable across up to 800 acres of wild Scottish highland. The transmitter itself would emit 60–120 Hz waves that could be picked up by submarines travelling at 16 knots up to 400 feet below the surface. Despite assurances from Mr John Lee, then Under Secretary of State for Defence Procurement, that 'every effort would be made to minimize the impact on the environment', many living in the area, including Mr Donald Stewart, former Scottish National MP for the Western Isles, were less than impressed. By November 1986 the site of the proposed transmitter had been fixed as Glengarry Forest in Invernesshire. At this point Simon Best sent information on the possible harmful effects of chronic ELF exposure to the SDP/Liberal Alliance MP for the constitutuency, Sir Russell Johnston (Best, 1987). This was forwarded to the MoD, on whose behalf Mr Archie Hamilton, MP, replied in January 1987 (Hamilton, 1987). Mr Hamilton rejected the possibility of harmful effects on plants or animals, citing two reviews of the ELF literature and stating that the most recent was one by the American Institute of Biological Sciences in March 1985. This, in itself, was somewhat disconcerting since two more recent reports, in July and October 1986, available to the public, had in fact been published (*Microwave News*, 1987, January/February). Either the MoD's exchange of information with its American counterparts in this area is not all it should be, or Mr Hamilton was receiving a somewhat selective view of the literature from his advisors. Mr Hamilton went on to point out that at the frequency the system will probably use (100 Hz), the NRPB is likely to propose (in a forthcoming document on protection from electric and magnetic fields below frequencies of 300 GHz, which was to be published in early 1987, now due Spring 1989), that no restriction on public access need be considered for electric fields up to 1300 V/m or magnetic fields up to 0.09 mT. As the proposed system is only likely to produce electric and magnetic fields of up to

30 V/m and 0.003 mT, respectively, the extra exposure should only be negligible.

In a further exchange, Best sent a copy of Comments by Cyril Smith (1986) on the NRPB's Consultative Document (NRPB, 1986) regarding the proposed new protection guidelines, which Smith had sent to the NRPB in September 1986 in response to their public invitation for comments. In his comments Smith discussed the phenomenon of electrically sensitive allergy patients and the importance of frequency and degree of coherence over the level of intensity, pointing out that an average 70 kg man could theoretically be sensitive to electric and magnetic fields as low as 8 μV/m and 300 fT, corresponding to a power density of less than 1 pW/cm^2. After the June 1987 General Election, Mr Timothy Sainsbury, Mr Hamilton's replacement, replied with comments from the Defence Radiological Protection Service (DRPS) (Sainsbury, 1987). While noting Dr Smith's comments, which included recommending the introduction of compensation for environmentally induced illness, Mr Sainsbury went on to say that the MoD had to look to the NRPB to provide the authoritative advice and that the radiation from its proposed system would be below the NRPB's current guidelines.

According to an April 1988 letter to Sir Russell Johnston (Freeman, 1988), the results of recent surveys of the area will enable the MoD to decide whether a proposed Demonstrator Aerial should be located underground, on the surface, or overhead. Once decided, work will begin on preparing a Notice of Proposed Development and an Environmental Impact Assessment for consultation with the Highland Regional Council. (On the basis of these proposals it is clear that the MoD has rejected the idea of the laser communication system the Americans were investigating, as mentioned above.) The letter indicated that the NoPD was unlikely to be submitted before Autumn 1988 or work to start on the site before 1990. As well as considering the initial results of Dr Szmigielski's two studies of Polish military personnel's exposure to NIR (mentioned earlier), such a time scale will allow the MoD to evaluate his current prospective study due for completion in 1989–90 before proceeding further – a not unwise deliberation.

Besides the possible effects on local residents, flora and fauna, their food and water sources, chronic exposure to the proposed transmitter's ELF radiation might pose a health hazard to men in the submarines themselves. The submarines' steel hull reduces the static component of the geomagnetic field but only reduces a fraction of the incident magnetic ELF field from such emitted radiation, which cannot be easily screened against. (The possibility and consequences of such low-level magnetic fields simultaneously triggering effects in all the operators in charge of the computers controlling the nuclear missiles, into emitting radiation able to affect the computers, hardly bears thinking about.) Although proving a health effect in this case might be difficult, it would probably be less so for servicemen involved with radar or other electronic equipment; the new 1987 Crown Proceedings (Armed Forces) Act, discussed below, now makes it possible for service personnel to sue for injury (or death) caused by fellow personnel while on duty.

Recent military EM applications

Protection from electromagnetic interference or eavesdropping is something the military has had to take very seriously in recent years. Reports of the EMFs given off by computers inside a building being picked up and decoded by equipment outside have meant very expensive screening for military installations, such as GCHQ in Britain (Drori, 1985). The NATO standard for such screening is called TEMPEST. However, the General Accounting Office (GAD), a US Congressional investigative office, recently found that poor management of the US Department of Defense's TEMPEST programme had cost millions of dollars in wasted expense and may have led to the leakage of classified information (*Microwave News*, 1986, June/July). GAD also accused all three services of failing to fully implement a January 1984 National Communication Security Instruction, setting out TEMPEST procedures, by June 1986, and recommended that a new TEMPEST-procedures security policy be implemented, with those responsible for enforcement brought together in a single body. One possible result of this inefficiency was the disclosure, in March 1985, that the Russians had succeeded in bugging a dozen typewriters in the US Embassy in Moscow, enabling them to eavesdrop electronically on letters ranging from routine memos to 'highly classified documents', for a year (White, 1985). Although technological advances have reduced the price of TEMPEST equipment, a shielded computer still costs more than twice an unshielded one, and it is estimated that US sales of TEMPEST equipment will exceed $1.5 billion for 1987, $10 billion in 1993 and possibly $19 billion in 1997 (*Microwave News*, 1987, May/June).

As the technology has developed, so electronic and electromagnetic surveillance systems have increased in sophistication. Intercepting microwave communications, which transmit phone calls by air rather than cable, is a relatively easy matter today, once armed with a receiving dish and knowledge of the channels and frequencies used. Large computers now monitor all international telephone calls and can be programmed to record conversations that contain selected words – such as, perhaps, Cruise, Soviet, IRA – and trace the calls. The United States has co-operated with the GCHQ station near Bude in Cornwall, as part of an Anglo-American agreement to monitor international private, commercial, military and diplomatic communications (Norton-Taylor, 1985). Very sensitive receivers can now pick up radiation from telephone calls and computers, even from within mobile vans (Witherow, 1986). Although this would give a listener only one side of the conversation, it emphasises the importance of TEMPEST-like screening where sensitive information is discussed by phone. As if that were not enough, laser devices focussed on a window or picture glass from up to a quarter of a mile away can detect the tiny vibrations caused by voices in the room; these can then be converted into transcripts of the conversations.

Users of car phones in Britain were recently warned that such communication could not be considered secure (Dawe, 1988). More sinister, however, are the phone-tapping possibilities offered by the new, computer-run telephone exchange, System X, now being introduced by British Telecom. According to a recent book (Fitzgerald and Leopold, 1987), one of whose authors is an ex-BT engineer, System X, developed by Plessey, who produce very sophisticated monitoring equipment for the MoD, will permit the monitoring of individual calls secretly and more easily through the use of voice and speech recognition. Moreover, since the 1985 Interception of Communcations Act does not cover 'automatic call tracing' provided by System X, there are virtually no legal safeguards. Whereas traditional phone-tapping involves a physical interference with the line at some point, System X uses digital signals the tapping of which leaves no physical presence anywhere and 'no discernible changes to the telephone circuit being tapped'. Thus, calls can be stored for later analysis and details on who called whom will be constantly and forever available. As the authors point out, all BT employees have to sign the Official Secrets Act, and BT now plays a 'vital integral role within the British Intelligence complex'. To get the tribunal that monitors phone-tapping in the UK to investigate whether a tap has been wrongly authorised, one must first be aware the tap has taken place; under System X this appears to be very difficult, if not impossible, to ascertain. According to a recent report (Hyder, 1988), a huge increase in phone tapping in the UK has taken place in the last decade, now totalling 30,000 taps each year at a cost of £10 million, without the knowledge or consent of Parliament.

But such possible surveillance pales in comparison with the information it is now possible to gather from spy satellites. From beneath the Pentagon in Washington, the National Reconnaissance Office (NRO), highly secret and bigger than the CIA, with an estimated budget of more than $2000 million, apparently controls America's fleet of spy satellites – 'apparently' because officially it does not exist; those who work for it are described as 'non-persons', their work 'black', that is, it must never be talked about (Lowther, 1986). According to a *YOU Magazine* report, it has offices and field stations in Britain and shares much of its 'reconnaissance' with MI5, though it apparently seeks permission before spying on friends, for example, before it photographed 30,000 Greenham Common women circling the base in 1983. Although Britain has abandoned the spy satellite it was to develop under its controversial Project Zircon, it is apparently still concerned to develop a replacement in order not to have to rely totally on the Americans, who are thought to filter some of the information that they relay to Britain.

The Russians, it is thought, have more spy satellites than the Americans and, though possibly not as advanced, are believed to be catching up fast. Thus each superpower is able to monitor the smallest details of the other's economic and military developments, from the state of the grain harvests and road construction to the opening of new missile silos and troop and ship movements. The US has more than 60 such satellites, of which the KH-11 (Keyhole) is the most sophisticated (Lowther, 1986). It orbits at an altitude of between 170 and 320 miles and sends back almost instant pictures. These, however, are not as good as those taken by 'Big Bird' which operates at between 103 and 167 miles up but drops its film by parachute every few days near Hawaii where it is picked up by aircraft. The third type of satellite, the KH-8, also drops its film by parachute and can descend to as low as 70 miles to get the best pictures, which can include detail down to newspaper headlines. Other satellites, known as 'ferrets', monitor radio, radar, and long-distance telephone traffic, as well as communications between other satellites and rockets in space (Evans, 1987). Indeed, the increasing distribution of high resolution, civil satellite photographs, for example from the French Earth remote sensing satellite, Spot, are causing concern among military experts due to their ability to reveal secret military sites (Lacoste, 1987). According to a recent book (Burrows, 1987), a new family of satellites now on US drawing boards will be able to hear and see everything important to Western security (and a few other things besides) everywhere on earth and in space, day and night, whatever the weather. Big Brother, it seems, has gone global and never sleeps.

These electronic 'eyes' and 'ears' of the Pentagon would, of course, be vital in the event of President Bush's Strategic Defense Initiative (SDI), popularly known as the 'Star Wars' programme, ever having to be activated. Research on this space-based, missile defense system is now well underway in both the USA and Britain, prompting concern over the possible health hazards of exposure to weapon systems using high-power, pulsed microwave or millimetre-wave radiation. As a result, the Walter Reed Army Institute of Research (WRAIR) is now carrying out research using two different high-power pulsed sources: two 200-million-watt

(MW), peak power units operating in the 2.5–3.0 GHz range, and a 10 MW peak power unit at 10 GHz (*Microwave News*, 1986, May/June). The Air Force School of Aerospace Medicine at Brooks Air Force Base, Texas, has already funded various research contracts, including one by Drs Om Gandhi and Abbas Riazi at the University of Utah, who have produced a paper, 'Absorption of Millimeter Waves by Human Beings and its Biological Implications'. The researchers apparently conclude that one of the problems associated with irradiation in the millimetre-wave frequency band is 'extremely high superficial SARs even for incident power densities of 5–10 mW/cm^2 recommended as safety guidelines' (*Microwave News*, 1986, May/June). They also strongly urged continued study of any ocular effects.

As to exactly how microwaves might be used in the Star Wars programme, a recent special report states that they are unlikely to be used as a 'hard-kill' weapon, more probably as a 'hard-jam' weapon to burn out the electronics of missiles, aircraft and radar (*Microwave News*, 1986, May/June). A further report claims that this has already been achieved by the Russians who have used high-power 'ground-to-space' microwaves to disable US reconnaissance satellites on more than one occasion, allegedly from a ground station near the Afghan border (*Microwave News*, 1986, November/December).

A classified briefing on the 'Possibility of a Soviet RF Weapon Program' was one of more than 70 papers and 100 posters presented at the '3rd National Conference on High-Power Microwave Technology for Defense Applications' held at Kirkland Air Force Base in New Mexico in December 1986, attended by some 600 scientists with special security clearance (*Microwave News*, 1987, January/February). Many branches of the DoD, as well as the SDI office, presented their high-power microwave weapons programmes to industry representatives. One session covered biological effects, with presentations of results by Army, Navy and Air Force representatives, as well as some university-based research.

Recent reports of Russian plans to exploit space by beaming solar power to Earth from orbiting platforms have raised suspicions that the main purpose is in fact military. UK astronomers Graham Smith and Lovell (1987) point out that the expected power density from such an infra-red beam at its collector site on Earth is likely to be 'orders of magnitude' greater than even the presently accepted safe limits for NIR. The population around each collector would need to be protected by a safety zone, whose effectiveness would depend on maintaining the beam's direction from the satellite to an angular accuracy of better than a 1000th of a degree. The weapon potential of such a beam thus becomes obvious. It also raises concern about the possible hazards from the far weaker but more widespread and chronic exposure of Europeans from 24-hour satellite TV broadcasts.

The possibility that the Soviet Union might be ahead of the USA in EM weapon systems has persisted at least since the discovery of the irradiation of the US Moscow Embassy in 1953. Such a fear was further boosted with the detection of a strange signal that first appeared on the air in July 1976, disrupting shortwave transmissions around the world, and which has persisted ever since. Nicknamed the 'Woodpecker', due to its very pronounced pulse repetition rate of 10 per second (i.e. pulse-modulated at 10 Hz), it emits a peak estimated power of 14 million watts per pulse at frequencies between 3.26 and 17.54 MHz, making it the most powerful, man-made non-ionising radiation ever broadcast. And its origin? According to one source (Becker and Selden, 1985), seven immensely powerful transmitters somewhere near Kiev in the Soviet Ukraine. The location is only some 20 miles from Chernobyl, giving the Soviet Union the dubious distinction of producing the largest man-made sources of both ionizing and non-ionizing radiation in the world. (Exactly what synergistic or reactor operator behavioural effects such close proximity may produce from interaction of the two types of radiation has yet to be determined, although one Soviet study of such synergism has found that NIR exacerbates the effects of ionising radiation (Tumanyan and Samoilenko, 1983).

The Woodpecker signal is so strong it can be picked up on a shortwave radio without the need of an aerial, and obliterates anything else on its wavelength. It is being broadcast all over North America, the UK, Western Europe, Australasia and the Middle East – but not in the USSR. It permeates everything and is re-radiated into homes via the power-lines of a country's national grid. According to Dr Robert Beck, a Los Angeles physicist and former member of an exclusive group of scientists recruited by the US Government to work on EM weapon possibilities, the signal has three likely functions: it may act as a somewhat crude over-the-horizon radar that could alert the Soviets to an American attack, if their spy satellites were disabled; it may act as a submarine communication system, since the signal is modulated in the ELF range; or its aim may be to affect the target populations psychologically and biologically (Becker and Selden, 1985). To many, including Dr Beck, the last is the most likely major aim. The signal certainly falls in the range known to have effects on animals and could well be psychoactive in man since 10 Hz is the top end of the frequency range of the brain's alpha rhythm. In addition, it generates a magnetic component that, according to Dr Beck, can penetrate anything – salt water, shielded rooms, etc. 'It's highly likely that this thing is causing neurological changes in certain people who are sensitive to this type of energy. ... Perhaps 30 per cent of the gross population can have neuronal alteration because of the presence of this particular electromagnetic interference' (Central TV, 1984). Dr Robert Becker, a researcher of long experience who was once funded by the Navy until his results drove them to withdraw, offers tantalising support for this view:

> Within a year or two after the Woodpecker began tapping, there were persistent complaints of unaccountable symptoms from people in several cities of the United States and Canada, primarily Eugene, Oregon. The sensations – pressure and pain in the head, anxiety, fatigue, insomnia, lack of coordination, and numbness, accompanied by a high-pitched ringing in the ears – were characteristic of strong radio-frequency or microwave irradiation. In Oregon, between Eugene and Corvallis, a powerful radio signal centering on 4,75 megahertz was monitored, at higher levels in the air than on the ground ... most engineers who studied the signal concluded that it was a manifestation of the Woodpecker. (Becker and Selden, 1985, p. 324).

Becker goes on to point out that Dr Ross Adey's research (Dr Adey, at Loma Linda Veterans Administration Hospital in California, is currently an advisor to the White House on EMR) suggests that the best method of getting an ELF signal into an animal is to make it a pulse modulation of a high-frequency field – which is exactly what the Woodpecker is. According to Becker, radiologist Raymond Damadian, who patented the first NMR scanner, has theorised that the Woodpecker signal is designed to produce nuclear magnetic resonance in human tissue, something which, on a chronic exposure basis, could considerably magnify the metabolic interference of electropollution or EMR weapons (Becker and Selden, 1985). Becker states that the pulse frequency that would be required to achieve this with the Woodpecker's signal range has been calculated as a band centred on 10 Hz – the frequency of the human alpha rhythm. He concludes:

> The available evidence, then, suggests that the Russian Woodpecker is a multipurpose radiation that combines a submarine link with an experimental attack on the American people. It may be intended to increase cancer rates, interfere with decision-making ability, and/or sow confusion and irritation. (Becker and Selden, 1985, p. 324).

He also admits to hearing persistent rumours that the USA has erected transmitters to neutralise the Soviet signal and to irradiate the Russian population in a similar way. If true, an electromagnetic war between East and West has been waging for perhaps a decade.

Although naturally thinking of his own countrymen, Becker might also have mentioned the other 17 countries in which the Woodpecker can be picked up, according to a report on its interference distributed at the 1987 World Administrative Radio Conference for High Frequency Broadcasting in Geneva in February 1987 (*Microwave News*, 1987, January/February). The Association of North American Radio Clubs' Woodpecker Project co-ordinated 97 short-wave listeners in 18 countries, and the report analyses the Woodpecker's transmission patterns and interference on broadcasting stations, as well as recommending that the conference pass a resolution condemning such interference. Judging by their past behaviour, the Russians are unlikely to take much notice; perhaps 'Glasnost' will improve matters.

With the atmospheric and other nuclear weapons testing in the 1950s and 1960s came the recognition that one of the chief threats in any nuclear war would be the immense electromagnetic pulse (EMP) of radiant energy – as much as 50,000 volts – that would be generated by a nuclear explosion, particularly one high in the atmosphere, which could knock out all electronic communications and computer systems over an entire continent. The potential damage from EMP spurred the US Air Force to develop a multi-million dollar testing programme to simulate EMP in order to determine its effect on the warheads and control systems of America's then 1000-odd Minutement ICBMs in underground silos (Brodeur, 1977). Brodeur (1977) recounts how the Air Force carried out extensive EMP tests on missile sites using both ground-based pulse generators as well as huge pulsers (known as 'big zappers') carried by helicopters. He also describes how the three branches of the Armed Forces, as well as NIOSH scientists, systematically delayed the setting up of safety guidelines to control the exposure of EMP radiation to those working on the systems, despite the occurrence of leukaemia and other cancers being reported in such servicemen in their early 30s and 40s (Brodeur, 1977).

As this situation persisted into the 1970s the only research carried out was by the DoD, who were in no hurry to set exposure standards for one very clear reason: they had realised the potential use of EMP as a weapon and were busy developing highly classified projects aimed at perfecting the use of EMP against nuclear ballistic missiles – the forerunners of those envisioned for the Star Wars programme. These included high-energy pulse weapons, charged-particle beam devices, and high-energy lasers. (The USAF's latest microwave device can produce more than 1 GW of power in short pulses, while a recent technique of heating the Earth's atmosphere with radiation in the 20–1800 kHz frequency could cause 'total disruption of communicatons over a large portion of the earth' (*Microwave News*, 1988, May/June).

By this time each armed service had their own EMP test facilities, which they continue to use today. The US Navy's system – EMPRESS

(Electromagnetic Pulse Radiation Environment Simulator for Ships) – was erected on the Patuxent River at Solomons, Maryland in 1972 and is capable of putting out a maximum pulse of 2½ million volts. But the Navy now wishes to replace it with EMPRESS II, which would be able to produce a maximum pulse of 7 million volts, with a pulsed electric field of 50 kV/m at 100 yards every 30 minutes. However, its proposed location – on Chesapeake Bay, Maryland – is meeting with fierce opposition from local inhabitants, pilots, Congressmen and Senators (*Microwave News*, 1987, January/February). Biologists and environmentalists have claimed that even the Navy's 'Supplemental Draft Environmental Impact Statement' (SDEIS), published in December 1986, is inadequate in its reported research and that long-term studies are needed.

Also omitted from the SDEIS is discussion of unintended EM ignition of nuclear ordnance and other explosive materials by stray EMR, ESD, or lightning – described together under the acronym HERO effects ('Hazards of Electromagnetic Radiation to Ordnance') – whereas a researcher of such effects has warned of the 'extraordinary risk of weapon accidents' in the surrounding bay communities (*Microwave News*, 1987, January/February). Patricia Axelrod, from Key West, Florida, who spent two years researching HERO accidents and risks, claims that at least 25 HERO accidents have occurred over the last 30 years (*Microwave News*, 1987, September/October), one of the best known accidents, attributed to electrostatic discharge (ESD), being the 1985 fire at a West German Pershing II missile site, which killed three servicemen and injured 16 others. Axelrod (who claims she is being investigated by the US Naval Investigative Service), and others are currently involved in a lawsuit to stop the DoD from using electro-explosive devices until detailed EISs on their siting near population centres are completed (*Microwave News*, 1987, September/October).

Other experts have warned that an EMP could cause false trips at a local nuclear power station only 20 miles from the proposed Chesapeake Bay site, with the potential to lead to a core meltdown in a worst-case scenario. Maryland's House of Delegates has joined with other objectors to block the Navy's intentions, while the EPA has also criticised their SDEIS, suggesting they relocate elsewhere. (One proposal by the Navy is Guantanamo Bay in Cuba!) Meanwhile, a lawsuit by a Washington-based environmental group has succeeded in forcing the DoD to shut down many of its EMP simulators pending completion of full EISs (*Microwave News*, 1988, May/June). And the US Senate has extended a ban on the DoD using EMPRESS II in Chesapeake Bay until the environmental and social costs have been fully investigated.

A further defence system in the USA that is arousing public concern is the proposed Ground Wave Emergency Network (GWEN). This refers to a communication system to withstand the EMP of a nuclear attack for which the military proposed to build 125 or more relay towers, operating at 150–175 kHz, at 150 to 200 mile intervals across the USA (*Microwave News*, 1987, January/February). The USAF has adopted a 50 V/m exposure standard for populations near GWEN transmitter sites but the proposals continue to meet with strong public opposition. Opponents have succeeded in some States in requiring the USAF to provide separate EISs for each site; many fear such sites will become the targets of nuclear attacks. Scheduled to be completed in 1989, the GWEN system will consist of 125 (some say many more) VLF relay nodes across the continental USA and a total of 400 receive and transmit stations (*Microwave News*, 1980, May/June).

All such defence and attack systems are, of course, almost totally controlled by vast computer networks, due to their complexity and need for speed of response. Recently, however, computer experts have realised that such networks are extremely vulnerable to a potentially devastating new threat – a 'virus' in one of the programs. This refers to a destructive electronic code inserted into a computer program by a secret agent, terrorist or even white-collar criminal. Both the USA's military computer nets and its highly automated banking system are vulnerable to 'catastrophic collapse', according to a Georgetown University report (Hanson, 1986). Indeed, in 1983 computer faults in US defence computers led to two false alarms of impending missile attacks every three days (Witherow, 1987). Soviet defence scientists are also very aware of the frightening possibilities; and at a private meeting of Nato computer experts in 1987 a consensus was reached that 'computer-aided disasters', due to design faults in military microchips, were 'inevitable' (Matthews, 1988). Dr John Collyer, of the MoD's Royal Signals and Radar establishment, is quoted as saying: 'Some time between 1991 and 1992 computers will start to kill human beings in a way that will be noticed by others.' He listed power stations, civilian aircraft and hi-tech cars as potential sites. Counter-measures are at last, however, being taken and a new Viper chip that can be proved mathematically to be free of design faults is attracting much interest among British organisations. However, such developments are still too novel radically to alter the situation in the short term and led a 1988 University of Lancaster report to conclude that nuclear war is now more likely by accident than design (Smoker, 1988). Perhaps recent breakthroughs in US and Soviet arms reduction agreements have more to do with the mutually recognised threat from computer-aided and HERO disasters to both world peace, and the nuclear industry in general, than is generally appreciated.

As the problem of EM interference (EMI) with military systems has increasingly been appreciated, the need for EM compatibility (EMC) between different electronic and computer systems has also become of vital concern to modern armed forces. A recent, devastating example of what can happen when EMC is overlooked or compromised is provided by the fate of HMS *Sheffield* during the 1982 Falklands War between Britain and Argentina. The destroyer was sunk by an Exocet missile because radar and electronic countermeasures that could have protected it were temporarily switched off by the operation of the ship's satellite communications systems (*Microwave News*, 1986, May/June). The Ministry of Defence confirmed a *Daily Mirror* story in May 1986 that a captain's telephone call had rendered the *Sheffield*'s anti-missile radar system useless, automatically blotting out the specific radar frequencies used by the Exocet. The Navy has now taken steps to ensure that such an incident does not recur, said the MoD. Easton, a US company with a UK subsidiary, makes EMC test rigs for the MoD. Such rigs cost about £500,000. Because modern planes 'fly by wire', i.e. by computer, the test procedure has to be very strict since the pilot is virtually powerless if the electronics fail.

In the USA, the US Air Force currently appears to have an EMC problem with their B-1 bomber, whose radar-jamming and radar-monitoring systems are incompatible (*Microwave News*, 1987, January/February). In 1984 the crash of a German Air Force Tornado is believed to have been due to interference with the aircraft's electronics after it flew too close to the high-power Radio Free Europe transmitter near Munich (*New Scientist*, 1984). How many civil aircraft crashes may have been due to some form of EMI may never be known but it is unlikely that none have been the result of this problem.

For the modern army, Marconi has developed the 'Isolator' shelter, which can shield sensitive battlefield computing and communications systems from EMI and EMP, as well as electronic eavesdropping. Up to 40 feet long, the Isolator is built as a sealed box from aluminium-faced panels, with metal-to-metal contact all around so that any EMI flows round and round the walls and does not enter the shelter (Williams, 1985). The military is also increasingly using fibre optics because of its resistance to EMP.

But the military is not the only business worried about EMI. The motor industry is increasingly building cars dependent on computer control or monitoring for many functions, making them vulnerable to EMI. One German manufacturer found that two prototypes failed at exactly the same spot on the motorway, which remained a mystery until it was found that it lay in the path of a local radio transmitter which was saturating the area (*New Scientist*, 1984). The potential hazards of cars and trucks that 'drive by wire' failing, at speed, on a motorway due to EMI is only just beginning to be appreciated by motor manufacturers and motoring safety associations. As yet they are unaware of the possibility of EMI from people (see Chapter 6) interfering with vehicle functioning. The average member of the public is still largely ignorant of the potential disasters built into his brand new piece of electronic wizardry on wheels. One further problem is that, whereas commercial broadcast transmitters and radar are fairly easy to locate and their whereabouts known, the locations of military microwave and other transmission systems are nearly always kept secret.

Secret or not, radiation from any microwave or radar source can be detected if one has the right equipment. Where that 'equipment' is mainly the human body, it is not so easy to know exactly what is happening. Since late 1985 the women at the peace camp at the American Air Force Base at Greenham Common in Berkshire have claimed that they are being irradiated from the base because of a range of symptoms that they have been unable to link to any other source (*Electronics Today*, 1985), In 1983 and early 1984 there was a very large military and police presence at the base when the Cruise missiles arrived. But, suddenly, around mid-1984 this presence had diminished considerably; a little later the symptoms began to appear. A report by Dr Rosalie Bertell, Commissioner for the International Commission of Health Professionals for Health and Human Rights, based in Toronto, details the violent treatment of the women by the police and others and lists the strange symptoms they have experienced: these range from skin burns, 'severe headaches, drowsiness, menstrual bleeding at abnormal times or postmenopausal, to bouts of temporary paralysis, faulty speech coordination and in one case apparent circulatory failure requiring hospitalization. There were two late (five month) spontaneous abortions' (Bertell, 1986). Contrary to the usual synchronisation of menstrual cycles that normally occurs in a community of women and which had occurred until then, their cycles from mid-1984 became highly irregular. Such a complex of symptoms fits well with EM exposure syndrome, according to Dr Robert Becker (Becker, 1987). Measurements have been taken around the base by members of Electronics for Peace using a wide range signal strength meter which showed significant signals up to 100 times the background level at one of the women's camps at a time they claimed to be experiencing ill effects. When the women created a disturbance near the fence, the signal rose sharply. Doctors from the Medical Campaign Against Nuclear Weapons, led by Dr Stephen Farrow, senior lecturer in epidemiology at University College of Wales Medical College, are compiling a report on the condition of those women whose symptoms are consistent with receiving NIR exposure (Parry, 1986). So far the MoD, who are responsible for security at the base, has denied that any form of electronic signal is being used against the women, but has not denied that an electromagnetic signal may be being used which, if below $10\,\text{mW}/\text{cm}^2$, would not, under current UK guidelines, be officially acknowledged as harmful. (MoD, 1989.)

Unfortunately, a precedent for deliberate peacetime exposure of fellow countrymen and women to noxious radiation by military or other authorities does exist. A chilling report by a subcommittee of the US House of Representatives details many experiments between 1945 and 1971 in which people, who had no hope of benefitting, were exposed to potentially toxic doses of radioactivity merely to satisfy scientific curiosity (US House of Representatives, 1986). Some had given 'informed consent' but whether they had been fully informed about the dangers of ionising radiation is doubtful. Those not given the option of consent were prisoners and hospital patients, including the mentally and terminally ill. Two examples illustrate the type of experiments carried out.

In one study over 100 Washington and Oregon state prisoners, between 1963 and 1971, had their testicles irradiated to discover what doses would sterilise them. The Atomic Energy Commission funded the projects at a cost of $1.5 million. No long-term follow-up occurred to guard against the risk of testicular cancers. In another study, from 1945 to 1947, 18 hospital patients, one of then five years old, and all with a short life expectancy, were injected with plutonium to measure how much the body would retain. The injections were represented as experimental treatments for the patients' illnesses. The subjects were given between 1.6 and 98 times the then permissible occupational dose. Many of the original diagnoses were later found to be inaccurate. The one redeeming feature of this appalling scandal, as the *British Medical Journal* reviewer Professor Hamblin points out, is that the United States has let such information become available; in many other countries it would remain an official secret (Hamblin, 1987).

A further example of blatant (ionising) irradiation of innocent people for military purposes is the continued French nuclear testing on Muroroa Atoll near Tahiti in the South Pacific. A total of 127 atmospheric and underground tests have been carried out there by the French since 1956. As a recent documentry by ITV and Television New Zealand (1987) showed, this has been paralleled by a growing incidence of cancers among the indigenous population and Polynesian workers at the base, who complain of receiving less protective clothing and inadequate medical checks compared to the French military personnel. Despite local and international protest the French continue to carry out tests, rejecting the evidence of harm to the people of the surrounding islands (which just happen to be some of the most beautiful in the world), while at the same time denying access to their own cancer data. A comprehensive account of the saga is given in a book by Swedish diplomat Bengt Danielsson (1986) and his wife. The environmental group Greenpeace have experienced at first hand French displeasure at their physical attempts to disrupt their nuclear testing. Not only did the French sink Greenpeace's *Rainbow Warrior* inside another country's territorial waters (Auckland harbour), but added insult to injury by recently returning, prematurely, to France those who had been convicted and sentenced to incarceration on a French atoll, despite the enraged protests of the New Zealand Government. One wonders if military research into non-ionising radiation weapons will ever engender such attempted interference, rejection and retaliation.

A further reason for believing that the Greenham women have in fact been irradiated is that the American military and police have certain frequency weapons that have been used for the control of crowds as well as individuals. Such equipment, listed in Dr Bertell's report, includes the Photic Driver, a glorified strobe light which emits pulses in the critical flashing range of 10–30 Hz; the Valkyrie, which enhances the effects of the Driver with sound pulses in the 4 to 7.5 Hz range; and the Squawk Box or Sound Curdler, used in Vietnam, and now used as a 'People Repeller' producing an output of about 350 watts. These were also listed in Manchester City Council's Police Monitoring Unit document (January, 1986) and are detailed in a general report on the Greenham Common irradiation claim by former radar engineer Kim Besly (1986). Until 1983 the Valkyrie was advertised in the British Defence Equipment Catalogue. However, the compilers apparently stated that it and similar frequency weapons were cut out of the catalogue after 1983 at the request of the British Ministry of Defence.

The US military also has an intruder detection system called BISS (Base Installation Security System) which operates by bouncing high frequency radar waves off a human body as it moved around a perimeter fence. The MoD acquired a similar British system in April 1984, though whether it has been installed at Greenham Common is unknown (Parry, 1986).

Recent revelations about the activities of the military and secret service establishments in Britain do not help to inspire confidence in the MoD's denial of any irradiation, especially in the face of the contrary evidence. When it is known that both American and British Governments sought out and used former Nazi scientists after the War, that the US military covered up the fact that their own soldiers were subjected to appalling experiments by Japanese 'doctors' during the last war (Williams and Wallace, 1989), and that certain elements in MI5 apparently sought to de-stabilise Harold Wilson's Government in the 1960s, as alleged by newspaper reports of ex-MI5 officer Peter Wright's book *Spycatcher*, it is perhaps not unjustified to be somewhat sceptical of the MoD's denials. It is conceivable that the Americans carried out such irradiation without telling the British MoD, but this is unlikely, given the huge embarrassment this would cause if revealed. The fact that nearly all the protestors are women whereas all the military personnel are men only adds another unpleasant dimension to the whole episode, which is underlined in the violence meted out to the women. Is this a case of personality changes being induced by NIR in the aggressors? Clearly, one may agree or disagree with the women's politics but attempting to control or dissuade them – or any other protest group – with harmful NIR has no place in a democratic state.

A recent report indicates that the MoD funds some 750 research projects at British universities and polytechnics (CAMROC, 1988). How many of these are exploring NIR effects is unknown. A team at York University's Physics Department, for example, has built and tested a 'Faraday magnetometer' under contract to GCHQ, to pick up very weak magnetic fields, possibly for use in remote eavesdropping (*The Times*, 1988). Another project, funded with $120,000 by the US Air Force, is research by Professor Edward Grant at King's College, London, on the effects of microwaves on human DNA (Chomet, 1986). Microwaves are, of course, used extensively in military communication systems. Grant and his colleagues (1987) recently failed to replicate experiments showing that aqueous solutions of DNA can absorb microwaves in the 1–10 GHz frequency band. Grant was unable to confirm any resonances or any form of enhanced absorption, as reported by US researchers, such as Dr Mays Swicord of the FDA in Rockville, Maryland, although others have suggested reasons for the failure (*Microwave News*, 1987, July/August). Grant is now looking at frequencies in the kHz range using frozen DNA, while others in the US are studying the biological significance of such possible resonances. Much of the US work on DNA absorption is being funded by the US Navy, while British and Swedish work is being paid for by the US Air Force. If it is confirmed that DNA does absorb microwaves significantly at certain frequencies, it will have profound effects on military operations.

Such university-based military research is not without its critics; Professor Steven Rose, Director of the Brain Research Group at the Open University, proposes a ban on all such research at British universities to prevent their 'creeping militarization', pointing out that in Britain 53 per cent of all scientific R and D money is spent on military research compared with less than 5 per cent in Japan (*The Times*, 1988).

The USA recently provided an example of how ordinary research, funded by other bodies, can be commandeered by the military. Chemists led by Dr Robert Birge (1987) at Carnegie-Mellon University, in Pittsburg, recently identified a family of compounds, retinyl Schiff base salts, similar to rhodopsin – the molecule basically responsible for vision –

which is capable of absorbing specific frequencies of RF and MW radiation (*Microwave News*, 1987, September/October). The potential implications and applications are huge and may help in comprehending a mechanism for frequency-specific biological effects, especially those in the eye, for example those claimed for MW radiation in cataract formation by Dr Zaret (see Chapter 9). However, they also promise to revolutionise the ability to make aircraft and other military hardware invisible to radar more effectively than present 'Stealth' technology. Once Birge realised that it should be possible to modify the salts so that they could absorb over the entire RF range, the military moved in and has shrouded his work in secrecy, being now classified along with other 'Stealth' research.

In the UK the 1987 Crown Proceedings (Armed Forces) Act has replaced Section 10 of the Crown Proceedings Act 1947 and finally gives servicemen the right to sue the MoD for injury or death incurred by other personnel while on duty. The Act was passed mainly as a result of the call for justice for the 20,000-odd British servicemen who were exposed to ionising radiation when they took part in the atomic testing in the Pacific and South Australia in the 1950s, although the Government has refused to make the Act retroactive which would have enabled many of them to seek compensation. However, members of the British Nuclear Test Veterans' Association are encouraged by a recently won test case giving one of their members the right to sue the Government for damages for cancer allegedly contracted while on such service.

Whatever the success of these cases, judging by the settlements achieved for American servicemen (usually out of court) mainly through the work of groups such as the Radar Victims Network and evidence linking cancer mortality and Air Force bases (Lester and Moore, 1982, 1985) (see Chapter 9), the new Act is likely shortly to produce the first case for damages brought by a British serviceman for health effects caused by NIR during service. And in the USA there is now a federal law which requires employers to give their employees details (and not misinformation) about hazards to which they may be exposed. (How long before a similar law is passed in Britain – or the EEC?) If this applies to military employers, the American military now faces the most profound quandary since the Russians first started irradiating the US Embassy in Moscow (recently reported to have re-occurred in early 1988) over what they must now tell their personnel about the hazards of non-ionising radiation.

CHAPTER 11

Old wisdom, new understanding

We must see to it that enthusiasm for the future does not give rise to contempt for the past.

Pope Paul VI (1898–1978)

The dowser, ancient trackways and stones

The best documented sixth-sense of man, ancient and modern, is the reflex of the dowser. The technique was probably known in neolithic times and certainly known in Ancient Egypt. The first reference to it in European literature dates from AD 1240, and reference to dowsing is to be found in Agricola's *De Re Metallica* of 1556. In 1639, Gabriel Platts described dowsing in the book, *Discovery of Subterranean Treasure*. In 1693, the Jesuit priest, Fr Le Lorrain, SJ, who was the Abbé de Vallemont and also the Professor of Physics at the College of Louis le Grand, described how 'the rod moves', when he placed a piece of lodestone (magnetic iron oxide) before a well-known dowser (Le Lorrain, 1693). This was published some 80 years before the polemic arose between Mesmer and another Jesuit, Fr Hell, SJ, which has already been referred to in Chapter 1. Clearly, the latter could have been aware of Fr Le Lorrain's writings through the libraries and traditions within his religious order.

> The controversy of the dowsers versus the scientific world is such that accounts of such experiences are practically excluded from the scientific literature. To find them, one must have the courage to explore the so-called (sic) literature of the dowsers and attempt to read it with a critical mind.

So wrote Rocard (1964) of the problems that dowsers have in getting a fair hearing from the scientists. There are those dowsers who do not feel any need to try to convince scientists of what to them is obvious. It is well known that Uri Geller engaged in financially highly rewarding prospecting activities in various parts of the world; these he described in a book by himself and Guy Playfair (Geller and Playfair, 1986).

One of the rare accounts of dowsing in modern scientific terms is to be found in the first of two volumes edited by Madeleine Barnothy (1964, 1969). These set out to 'bring together all the active fields of biomagnetic research and at the same time to provide a theoretical and practical background to all scientists who wish to engage in investigations'. Rocard (1964), describing the limiting sensitivity of dowsers to magnetic fields, reports that a dowser walking with uniform speed at his normal rate of about 1 m/s and with his rod in the dowsing position, has his reflex started when he moves through a region where the Earth's magnetic field has an anomaly giving a field gradient of 30 to 50 nT/m; there is a latency period or time lag of the order of 1 second before the dowsing reflex is observed. If the gradient increases to 200 or 300 nT/m, the detection becomes more accurate; if it falls below 10 nT/m, the detection is wholly inaccurate.

For a dowser moving at a much higher velocity than 1 m/s, for example in a plane or car, the dowsing reflex threshold is found to depend on the latency time rather than magnetic field gradient, so the relevant threshold is a time variation of magnetic field which exceeds 30 nT/s. This represents an induced voltage of 30 nV around the region through which the magnetic field is changing and is one millionth of the voltage necessary to trigger a nerve impulse. These values were determined by having the dowser walk near a large coil which could generate a controlled magnetic anomaly, but without the dowser knowing whether the current was on or off during any given trial. A strong, irresistible signal is only obtained if the dowser has to pass in succession two coils about 3 m apart; this lengthens the duration of the influence.

It appears that the dowser may not detect the still water in a pond nor the running water in a river, but can detect water filtering through porous media, and water in permeable layers adjacent to beds of clay. Rocard calculates that, from the effects of electrofiltration and of clay electrical potentials, magnetic gradients of 10 nT/m can be justified, but higher values would be very difficult. It is possible that dowsers detect a structuring in water layers or in water present as dampness in soil and stone rather than the water itself. Such water structuring is proposed to account for the clinical effects from diluted allergens and homoeopathic potencies (Smith *et al.*, 1985).

The dowser can be made to err by the presence of objects encased in iron which give anomalies of 200 to 300 nT/m, by certain rocks such as basalt which become magnetised after being struck by lightning, and by the reduction of non-magnetic iron oxides in the soil to a magnetic state, either by fire or organic decomposition.

Rocard considers that it is more difficult to determine the reality of a dowsing signal with a pendulum than a rod, but believes that both detect approximately the same magnetic gradient. Brown and Behrens (1985) describe in considerable detail how to go about pendulum testing and the various experimental conditions which assist or interfere. They have also extended the technique by using an electrically resonant antenna as a rod pendulum or on a thread, as the bob of a pendulum. They claim that these resonant devices enable radio and microwave transmissions as well as body radiations to be detected and their frequencies determined, and they give instructions for dowsing commercial transmissions and even police microwave radar speed trap guns.

While a pendulum of soft iron will circulate in front of any part of the body under stress, a rod of copper will only circulate in front of a part of the body under stress if it is supposedly resonant with emitted electromagnetic radiation. Brown and Behrens list frequencies calculated by assuming that the physical length of the resonant rod is one whole wavelength. The values obtained for substances compatible with the body come in the range 38 GHz to 78 GHz, and for stressed body organs and incompatible foods and other substances the resonances come in the range 8 GHz to 27 GHz (except for two very narrow bands near 15 GHz and 23 GHz which are reported to be compatible). Since they find that a calculation based on the whole length of the wire or rod pendulum gives the correct frequency for radio stations and radars, their method of suspending the rod must damp out the possible quarter-wave and half-wave resonances, unless these other possible modes are not detected for some reason.

An electrically sensitive allergy patient who was able to use a pendulum for dowsing was tested for electromagnetic sensitivities as described in Chapter 6. In this case it was possible to detect the patient's neutralising frequency by observing the reaction of a pendulum which the patient held. An interesting result was that the eye–hand link appeared to be necessary for this pendulum to function; it did not respond when the patient's eyes were closed. When demonstrating the electrical provocation and neutralisation of an allergic reaction (Rea et al., 1986) during a workshop session at a conference, some participants reported afterwards that their own pendulums had reacted as the electrical oscillator was adjusted in frequency.

Dr Smith and his students found that about one-third of a group of persons tested could sense a steady magnetic field as a change in the feel or texture of a surface (a rubber diaphragm is the sensor in de la Warr apparatus). The threshold was at about 700 µT (7 Gauss or 14 times the strength of the Earth's magnetic field) for a half (50 percentile) of those who could sense magnetic fields by touch; but there was also a latent period of 20 seconds (at threshold) before the effect appeared. This field is stronger than most magnetic fields to be found in the natural environment, with the exception of lodestone, metallic iron and steel. However, it is necessary to stroke the magnetic surface to be able to feel its texture; this motion of the hand is like the walking of the dowser and it puts the threshold for this effect at the same rate of change of magnetic field as the dowsing threshold. It is interesting to note that researchers who published the results of experiments which failed to find any evidence of 60 Hz magnetic field perception, had programmed their computer to 'time out' a subject who had failed to make any choice between 'field present' and 'no field' states for 10 seconds, after which a new trial was automatically started (Tucker and Schmitt, 1978).

The above is about as far as one can go using measurements to try to examine what magnetic senses ancient man must have possessed. From now on it is necessary to become one of A.J.P. Taylor's (1967) 'literary artists'.

Tom Graves (1978, 1986), in a well referenced book, demonstrates how dowsers can detect some form of natural energy pattern associated with ley lines and megalithic stones, barrows and pre-Reformation churches. He starts from the work of Alfred Watkins and Guy Underwood and builds a comprehensive picture of the Earth's energy patterns as detected by the dowser. He appreciates that there is a hen-and-egg problem in determining which came first, the energy patterns or the structures built there? The patterns are classified according to the strengths of signal detected by dowsers and the nature of the parallel groupings of the line patterns. The strongest groupings are termed 'water-lines'; the so-called 'track-lines' and 'aquastats' are more weakly grouped. There also seems to be evidence of complicated spiral patterns (Brooker, 1983); these could function as resonators and antennae if they happen to be regions of high electrical conductivity or dielectric constant (Lakhovsky, 1939).

Since it appears that human beings can emit electromagnetic signals which can affect water, some of these patterns detected by dowsers could be made by people. Graves mentions recent work showing that the patterns found by dowsers extend to other types of 'site' including: crosses; crossroads and junctions; 'heel-stones' in roadways; local boundaries and field divisions, which were perhaps marked out and reinforced by the annual Rogation-tide processions; stocks; gallows, perhaps reinforced by 'necrotic radiation' (see Chapter 12); pre-Reformation churches, many of which are orientated according to the magnetic meridian at the declination appropriate to the year of building (Searle, 1974).

The dowsing reaction has an element of individuality. Graves notes that in the case of churches, one person reports that two or more dowsable 'streams' cross over each other at different depths directly beneath the high altar; another person describes their dowsing reaction as if there were 'domes' of rising water beneath the church altars, fonts, chancel steps and doors – all these are sites of past human activity, stress and emotion.

From the scientific point of view, one must be a 'fly on the wall', remembering, with Alice in Wonderland's caterpillar, that words mean what their users want them to mean – no more, no less. However, it is possible for most persons to learn the techniques of dowsing with some degree of sensitivity. Cyril Smith gratefully acknowledges a day in Germany during which an engineer, Hubert Riesch, taught him how to dowse using previously mapped out dowsable features in the car park of the Benedictine Monastery and Abbey Church of St Ottilien, near Munich. One of the monks there, Pater Frumentius Renner, has investigated the effects of local geopathic stress on the perceived quality of the organ music in the Abbey Church. We discussed the relation of cracks which had appeared in the walls of one of the newer monastery cloisters to geopathic stress lines, and noted that there were strong, well defined and highly localised stress lines between regions of canker on certain trees around the car park.

Attributes of flow are given to the 'lines' which a dowser picks up. This seems to be figurative in respect of the bulk motion of water, which is reportedly not usually detected by dowsing, but there is experimental evidence that these 'streams' can be physically redirected, using techniques available to dowsers. The concepts of streams seem closer to electromagnetic conduction of energy along a line of structured water (perhaps a water-helix) than to the flow of water in bulk. The early theories of electricity and magnetism invoked models of fluid flow, hence the term 'flux'. Venceslav Palnovsky (1986), of Prague, has found that he can detect dowsable water veins by measuring the fading of ultra-short-wave radio transmission (5–15 cm wavelength) on a commercial receiver. He concludes that the dowser is a source of electromagnetic radiation in this region and detects its reflection back from underground anomalies, or the disturbances in the environmental electromagnetic radiation which the anomaly generates.

Dowsers also distinguish 'good' 'water-lines' from 'bad' ones ('black-lines' and 'black-streams') which are associated with disease (Beadon, 1980). Graves draws parallels with the Yin–Yang, ch'i–sha of Chinese philosophy and acupuncture practice. One person described unpleasant sensations persisting in the house after an electrical short-circuit had occurred beneath it during work on the London Underground railway, supposedly redirecting a 'black-line' so that it passed beneath the house.

Graves describes as 'energy bands' regions on the surfaces of ancient standing stones and buttresses which give distinctive responses to interrogation by dowsing; these also vary in strength with the lunar phase cycle. This feature is consistent with the astronomical alignments reported for standing stones and henges. He later describes an experiment in which two experienced dowsers were able to use their pendulums held in a neutral position over a water-line as a Morse Code-type communication system over distances of a few hundred yards; the main interference with such a system was said to be the background of natural pulsations associated with the water-lines. This represents a further possible reason for the erection of standing stones and a justification for carting stones over great distances; they may have enhanced the stability and sensitivity of ley-line communications systems. Perhaps the 'stone' Stonehenge and its 'wooden' predecessor combined the functions of observatory with communications centre for the time and season checks. Graves compares the 'needles of stone' – Britain's standing stones, stone circles, barrows, lone-pines and ancient churches – with acupuncture needles, and the beacon hill fires with the burning of moxa cones, in a gigantic earth-acupuncture therapy concept, having potentially both defensive and offensive strategems.

Major progress in the scientific investigation of the phenomenon of dowsing has been described in a book by Dr J.Havelock Fidler (1983), a retired agricultural researcher. In brief, he has devised a technique for calibrating the swing of the dowser's pendulum which has been extended so that the calibration can be carried out on site. This has enabled him to calibrate the dowser and to allow for the various circadian (possibly even lunar phase) variations in performance. There is also a definite male/female difference. Next he has been able to quantify the units of dowsing reaction to a stone or other object, which he calls its 'charge' and measures it in defined units which he calls 'petrons'. There is a line of interaction between two stones which can be detected by dowsing – this he calls a 'petrostat'. He has produced an empirical equation relating the percentage reduction in strength of a 'petrostat' to the separation of the stones generating it. He calibrates a stone in 'lithons' – the product of its mass and the number of 'petrons'.

He has shown that a stone can be 'charged' by holding it in the hand and hammering it or throwing it hard at a neutral wall; it also takes on the appropriate male/female characteristic of the person working it. However the 'charge' decays exponentially unless 'fixed'. This can be done by hammering it (analogous to homoeopathic potentising?) or by placing it in a fire and leaving it overnight. He, too, thinks that the Rogation-tide processions, with their beating the ground around the 'bounds' with rods, would have left and reinforced the territory markers around the parish boundary.

At the mind–matter interface, he has measured psychological 'ley lines' between two persons. These were only present when the two persons were each concentrating on the other. The process of map dowsing also comes at this interface; the map serves to concentrate the mind on a particular remote location and the pendulum indicates subconscious mental perceptions to the dowser. We need to know much more about space, time and the mind–body interface before we can even locate the boundaries which must circumscribe any scientific explanation in terms of physical 'nuts and bolts'. There is work going on in this area, particularly in Eastern Europe, some of which was reported at the 6th International Conference on Psychotronic Research, Zagreb, 13–16 November 1986.

Geopathic stress

The Chinese have a concept – Feng-shui (Graves, 1978) by which the 'living energy' of an area, 'chi'i', needs to be able to propagate along clearly discernible pathways, else it stagnates and becomes the noxious 'sha'. These pathways can be interfered with and blocked by the activities of man. Last century, the Chinese were continually concerned by the Westerner's development of railway and telegraph lines upsetting the local residents' Feng-shui. It is possible that the 'living energies' and 'earth fields' correspond in some part to electromagnetic energy of an extremely high coherence. This can produce effects quite different from the usual energy concepts based on random, disordered energies, such as heat and light.

The speeding trains on railways and vehicles on motorways are considered to distort the earth energy fields in a transient manner; activities such as quarrying, earthworks and mining, and the erection of overhead power lines are claimed to produce a permanent interruption of the energy flow. Graves maintains that:

> Basically, pylon lines split the energy-flow, allowing part of it to continue on its way, but sending the remainder down the pylon line itself. The proportions 'stolen' by the pylons vary enormously, for no known reason. At each bend in the line of cables some of the energy that originally ran down the overground 'spins off', effectively forming a new low-powered overground. The result is that in some areas ... the web of pylon lines,

large and small, produces large numbers of 'unofficial' overgrounds, allowing energy of the wrong kind to arrive at the wrong place at the wrong time and probably the wrong direction. The result, in other words, is not just a mess, it's absolute chaos. In some cases and areas it may be possible to divert the major overgrounds upwards so they are above the power lines; but in others the dowsers I talked to felt that the only satisfactory solution would be to put all the electrical power cables underground. Even given the enormous cost of doing so, they reckoned that it would still be worthwhile in every sense to do so, because of the pylon's hidden effects on the health and fertility of the land.

Dowsers have developed an 'Earth Acupuncture' procedure for re-structuring the energy flow in a region and isolating it from flows of 'sha', negative and destructive energy. This involves placing stakes in the ground at places selected by dowsing. Initially these are wooden stakes with copper wire wound round the top of each, reminiscent of Lakhovsky's coils around his plants. These stakes might eventually be replaced by an arrangement of copper-sheathed, iron stakes to permanently re-structure the energy flow in the region and give it a feeling of deep peace and quiet – like an old church. Indeed, that special sense of stillness in old stone churches may in part be due to their ability to shield disturbing electromagnetic fields. Using a magnetometer, Brooker (1983, 1988) has produced evidence that ancient stone circles – he tested the famous Rollright Stones, in Oxfordshire – could have acted as magnetic refuges for ancient man. This might have aided the development of special states of consciousness. Stone churches may also act in this way, perhaps promoting resonance amplification through their special geometries and orientations. The Cathedral at Chartres, in France, is one of a number of churches considered to possess special qualities or powers due to its unique design and geometry (Charpentier, 1983).

Conversely, Aschoff (1986) has shown correlations between disease locations and physically measurable parameters such as magnetic fields, air ionisation and ionising radiation particle counts. He has proposed that some geopathic zones may correspond to geological faults in the Earth's crust, leading to an increased neutron flux emerging from the core and, if the faults have filled with water, giving a localised enhancement of highly interactive slow neutrons. A neutron decays into a proton and an electron, and in the process magnetic flux quantisation must be conserved; as discussed in Chapter 4, living systems may be able to respond to changes of a single quantum of magnetic flux.

A recent translation of a 1932 book by von Pohl, of which an English translation by Lang appeared in 1987, documents his substantial research linking geopathic stress to cancer development and many other diseases.

Such a connection is particularly accepted in Germany where the findings of German doctors recently prompted the funding of a major research project by the West German Government (Best, 1988). In Britain geopathic stress and its effects are being studied by the Dulwich Health Society which has published methods of assessing and preventing exposure to it as well as documenting case histories (Gordon, 1988). Recent geopathic stress research is discussed further in the Postscript.

Biblical and Talmudic writings on water

The Holy Bible (Genesis 1:1–20) assigns an important role for water and electromagnetic fields (light), in that order, thus, '... the Spirit of God was moving over the face of the waters. And God said let there be light ...' A similar importance is given to water in the Holy Qur'an, 'We made from water every living thing' (Sūra 21:30); 'It is He Who has created man from water' (Sura 25:54). There are Biblical and Talmudic prescriptions for ritual bathing (Leviticus 15:116–118) and descriptions of the contaminating effects of the carcasses of unclean creatures (Leviticus 11:24–40), which may, however, be cleansed by the prescribed washing of the person and clothing that has come into contact with them. In the case of earthen vessels, ovens and stoves, these are to broken in pieces to prevent further use.

> Nevertheless [Leviticus 11:36–38] a spring or cistern holding water shall be clean; but whatever touches their carcass shall be unclean. And if any part of their carcass falls upon any seed for sowing that is to be sown, it is clean; but if water is put on the seed and any part of their carcass falls upon it, it is unclean to you.

The clinically observed effects in allergic subjects produced by water exposed to allergens or electromagnetic fields – and even then much diluted (Smith *et al.*, 1985) – implies that it is now worthwhile to look more deeply for a scientific basis to the Biblical washing and bathing prescriptions (Smith *et al.*, 1986).

Preuss (1978) writes,

> For certain categories of impurity, the Bible prescribes the requirement to bathe in 'live (flowing) water', which tradition considers desirable for *every* ritual bath. 'Live water' is that which flows from wells, but also the water of rivers (other than during the rainy season and during the time when the snows melt) and the seas. A substitute for it is offered by the rainwater which gushes forth from the *fountains of the great deep* (*mayenoth tehom rabba*) (Genesis 7:11) in cases where it is collected in

a reservoir, and if at least 40 *seahs* (approximately 800 litres) are present; that is as much as is required for a full-grown person to immerse himself in. The column of water should be three cubic cubits, that is cover a floor area of one square cubit and have a height of three cubits. The basin (or reservoir) itself must naturally be large enough to hold not only the water but also the bather. From the reservoirs which are ordinarily found under open skies, the rainwater can be led through a pipe, *tzinor*, which may not be made of metal, however, into the true bathing basin, the *mikveh*. Drawn water in and of itself is absolutely unusable; however, one may add therefrom to well water or to the minimally prescribed quantity of rainwater. It is similarly not permissible to bathe in a utensil such as a bathtub. Scripture states (Levit. 11:36–38): '*Only a well or a cistern, a gathering of water (mikvey mayim) is clean*; that is, it cleanses'.

Preuss continues:

The ritual immersion bath was naturally required not only in summer, but also in winter, and for that season the temperature of the water was of utmost importance. For the High Priest, one warmed a bath on the Day of Atonement, in case he was old or weakly, by adding hot water, or according to another interpretation, by placing pieces of iron, which were made red hot, into the water. This was thus the opposite of the old Germanic stone baths, in which the hot water was poured on to glowing stones in order to produce steam. Since a bath in well water was not always available, and even where available not usable in the cold of winter, the communities in which no well (underground) water was obtainable, or was obtainable only with difficulty, used to place basins under the open sky to collect rainwater, and warm the contents thereby pouring hot water therein. But even rainwater is not always available in the desired amount – every bath, as already mentioned, requires approximately 800 litres of water – so that, *for this reason*, the basin could not be pumped dry as often as one would have liked.

The Biblical precept which applies only for pollution: *he shall wash his entire flesh in water (Levit. 15:16–18)*, is extended to *every* ritual bath. It is only valid if there is no separation (*chatzitzah*) between the body and the water. For this reason, not only must all clothing and jewelry be removed, but the body must *first* be rid of all dirt (even under the nails), accidentally adherent blood, etc. From time immemorial, one, therefore, took a (warm) cleansing bath *before* entering the ritual immersion bath.

The regulation that *every* part of the body surface come in contact with the water has the result that one must also give consideration to the maintenance of the cleanliness of the *water*. Otherwise, if any object, no matter how small, accidentally adheres to the skin (for example, a hair floating in the water) it serves as a separation between the body and the water and thus renders the immersion invalid.

The first comment which should be made is that the 800 litres of water required for the bath is large (i.e. ten times) compared with the amount of water in a standard 70 kilogram (approximately 70 litre) man. This may prevent an immersed person imparting any effects into the bath water. Likewise, 'clean' water may be diluted with water from other sources in time of shortage. In the case of allergy patients, it does seem that they are able to 'overwrite' their own electromagnetic signature on a 5 millilitre tube of water or saline held in their hand while reacting allergically; they describe the tube as becoming 'drained of its effectiveness'. A similar result is obtained by 'overwriting' a tube of water exposed to a neutralising frequency with a frequency which provokes an allergic response. This is also consistent with the ability of a large cistern (or the sea) to remain clean in spite of contact with the carcasses of unclean creatures which must, perforce, be inhabiting the sea and dropping into underground cisterns, such as can be seen in Masada, Herod's hill-top fort on the shores of the Dead Sea. Many patients find that bathing in the sea or even standing on damp grass alleviates their symptoms; again, this is probably an electrical 'grounding' phenomenon involving contact with a large conducting object (the sea or land) at constant electrical potential.

Second, the water filling a bath has to be 'living'. There are allergy patients who are unable to tolerate water from the majority of sources available today (Smith *et al.*, 1985). If all else fails, they can make non-spring water acceptable by burying it in glass bottles in the ground (for example, by digging a hole in the garden) for three days. Two days is not usually enough, according to the patients. A glass bottle is probably equivalent to a stone or glazed tile cistern, but we have yet to discover what this treatment does to the physical properties of the water. The ancient Chinese found that they could potentise remedies by burying them in the ground. One possible scientific explanation is that, because of the electrical characteristics of soil, the environmental electromagnetic field energy spectrum to which the water would otherwise be exposed will be modified as the energy penetrates the soil; only the ELF frequencies, especially the Schumann radiation, will penetrate appreciably. Even ultra-weak magnetic field fluctuations in the 0.01 Hz to 10 Hz region with amplitudes of 5 nT to 50 nT have been found to produce effects in human subjects.

Third, the collection of rainwater is deemed adequate if it is led to and from the reservoir by a non-metallic pipe. This strongly suggests that electrical phenomena are involved. The technology (Hodges, 1970) of copper, and its alloys with tin (bronze), had been developed by 3500 BC and was accompanied by and engendered the development of 'cities' and groups of craftsmen. Gold and silver, which occur naturally in the metallic form, had interested man before 4000 BC. Lead, as a metal, had been known from perhaps 3000 BC. Iron, and the iron sword and ploughshare, date from about 1000 BC. Of these metals, lead is the most likely metal to have been used for piping, as it was later in the Roman Empire, and it is of little use for anything else, being too soft and not decorative. The Mesopotamians discovered, before 1000 BC, how to make a lead glaze which matched the thermal expansion of pottery and therefore did not craze on cooling, but the Talmudic prohibition was clearly against metal (per se) and not against the toxicity of lead; in any case, drawn water would have been kept in unglazed pottery vessels where the evaporating seepage would have had a cooling effect on its contents in the hot, dry climates; such water would have been absolutely unusable for ritual washing.

In about 1300 BC, the (Bronze Age) Israelites under Moses made their desert journey and at Sinai they came to know the God who had made a Covenant with them. It was at this time that the customs which had marked them off from other peoples were first regulated into a body of religious and civil law. Following the 50 years' captivity in Babylon, ended when the (Iron Age) Persians defeated Babylonia in 538 BC, the return from exile was accompanied by a codification of Jewish Law as recorded in the Book of Leviticus and finally recorded in the present form of the Pentateuch only by 350 BC. By 1500 BC, the skill of the craftsman had reached the limits of the unaided human hand and eye; there were no major developments for the next 3000 years, not until the invention of the microscope extended the range of human vision – and mind.

The prescriptions regarding seeds for sowing imply that so long as the seed is dormant (dry), it will not be contaminated by a carcass, but if water touches the seed, perhaps for germination before planting out, then this seed becomes unclean. It has recently been found that small amounts of a biological stressor (e.g. formaldehyde) can sensitise growing cucumber seedlings to other chemical stimuli (Slawinska and Slawinski, 1986). Formica is the Latin for 'ant', a winged insect that goes upon all fours and is listed as an abomination (Leviticus 11:20–23); the formic acid in the sting is the acid corresponding to formaldehyde.

The 'live water' of the rivers refers to normal levels and excludes times of flood and melting snow when the rivers would be carrying the general accumulation of debris from their beds and from the snow as it melts. The countries of that part of the world have much high ground and heavy snowfalls in the winter, which, of course, preserves in 'deep-freeze' conditions all the biological contamination it has accumulated, as mountaineers using melted snow for drinking water have found to their cost.

The substitute for 'live water' offered by 'rainwater which gushes forth from the fountains of the deep', suggests that water which has flowed underground, as one finds particularly in limestone areas, has become acceptable even though it may have only been underground for a short while, provided that it is collected in a reservoir and used in sufficient quantity. Scientifically, there may be some critical minimum dimensions for such a reservoir. This is reinforced by the fact that one is allowed to dilute the 'living water' with drawn water and heated water without rendering it ineffective for ritual purposes.

Water has a very high dielectric loss, so there should be no electrical resonance in an aqueous environment. But Edwards and colleagues (1984) have found extremely intense and sharp absorption resonances in the microwave region for the DNA extracted from *E. coli* relative to that of the aqueous environment, confirming the theoretical predictions of Prohofsky and co-workers. Genzel, Edwards and Powell (1986) have proposed a longitudinal acoustic mode model which can account for all the experimental facts. The physical properties of 'structural water', that is, water in close contact with biological systems, are regarded as being between those of liquid water and ice and capable of giving broadband absorptions, but the above resonances are too sharp to be so attributed. Van Zandt (1986) has also constructed a simple mathematical model which is so successful at describing such DNA resonances in water that the journal *Nature* (Maddox, 1986) headed its report of Van Zandt's work, 'Physicists about to hi-jack DNA?' This may be the beginnings of 'Theoretical Biology', but there is still a long way to go.

When a single drop of an allergen at a dilution which affects a particular, hypersensitive, allergic person is placed on the skin, the whole body will react within ten seconds and all the reaction that is going to be obtained will have become apparent within a minute. This is an extreme situation, but probably 15 per cent of a given population function below 100 per cent capability because of some allergic responses; these are more common among women between the ages of puberty and menopause, and are regarded as hormonal in origin. The dramatic effects that even a single drop of allergen can have on sensitive persons is clear justification for the minutiae of the pre-cleansing instructions prescribed in the Talmud.

Metal jewellery provides the equivalent of microwave resonant circuits in contact with the body which would interfere with neutralisation; allergy sufferers often wear copper bracelets or belts. Gemstones also seem to be able to affect allergic subjects; in this connection one should note that living systems emit very coherent radiation, albeit at very low intensities, right up to the ultra-violet part of the spectrum (Smith *et al.*, 1986). A cut (synthetic) ruby is able to function as the active element of a laser, so a cut gemstone ought also to be able to function as a resonator or amplifier of natural electromagnetic oscillations in the body. The blood and hair of sick persons appears different to that of healthy persons when recorded by Kirlian photography, hence the importance of ensuring that no single trace of diseased tissue remains in contact with the body, thereby preventing the access of the 'living water' to the whole body surface.

Enough has been written to show that these subtle effects are now worthy of further investigation. The properties of 'living water', in a bath of the dimensions and materials of a *mikveh*, should be investigated as a universal resonance damping medium for allergic responses. If this 'living water' is exposed to the electromagnetic fields emitted by reacting allergic persons or electrical oscillators, the question as to whether the water will still retain its effectiveness for neutralising further allergic responses, even after a strong allergic response has been neutralised, should be investigated. This would lead to scientific criteria for water able to neutralise allergic responses. Even so, the construction of an 'elegant ritularium' (Preuss, 1978) is likely to be beyond the resources of many allergy sufferers.

There are many accounts of healing to be found in the Bible, and particularly in the New Testament. The general impression that one gets is of a Creator who prefers to let things happen by secondary causes in the universe, rather than to keep tinkering with the basic mechanisms. Thus, if any of the matters discussed in the present book are at all relevant to the detailed processes whereby, for example, healing by the laying on of hands can be accomplished, this merely emphasises the need for an answer to the question, 'What was the purpose of the healing?' – not, 'How was it done?' Science is unable to answer the question 'Ought I?' If a person laying on hands or merely electromagnetically coupling to another's 'aura' (personal electromagnetic field region) is transmitting healing frequencies, then that would be beneficial for the recipient, i.e. morally good. However, it is conceivable that an evil person could deliberately couple harmful or disease causing frequencies by the same physical mechanism; the same science but the opposite morality.

Astrology re-assessed

Kepler's original work on planetary motions (1609) was carried out with the proof of astrology in mind (Field, 1984). But material causes have been as unpopular with astrologers in recent years as they have been *de rigueur* with physicists. Yet, as if to disquiet them both, correlations of planetary positions with the births of eminent professionals and even with chemical reactions (Kollerstrom, 1984), have been reported by Gauquelin and permit a possible mechanistic explanation based on known electromagnetic effects.

Since Kepler's time scientific interest in the propositions of astrology has declined, being now regarded by the majority of today's scientists as unworthy of serious consideration. However, in the last 30 years the monumental work of psychologist Dr Michel Gauquelin, begun in 1950 at his laboratory in Paris, has attracted serious academic scrutiny (Gauquelin, 1976, 1980, 1982). Michel Gauquelin has produced a large body of data supporting a relationship between planetary positions (Moon, Venus, Mars, Jupiter and Saturn to date) and the births of certain groups of eminent professionals. (He was later assisted by his wife, now Françoise Schneider-Gauquelin (F. Gauquelin, 1982).) Gauquelin first published his findings in French in 1955 (Gauquelin, 1955, 1960), an abbreviated English translation of which has just been published (Gauquelin, 1988a).

Specifically, he has found that different planets occur significantly more often, or in certain circumstances significantly less often, in the birthcharts of famous professionals very near to either of two traditionally sensitive points in the horoscope, or birthchart. These positions are, one, just after a planet has 'risen' over the 'Ascendant' (the Ascendant is where the projected Eastern horizon for any locality cuts the ecliptic or plane of the Earth's orbit) and two, just after the planet has reached its upper culmination at the 'Midheaven' (the Midheaven is where the upper meridian, or plane passing through a given terrestrial location, and the Earth's axis, cuts the ecliptic). For example, Mars was found to fall in either of these sectors significantly more frequently than would be expected in the birthcharts of sports champions, whereas in those of eminent scientists the planet involved was Saturn.

These and the other associations observed usually involved the planet traditionally linked with the profession in question but were only found with those professionals achieving a high degree of eminence in their respective fields. Similar results were not obtained with the corresponding non-eminent professionals. The significance of Gauquelin's results reached a probability of 1 in 10,000 in many cases and, in one case reached a probability of 1 in 1,000,000, as shown in Table 11.1.

His combined results are based on a total of over 16,000 famous professionals from five European countries in which, unlike Britain, reasonably exact birthtimes have been noted on birth certificates since 1920.

Gauquelin was able to reproduce his results with samples from different countries. A highly sceptical committee of leading scientists, the Belgian Committee for the Scientific Study of Paranormal Phenomena, also successfully replicated his findings using an independent sample of 535

Table 11.1 Frequency of planets in sectors 1 and 4 of the diurnal circle for famous professionals (after Table 1, Gauquelin, M., Correlation, 4(1), 1984: 8–24)

Group	Planet	Computer results (rise/set sectors)			
		Exp.	Act.	Diff.	Prob.
2088 Champions	Mars	358.5	435	+76.5	.00002
3647 Scientists	Mars	626.2	703	+76.8	.001
	Jupiter	602.5	547	−55.5	.05
	Saturn	598.0	685	+87.0	.0001
3438 Soldiers	Mars	590.3	662	+71.7	.002
	Jupiter	575.1	686	+110.9	.000001
5100 Artists	Mars	875.7	773	−102.7	.0002
	Saturn	828.0	744	−84.0	.003
1409 Actors	Jupiter	234.0	273	+39.0	.01
1003 Politicians	Jupiter	166.4	202	+35.6	.002
1352 Writers	Moon	225.4	288	+62.6	.00001

Total number of sectors = 12. Sectors 1 and 4 are just past rise and culmination respectively.

Exp. = expected frequency, Act. = actual frequency, Diff. = Act. − Exp., Prob. = significance level of the difference by two-tailed Critical Ratio test.

The soldiers include aviators. The artists consist of painters, the 1409 actors shown, writers and musicians (military musicians are excluded).

Belgian sportsmen (Comité Para, 1976; Dean, 1977). Further tests by the even more sceptical and hostile American Committee for the Scientific Investigation of Claims of the Paranormal (CSICOP) produced highly controversial results involving accusations of fraud and cover-up on the part of CSICOP (Rawlins, 1981; Curry, 1982) but which were ultimately seen to vindicate Gauquelin's findings (Abell et al., 1983).

The possibility that Gauquelin's findings might be explained by an electromagnetic mechanism was recently explored by Dr Percy Seymour, a British astronomer at Plymouth Polytechnic, at the 5th International Astrological Research Conference in London in 1986. Invoking the phenomenon of resonant amplification, Seymour proposed a model in which the planets resonate with the Sun's magnetic canals. These are caused by differential rotation, which affects the solar activity, which affects the geomagnetic field. This, in turn, is considered to affect the propagation of human nerve impulses. McGillion has outlined a plausible involvement of the pineal gland in such effects, with its sensitivity to weak magnetic field changes (McGillion, 1980), while Landscheidt (1989) has produced considerable evidence supporting a strong causal link between the planets, solar activity and terrestrial events. Seymour develops his theory more fully in his recent book (Seymour, 1988).

The likelihood that electromagnetism may, at least in part, explain his results is reinforced by Gauquelin's additional discovery of what he terms a 'planetary hereditary effect', which is based on 30,000 French parents and children. Starting in 1961, he found that if one or both parents had been born when either the Moon, Venus, Mars, Jupiter or Saturn was just past the Ascendant or Midheaven, the same planet or planets occurred very significantly (with a probability greater than 10 parts in a million) more often in one of these positions in the charts of their children (Gauquelin, 1966, 1982, 1983, 1986, 1988b). Although a fully satisfactory replication remains to be done, a further interesting finding was that the correlation was observed to increase on geomagnetically disturbed days. Using the index Ci as the magnetic character index on a scale of 0.0 to 2.0, the planetary effect was twice as strong when a child was born on a day when Ci was equal to, or greater than, unity.

In his comprehensive critical assessment of astrological research, Dean (1977) says of Gauquelin's results, '... they provide, for the first time, rigorous and objective evidence about the basic fundamentals of astrology'. In his book with Nias (1982), Professor Hans Eysenck, the renowned psychologist and personality theorist and one of the few psychologists to have studied the Gauquelin research in detail, refers to their findings as 'inexplicable but they are also factual, and as such can no longer be ignored'. Taking the Gauquelin findings a step further to examine any mediating psychological variable, Eysenck (1975) predicted certain links between the personality descriptions of eminent professionals culled from biographies by the Gauquelins and correlated with dimensions on his Eysenck Personality Questionnaire (EPQ). In particular, he predicted Saturn linked with introversion and Mars and Jupiter with extraversion. And, as predicted, introverted eminent professionals were found to have been born significantly more frequently when Saturn had just risen or had just passed its culmination; extraverts were born when Mars and Jupiter were in these positions. (Gauquelin *et al.*, 1979). Similar results were obtained with an American sample (Gauquelin *et al.*, 1981). These findings suggest that it is personality which is related to planetary position at birth rather than profession, and that the profession is related to the planetary position through the intermediary of personality. All of which suggests that eminence may be as much a matter of personality as innate ability. Although the factor of eminence seems to be crucial for obtaining the correlations with professionals that Gauquelin has found – a criticism against their more general application – recent research by Startup (1984a), who obtained the first PhD in the UK for research into astrology (Startup, 1984b), and Stark (1986, 1987) has provided preliminary confirmation of similar planet–personality correlations with ordinary people.

Professor Eysenck has recently formed his own Committee for Objective Research in Astrology (CORA) (Eysenck, 1987) to advise those wishing to do research in the area, as well as to comment on published research – for example, see his criticisms (Eysenck, 1986) of some much publicised negative results by Carlson (1985) that appeared in *Nature*. With the plausible electromagnetic explanatory model of the Gauquelin's results offered by Seymour, mainstream scientists may now perhaps feel a little easier about examining astrological claims and results as a legitimate area of study.

Brooker's discovery of a sweeping geomagnetic field

Living systems tend to have built-in redundancy, that is, several systems capable of performing the same function, as a protection against one system failing. What is probably Nature's second directional navigational aid has been found by a retired BBC engineer, Mr Charles Brooker (Smith *et al.*, 1986; Smith, 1988; Brooker, 1988) mentioned at the end of the dowsing section above. In experiments to try to cancel out weak magnetic fields and field gradients which dowsers could detect, he found that, although the fields and field gradients could be reduced to zero, as measured by a magnetometer, with a suitable set of current-carrying coils, the dowsers could still detect the objects producing the original field perturbation. He then realised that the only magnetic field which his coils would not cancel was a uniform magnetic field travelling in space at a constant velocity. He constructed a modified 'Earth Inductor' experiment in which a coil is rotated in the Earth's magnetic field and the voltage generated is measured. His modification was to include a second commutator so that the voltage generated in the part of the coil travelling in the direction of the Earth's rotation was measured separately from that generated in the part of the coil moving against the motion of the Earth. These two voltages were different by an amount corresponding to almost the full velocity of the Earth's rotation.

He found that Michael Faraday had recorded in his Diaries (Faraday, 1855) experiments which showed that a magnetic field does not rotate when the magnet producing it is rotated about its axis. This is not so unreasonable; think of the magnetic field generated by a coil rotating about its axis. The effect of the rotation would be a minute increase or decrease in the current in the coil and hence the absolute value of the magnetic field strength. Only in a moving plasma are the lines of magnetic flux dragged along. Brooker's claim needs urgent verification.

Future possibilities for 'alternative medicine' and 'health engineering'

Homoeopathy (see Chapter 7) often seems to be missing the possibility of fine tuning the therapy by the fact of using a limited range of potencies instead of titrating the potency for the individual patient. However, this is becoming more practicable with the recent electrical devices which can determine as well as prepare the correct potencies, although it seems that the operator is an essential part of these systems. One of these (Brügemann, 1984) makes therapeutic use of the complex oscillation spectrum of a living system. Frequencies normally present in a healthy system are measured; where they are deficient, they are reinforced electrically or homoeopathically.

The senior author is frequently asked whether mass-medication is possible using electromagnetic radiation. In the light of the above work, the answer must be, yes! It is now possible to obtain highly coherent microwave oscillators (and masers and lasers) which emit radiation of a short enough wavelength to be formed into a narrow beam and are coherent enough to be modulated at the frequencies corresponding to homoeopathic potencies. It is then only necessary to remember that the effect of a homoeopathic remedy on a healthy person is to stimulate the (proving) symptoms that the remedy cures in the sick. Excessive exposure to such radiation (which would act as an allergen) would be likely to hypersensitise those so exposed who would then react allergically to subsequent triggering signals in the environment. This may also be the mechanism by which certain crowd behavioural phenomena are triggered, since people can also emit coherent electromagnetic radiation and selectively sense the radiation from others, according to recent Russian work mentioned in Chapter 3.

In principle, this is no different to mass medication by the fluoridation and chlorination of water supplies. It could be of value in the treatment of widespread epidemics or radiation-sickness. Homoeopathic potencies of radium bromide have been used for the latter and there is no reason to suppose that they cannot be simulated electrically.

Modern expensive 'high-tech' medicine can give health to some of the people some of the time, some of the people all the time but no country can afford 'high-tech' health for all its people all of the time. In Western countries, health care consumes more than a twentieth of the gross national product. Yet, medical research tends to assume that all problems of health and disease can be solved if only enough money can be thrown at them. Many tests are performed on patients which are not for the benefit of the patient but are intended to protect doctors and institutions in case of litigation, where costs and awards, like medical defence insurance dues, are escalating rapidly. Many drugs and treatments are prescribed unnecessarily and these go on to produce undesirable side-effects. Within the past century, medical science has raised the life expectancy at birth by 20 years, but that at retirement age by less than a year. Much of the former improvement, anyway, was achieved by improved social conditions and public health measures.

Following the Prince of Wales' remarks to the British Medical Association in 1983 there has been an increased interest in alternative, or complementary, medicine amongst the medical profession and the general public (*Practitioner*, December 1986). Some of this is a trend away from the concept of the patient as a collection of parts which will work again if the faulty component is found and replaced. Holistic medicine considers the patient as a whole, is prepared to consider that several factors may be involved and assumes that the patient's own co-operation in health care may be needed. The holistic approach is not restricted to any particular system of medicine.

There is no method yet available for the objective assessment of the state of (holistic) health of an individual and offering the possibility of advice on life-style and health care through the detection of biological stress before a disease state is reached. Physiological measurements can monitor progress in athletic training programmes but these relate to specific parameters only. What the patient needs is a 'road test' of the body and its driver (the mind), not the oil and water checking.

The trouble with preventative medicine is that it will not sell anything unless the patient can be convinced of the accuracy of its predictions (it-can't-happen-to-me syndrome) and the future efficacy of its demands on present life-style.

CHAPTER 12

The last frontiers

All that lives must die, Passing through nature to eternity.
William Shakespeare (1564–1616), *Hamlet*

The limits of sensory perception – set by the laws of physics

It could be best felt when it could not clearly be seen.
Thomas Hardy (1849–1928)

For one material system to influence another material system requires energy, the limiting amounts of which can be quantified as described in Chapter 3. Now, much has been written (Popp *et al.*, 1979) on the relation between the thermodynamical concept of entropy (a measure of the disorder in a system at a specified absolute temperature) and information but, if there is to be a bridge between mind and body, spirit and matter, it must be possible to enter into the world of physics from outside time and space and without any energy requirements.

Supposing, as theologians maintain, that knowledge, or information, has an objective existence outside the constraints of space and time and it is possible for a system to become more ordered as the result of an input of information. The two extremes are, respectively, a perfectly random material system with no ordering but a mean kinetic energy corresponding to its temperature, on the one hand, and on the other, a system of pure information and order that is not material and not containing or carrying energy.

In the material world, all systems combine these two quantities in varying degrees. Mathematically, they may be treated as a complex quantity (one combining real and imaginary parts); the real component will represent the random energy, the imaginary component the pure information, as shown in Figure 12.1. The mathematical laws governing complex quantities will apply so that multiplying the 'real system status' by its complex conjugate will give the random energy content (U as shown in the Figure). The slope of the line is a measure of the temperature.

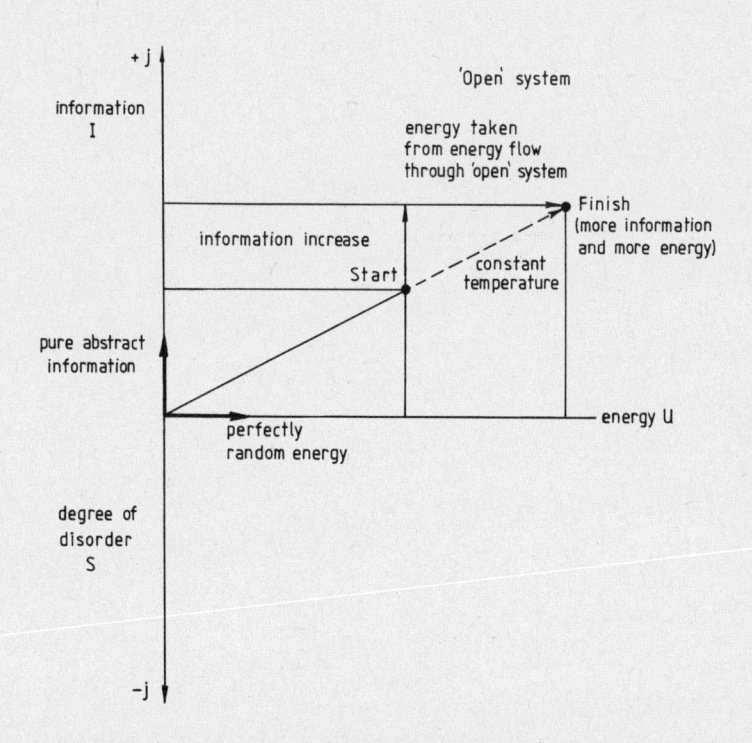

Fig. 12.1 This figure represents information and energy as two distinct, but inter-related, quantities which combine according to the rules of trigonometry rather than arithmetic. They are pictured as what are called 'complex' numbers that is, they are the combination of a 'real' part (R) = energy, and an imaginary part (I) = information. This would be written mathematically as (R + jI). The quantity j is defined as being the square-root of minus one. Thus $j^2 = -1$ and $j^4 = (-1)^2 = +1$. Multiplying by j has the effect of rotating the line (called a phasor) by 90 degrees. Reversing the sign of the j-term gives mirror reversal and what is called the complex conjugate, (R − jI). Multiplying by this gives the energy at zero information content, i.e. square of the length of the line (phasor), or $(R - jI) \times (R - jI) = (R^2 + I^2)$.

If the system is 'thermodynamically closed', as in Figure 12.2, an increase in the information will result in a fall in the temperature, shown by the line (phasor) being rotated towards lower random energy.

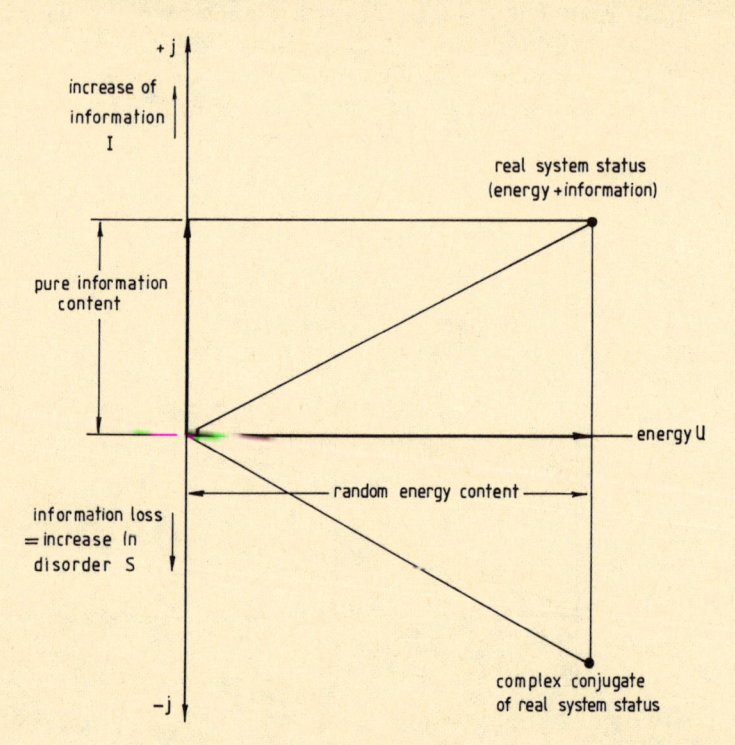

Fig. 12.2 This figure represents the situation where a system is isolated from its surroundings. The only way it can accommodate an increase of information is to cool down, as shown by the rotation of the line.

If a 'thermodynamically open' system, as in Figure 12.3, is given information, the energy required to keep the temperature constant will be taken from the flow of energy through the system. The line (phasor) remains at a constant angle, i.e. at constant temperature. This must be the way a living system interacts with information and ordering. For a physical system to be influenced by a zero amount of energy, an increase in information must be used to absorb more random energy raising the system above its thermal environment as shown in Figure 12.3.

In electronics this can be realised, as near as is possible with a practical system, by the 'super-regenerative receiver'. This was invented in the early days of wireless, when vacuum tubes (valves) were scarce and radio amateurs wanted the most sensitive receivers possible. It is not now

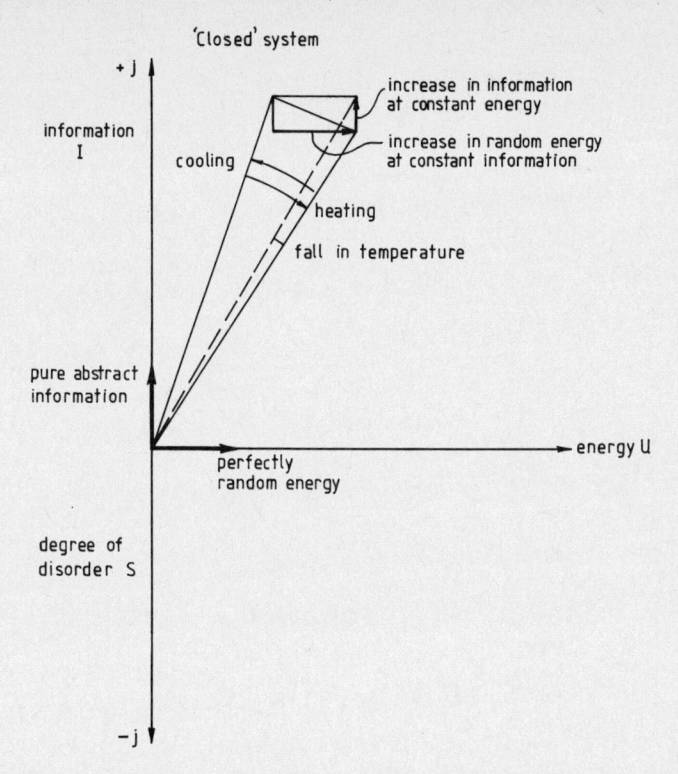

Fig. 12.3 This figure represents a system which is kept at constant temperature but where the information increase is used to absorb energy from that flowing through the system so as to restore the temperature, but thereby taking the system away from thermal equilibrium with its surroundings, as is characteristic of living systems.

used because the circuit radiates electromagnetic energy as well as detecting it. In this circuit, an oscillation is allowed to start and build up before being 'quenched'. The instant at which the oscillation commences to build up and the rate at which this happens depends upon the most minute amount of information present, superimposed on the electrical noise of the circuit. A 'super-regenerative' circuit could be used to determine the limitations of man's ability to influence electronic circuits and be influenced by them, since it also radiates. Such experiments would show whether the sensitivity of a living system can exceed the limitations set by the laws of physics.

Pethig (1973) has estimated the total number of chemical (redox) reactions involving electron transport along each metabolic pathway in the body, and concluded that a total current of the order of 200 amps is involved. Since the energy band gap of a protein is about 5 eV, this current represents an electrical power of about 1 kW and is about the body's maximum output, somewhat higher than the basal metabolic rate. A man with arms upstretched would approximate to a quarter-wavelength dipole antenna at a frequency of 30 MHz (10 metres wavelength), the highest frequency which can reliably be reflected around the world by the ionosphere. If a man could synchronise all his chemical reactions to produce the energy of metabolism at a frequency of 30 MHz, he should be able to communicate with a hypersensitive man anywhere in the world, just using electromagnetic radiation. On an inverse square law basis for the propagation of electromagnetic radiation, the range for a transmitted power density of $1 kW/m^2$ to be received by a sensor capable of detecting $0.7 pW/m^2$ is 3.7×10^7 m (almost twice that needed since the mean circumference of the Earth is 4.0×10^7 m).

Thus, the dimensions of the world provide the limit for single man-to-man communication on Earth. To get further, or reach less sensitive persons, would require a more powerful source of radiation. This might be achieved either by using a group of persons to transmit, holding hands to synchronise their respective power outputs (as can happen in surrogate kinesiology). Sunlight at glancing incidence (sunrise or sunset) shining through the aura of a man, a group of men, or perhaps standing stones, might become modulated by non-linearities in their surrounding water vapour (analogous to the 'Luxembourg Effect', in which the ionosphere was found to become perturbed by that powerful radio transmitter of the 1930s), so as to enable the sunlight to propagate messages ahead on the Sun's rays in the manner of a forward-scattering radar. One wonders whether such an activity was possible from places like Stonehenge where the alignments favour some sunrise phenomenon.

This concept becomes even more pertinent as a result of the success of experiments before, during and after the flight of the astronauts in Apollo 8. In these, all the physiological functions of these astronauts were quantitatively monitored from the Earth by the detection and analysis of signals from them. These were received through the walls of the space capsule except when the capsule was in the moon-shade even though on the Earth-side of the Moon (Hieronymus, 1968), implying that the sunlight scattered from the capsule was being modulated from within.

Professor Robert Morris (1986), currently the first Koestler Professor of Parapsychology, at the University of Edinburgh, has discussed the way in which, in recent years, parapsychology has commenced to build connections between its own body of knowledge and the knowledge bases of more orthodox areas of endeavour. He is particularly concerned with human-equipment interactions and lists nine working hypotheses relating mainly to persons abnormally good or abnormally bad at human-equipment performance. He is currently devising experiments to test some of these hypotheses in his laboratory.

Man–machine interactions, from the theological arguments advanced later, ought to come clearly within the realms of physics, as ought interactions between man and animals, like the shepherd and his sheep dog or a horse and its rider. In 1975, Del Blanco and Romero-Sierra, working in Canada, found that both man and the rabbit produced microwave signals at 8.95 GHz which were superimposed on, and well above, the thermal background noise corresponding to the body temperatures. Measurements were taken of signals from the abdomen and the hand of a man and from the head of a rabbit. The magnitude of the signals corresponded to different states of stress. They concluded that since the signal can be emitted by an animal and detected by conventional electronics, it is possible that animals can receive such signals as well – in effect communicate by radio. They do not suggest a mechanism, but they do 'call the attention of the reader to an interesting hypothesis in which DNA molecules are regarded as RF signal generators, RNA as amplifiers, the cell wall as a noise filter, and enzymes and amino acids as effectors of signals'. The present writers think that a 'holistic' approach may be more realistic.

Extrasensory perception

Only when the boundaries marked out by the laws of physics have been reached can it be ascertained whether there is a frontier with something beyond, whether we have reached the edge of the world, or whether we have been right round the world and returned to the starting point. Only when there are interactions between two 'spirit systems' (living systems having a dimension outside space and time) should it be necessary to consider the direct acquisition of information, knowledge and intelligence and their subsequent interactions with material parts of the systems. Whether the computer can function as a material extension of its spirit dimensional master must be left unconsidered.

To be able to discuss extra-sensory perception it is first necessary to ascertain how far our senses could possibly take us before the fundamental limitations set by our present understanding of physics are reached. Anything beyond this must only provisionally be labelled extra-sensory unless, or until it can be shown otherwise.

An account of Russian and East European work on Extrasensory Perception (ESP) has been given by Ostrander and Schroeder (1970). They note a Russian experiment which suggests that ESP can be 'bugged'.

When one subject, Kamensky, was attempting to send pictures telepathically from Leningrad to another subject, Nikolaiev, in Moscow, unknown to them was an interceptor, Milodan, in a different building in Moscow. Nikolaiev got good images on three out of five images, Milodan also got good information on two of them. This raises the question as to whether one person can, through the interaction of the body's electromagnetic field on another person, read magnetic signals from that person's brain currents; or even more importantly, is it possible for one person's aura field to access and scan another's memory locations? The magnetic field sensitivities of the human can be such that the magnetic fields due to the brain currents are significant throughout the body, and thus should be strong enough for perception by a person close by. In the UK physicist Michael Shallis, at Oxford University, has carried out successful ESP experiments with some of Dr Jean Monro's allergy patients who, when in a highly reactive state, appear to exhibit enhanced ESP ability (Shallis, 1988).

Any highly sensitive biosensor has the possibility of becoming unstable and oscillating. It is likely to oscillate at the frequency of its maximum sensitivity. Objective tinnitus is one example. If the eye becomes electrically unstable, it ought to oscillate in the visible region. Thought images have allegedly been made by a person looking into the lens of a camera. With the eye and the camera focussed to infinity, any luminous image on the retina would be focussed on to the film in the camera. The only thing to be determined is whether mental concentration on thought images can generate luminous images on the retina under any circumstances.

From what has been presented so far in this book, highly coherent electromagnetic radiation must be a strong candidate for consideration in respect of those manifestations of 'energy' which do not behave in the manner expected of energy in simple classical physics. Saxton Burr (1972) has written about the possibility of 'fields of life' (L-fields) which are electro-dynamic and measurable; he considers that they may be small electrical potentials of the order of millivolts.

Psychic research still thrives in the Eastern part of Europe, as witnessed by the 6th International Conference on Psychotronic Research. Held in Zagreb from 13 to 16 November 1986, it attracted more than 200 participants, mainly from Eastern Europe. The term psychotronics was coined to distinguish from the vague term parapsychology, and to relate to the phenomena of the psychic and nervous systems of man and living systems in general.

Since ancient times, the Hindus have spoken about the existence of a 'third eye'. This is taken to be an organ (the pineal gland) or some part of the body (the finger tips) other than the retina which can be used even by blind persons for the perception of light, colours and shapes. There were several papers at the above conference discussing this phenomenon. However, now it is known that the stimulation of acupuncture points can be effected by laser and by microwave radiation, this phenomenon may well now have to be placed within the boundaries of existing physics. If the acupuncture meridians become electrically unstable, the wide range of stimulants suggests an equally wide range of emissions.

Dr Andrija Puharich (1962, 1986) also presented a paper in Zagreb. He discussed various forms of medical healing practice in which the frequency of 8 Hz appeared to be of importance as an agent of self-organisation and the generation of novelty. According to O'Keefe and Nadel (1978), 'It appears that one of the functions of hippocampus theta frequencies is to maintain large areas of the hippocampus (and perhaps other parts of the brain as well) in the same or related phases of excitability.' The narrow band of theta frequencies between 7.5 and 8.5 Hz, is said to be 'responsible for the suppression of ongoing-behaviour upon receipt of signals of novelty, punishment, or omission of anticipated reward and for the processing of new information under these conditions.'

When the bio-control system is faulty, as is probably the case with multiple-allergy patients (Chapters 6 and 7), then ultimate extremes of electromagnetic sensitivity may be observed. The strong emission of electromagnetic signals is then also likely. This is also when patients may experience what appears to be paranormal phenomena. A patient who, in the course of giving a medical history, indicates having had psychic experiences is very likely to be electrically hypersensitive. It is also notable that eight times more women between the ages of puberty and menopause present with extremes of environmental sensitivity. After menopause, the ratios become equal; before puberty boys outnumber girls by three to one (Thomson, 1985).

Perhaps there is a biological advantage in high sensitivities for those more intimately concerned with life and survival, growth and development. It has been suggested, by a monk, that the monastic life tends to lead to an increased development of the feminine side of the human male–female duality in the natures of those who live the monastic religious life and that the soul is always 'feminine' to God. This places a very different emphasis on the traditional 'feminine' attributes. Male aggression and the male dominated hierarchies of the world's churches may be in greater need of Mariology and the St Teresas of the world than they realise.

David McClelland, a psychologist at Harvard University, has found a 'Mother Teresa Effect'. After watching a BBC documentary film about Mother Teresa, the majority of audiences of Harvard students were found to have enhanced immunoglobulin A (IgA) in their saliva (Colligan, 1987). Although half the audiences disliked the film and Mother Teresa, these were just as likely to have enhanced IgA in their saliva. McClelland remarked that even the disapproving people were unconsciously responding to the strength of her tender loving care and that this boosted their immune systems. The effect disappeared within an hour of seeing the film. This raises two questions: first, whether the coherence in space and time of the features and voice of a person can have a direct electromagnetic effect, and, second, whether there is here evidence that ideas – in this case of tender loving care – can enter the body's regulatory systems to produce changes in the immune system. This may also be the mechanism whereby the spiritual dimension, at such places as Lourdes, enters the material dimension through the sick.

Spirit and matter

Science without religion is lame, religion without science is blind.
Albert Einstein (1897–1955)

Abbot Vonier (1953) considers modern science to have done theology a very great service in demonstrating the characteristics of the physical world, even to the point where the stability of Nature's laws has become almost a fetish, but at the same time it has failed to see God in Nature because the laws of Nature seem to account for everything. Yet, nothing is brought home to us so insistently in the present life as the enormous disproportion between reality and our knowledge of reality. Man is born to know, he writes, as the beast of burden is born to labour, but knowledge comes to man gradually through life. Man, in common with all living systems, has some 'principle of life' and sensation which ceases to function at death. This must mean at the death of the person because viable organs can still be transplanted and become a part of another person after the donor's decease.

The real distinction between man and the rest of living systems is that man's 'principle of life' (the technical term is 'soul') has the powers of intellect and the powers of willing things to happen; these are the powers of a 'spirit'. This activity requires knowledge and, if it is to continue outside space and time, knowledge must have an objective existence irrespective of the material systems in which information is gathered and stored during life in this world. Man's body is the gatherer of his information, the seeds of knowledge which must be stored in a form that the intellect can read and consider, and the Will, will.

The concepts of 'spirit' and 'spiritual substance' involve 'total freedom from the laws of space and time; the total absence of all that is matter [and presumably also energy], of all organic life, complete lack of sensation or sensitive life generally.' This is internally consistent, because any system which is outside space and time ought to be able to have perfect coherence (zero bandwidth) and consequently be able to interact with any temporal material system with zero energy requirement, possibly through the principles outlined at the beginning of this Chapter.

The traditions of theology give the concept of 'spirit' and matter as being completely incompatible in their modes of acting. 'The human body is raised to higher sensitive activities through the presence of a spiritual substance and, in return, the soul is perfected in will and intellect through those highly developed bodily senses.' An objective existence for knowledge and for the existence of entities capable of comprehending knowledge and of acting upon it, is implied. The manner in which any such entities are able to interact with the physical world comes within the competence of physics and must be of particular relevance to any mind–matter interaction. When the possible modes of interaction have been identified, it may then be possible to establish that an interaction took place on a specific occasion. The purpose of any such interactions may be 'good', 'bad', or 'indifferent'; to establish this requires a set of criteria for distinguishing 'good' from 'evil'. In the Bible, there are clear accounts of demonic possession of persons and of exorcism. In terms of the mechanisms proposed herein, this would be the informing and control of the material functions of a body by an alien intelligence, rather in the manner that a virus takes over the regulation of a cell. It was once remarked to the senior author by a monk that this is now a much less common occurrence than in the early days of Christianity, but that it still used to be common in remote regions and lands in which the Mass had never been offered.

Electromagnetic radiation and the afterlife

Abbot Vonier (1953) observed that,

> There are few things in theology that are of greater personal interest to each of us than the conditions of existence for the human soul the moment it departs from the body. ... The destruction of the organism makes the soul lose its hold on the body. Being a spirit, its only tie to the body is its activity in the body. ... The spiritual substance which we call the human soul has both spirit-functions and soul-functions. ... The spirit's causative power, actually exerted on a fit material subject, is the only link that keeps the spirit tied to the body. The moment the soul's causative influence on the body ceases from lack of an appropriate subject, i.e. normally constituted organic matter, the soul turns back on itself, and enters, that very moment, upon the pure spirit state. ... A spirit not only moves freely in space, but he is absolutely superior to space ... duration

[for it] has nothing in common with the best and division of human time ... its activity is all intellect and will ... a spirit by his very nature knows all those thing that are inferior to him, with the exception of the free acts of rational creatures.

At the moment of death, the acquisition of sense information must cease and the body's material information storage locations are about to cease functioning. If this 'information of a lifetime' is not to be lost for ever, it must be accessed and 'dumped' in a form appropriate to the knowledge-handling facilities of the soul in its spirit-state. Perhaps the soul in this state is able to 'read', from outside space and time, the information contained in electromagnetic radiation propagated from within space and time. It is to the transition point between life and death that a paper entitled, 'Electromagnetic Radiation and the Afterlife' (Slawinski, 1987) addresses itself. 'Nature abhors hard boundaries' so, if there is any essential complementarity to knowledge as a whole, the natural sciences and the supernatural sciences still have much to learn from each other, especially from within their interdisciplinary regions.

In the 'wet' account of the Creation as given in the Book of Genesis, light is given an important role. Slawinski (1987) attempts to sketch some of the boundaries between the literal and the figurative in the possible roles for 'light', which is, of course, only one octave in the spectrum of electromagnetic frequencies. The manner in which electromagnetic fields are ordered is a feature which distinguishes living from non-living matter. In general, electromagnetic fields are associated with those forces which act over greater than nuclear distances, in systems which involve masses too small to be gravitationally significant. Furthermore, there is an essential duality between electromagnetic frequencies and chemical structure. In living systems there is a coherence or ordering imposed on the essential randomness of the inanimate. There is now much literature describing the emission of coherent electromagnetic radiation (light and other wavelengths) from living systems; it appears to be an essential part of the bio-communication systems which control the homeostatic status of a living organism. A living cell needs a communication channel with the bandwidth provided by a coherent optical (light ray) carrier frequency in order to be able to communicate in real time all the information necessary for its detailed 'housekeeping' operations (Dr F.-A.Popp, 1986, personal communication). Slawinski also considers, by implication, the question as to whether the ordering which appears in coherence can have an existence like knowledge and be independent of the particular material or radiating system exhibiting that property of coherence.

At death, the whole entity of a person's 'acquired' information field must become separated from the body which is about to commence decay, if it is to retain any objective existence in the material world. This may be as the so-called 'death flash' or other 'out-of-the-body' experience. There is the possibility that information could be 'written' into environmental water, such as that retained in the stone or brick of a building. The necrotic radiation, if this is indeed an electromagnetic field phenomenon, could be the origin of such memories in locations for events which happened there. The possibility of 'fixing' a dowsable 'charge' into stones by cremation (Havelock Fidler, 1983) supports this view. Effects corresponding to the frequencies of electromagnetic fields can be precisely retained by water for extended periods (Smith *et al.*, 1985). If this is the case, then a reacting hypersensitive allergic subject should be able to 'read-out' this information at a later time, just as if they were accessing a magnetic tape or a hologram. A dowser might describe it as a 'water-line', 'track-line', 'aquastat' or 'black-line'. This information might also be holographic in nature and be interpreted as an actual presence at that point in space and time, that is the person might 'see a ghost'. This is close to Slawinski's (1987) coherent, non-corporeal consciousness field, with its innate creative action for light, giving the possibility of creating a substantial replica (apparition?), or an 'exact' re-creation. The regular array of cells in a biological system, or crystallites in stone, is similar to that mathematical function (the Shah Function, which is its own Fourier Transform) which could generate a holographic image of itself if illuminated by coherent radiation.

The more one studies Nature, the more clearly one sees the known physical laws being used with greater and greater precision and more and more sophistication. Much more in the Universe than we suspect may be run on the basis of 'secondary causality', without any need for the continual intervention of a deity, thereby making the original light-mediated Creation, as described in Genesis, even the more awesome.

Conclusion

> What a piece of work is man! How noble in reason! how infinite in faculty! in form, in moving, how express and admirable! in action how like an angel! in apprehension how like a god! the beauty of the world! the paragon of animals!
> <div align="right">William Shakespeare (1564–1616), <i>Hamlet</i></div>

> Man with all his noble qualities, with sympathy that feels for the most debased, with benevolence which extends not only to other men but to the humblest living creature, with his god-like intellect which has penetrated into the movements and constitution of the solar system – with all these exalted powers – still bears in his bodily frame the indelible stamp of his lowly origin.
> <div align="right">Charles Darwin (1809–82), <i>The Descent of Man</i></div>

Electromagnetic Man is marked and permeated both with the stamp of the duality between the chemical matter and coherent electromagnetic oscillations of his living body on the one hand, and with his body-spirit duality on the other.

From the evidence now available, it seems that living systems are able to make use of the whole of the electromagnetic spectrum for communication and control activities, from the ultra-violet to the sub-Hertz and with sensitivities limited only by the laws of physics. The oscillations must be highly coherent in both space and in time. The maximum degree of coherence in time which can be of significance is that corresponding to the life-time of the organism itself; for this the bandwidth of the frequency spectrum will be of the order of the reciprocal of the life-time. The degree of spatial coherence must be at least that corresponding to an organism's spatial dimensions; but, man's coherence may well extend outwards in space and time to encompass the total sphere of his influence through the spiritual dimension.

A living system under good homeostatic control can probably choose when, whether and how to make use of the extreme sensitivities potentially available to it for bio-communication. Does being under good spiritual control facilitate extremes of sensitivity in communication outside the material world?

The clinical effects which can be produced by water exposed to chemical allergens or magnetic fields require explanation, as do the other remarkable properties of water and particularly the 'living water' of the Bible and Talmud. The ice crystals obtained by freezing water in a magnetic field are asymmetrical with respect to the field direction. The varied crystal patterns obtained by crystallisation of solutes from homoeopathic potencies must be the result of physical processes because there can be no chemistry in potencies diluted beyond Avogadro's Number. Professor Jacques Benveniste and his colleagues in several other laboratories around the world have found immunological experiments to be affected by dilutions carried out to homoeopathic potencies (Davenas et al., 1988). This work has produced quite remarkable and pathological reactions from the scientific establishment which, taken in the historical context presented earlier in this book, say something very profound about human nature in all centuries.

The only symmetry suitable for structuring water by a magnetic field is a helical or toroidal symmetry. The basic symmetry remaining after the cavitation produced in homoeopathic potentisation should be that of a dodecahedron, a twelve-faced spherical cavity formed from pentagonal rings of water molecules. The combination of these criteria leads to a pearl chain of dodecahedron cavities around the surfaces of which electrical currents arising from coherent jumping of the hydrogen bonds would circulate in solenoidal paths. Quantitative measurements of structuring in aqueous media is an urgent topic for research as it would provide a detailed and predictive physical basis for homoeopathy, acupuncture and some other alternative therapies. It is known that chemical reactions can be speeded up by stirring and by the application of ultrasonics. The procedure of succussion may also produce a phase change within the water structure. This possibility has implications for electromagnetic interpretations, for example through 'water of crystallisation' in silicates, for phenomena associated with dowsing, ancient stones and the effects produced by hammering stones.

The realisation of the essential duality between electromagnetic frequencies and chemical structure, as exemplified in chemical analysis by spectroscopy, makes electromagnetic hypersensitivity less remarkable.

Because of this duality, one should not really be surprised to discover that Nature has made use of as many combinations of frequencies as she has of atoms in the wonderful atomic architecture of organic chemistry and biochemistry.

Energy calculations only depend upon initial and final energy states of a system and are independent of the physical processes by which the transition between states is achieved. For a magnetic or electric field to be effective in establishing an ordering, it must be able to overcome thermal fluctuations which would cause the ordering to diffuse away. The energy contained in a field is proportional to the volume it occupies. Equating the thermal energy and the energy density of the field gives an estimate of the minimum volume over which such ordering could be established by any given field. Conversely the threshold field sensitivity for an organism of given size can be deduced. These threshold fields can also be related to the incident or emitted power densities by multiplying the energy per unit volume by the velocity of propagation of the energy. The minimum incident power density for a biological cell just a little larger than 10 μm corresponds to $100 \, W/m^2$. This happens to be an international exposure safety level for microwave radiation, which was chosen as being unlikely to give rise to injury in human and biological systems, which is of course based on the premise that only thermal injury can occur.

However, if a complex biological system is able to absorb or emit radiation in a coherent way involving the whole organism rather than its component parts, then effects of emission and absorption at the very much lower field strengths should be expected, as shown in Table C.1 (Smith *et al.*, 1987).

In the course of measurements on various magnetic field effects in

Table C.1 Threshold fields within the volume of the biological system, corresponding to an energy of kT at 310 K

Biological system	Single cell	Hen's egg	Standard man
Size of system	10 μm	70 g	70 kg
Threshold (electric field)	100 V/m	250 μV/m	8 μV/m
Threshold (magnetic field)	3 μT	9 pT	300 fT
Threshold (power density)	$80 \, W/m^2$	$600 \, pW/m^2$	$<1 \, pW/m^2$

biological systems, it was noticed that in many cases the onset conditions corresponded to the magnetic field strength at which a single quantum of magnetic flux would be linking the apparent cross-sectional area of the cell as measured with an optical microscope. It has been pointed out by Fröhlich that theoretically, magnetic flux is always quantised. In most physical systems, magnetic flux quantisation is not detectable. The quantum of magnetic flux has the value $h/2e = 2.07 \times 10^{-15}$ Wb, and represents another fundamental limitation to sensitivity. Furthermore, any system which is able to make use of magnetic flux quantisation also has the 'Josephson Effect' available to it, since this depends directly on magnetic flux quantisation. In turn, this implies the availability of a conversion between frequency and voltage of 500 MHz/μV.

The fundamental physical limits to the ultimate sensitivity that any given living system can have to electromagnetic fields is actually approached in certain cases. These include not only human vision and hearing, but also the electrical sensitivities of certain fish. Multiple-allergy patients who have acquired hypersensitivities to many environmental and nutritional factors may also acquire this theoretical limiting sensitivity to electromagnetic fields as a part of their general allergy package. Their allergic reactions may be provoked by any frequencies from at least milliHertz to gigaHertz and at extremely low intensities. Electrical hypersensitivity is not likely to be found in any patient who does not already have a number of environmental, chemical or nutritional allergic responses. If these can be cleared up by suitable treatment, the electrical hypersensitivities tend to clear up too. This strongly suggests that some chemical pre-sensitisation is a necessary precursor. Chemicals particularly suspect include organo-chlorides and formaldehyde. It is fortunate that the formaldehyde microwave resonance line at 14.489 GHz is reserved for radioastronomy. This means that there should be no transmissions on this wavelength since these would interfere with the possibility of detecting formaldehyde in outer space. Since all matter, living and non-living, is made from chemicals, and feeds on chemicals, it is necessary to find out precisely which molecules (i.e. the spatially and temporally coherent arrangements of the atoms) may be causing the problems for hypersensitive persons. The practicability of selective pesticides means that such molecules, and coherent frequencies associated with them, will be organism-specific. Geophysical and climatological bio-effects, allergic, behavioural and social problems all require to be re-examined in respect of electromagnetic hypersensitivities.

Coherent frequencies have been found to be very patent-specific. It is possible to neutralise electrical hypersensitivities by reinforcing certain coherent frequencies which are specific to a particular patient. It appears that those frequencies corresponding to a disease state take longer to establish and must therefore be more coherent than those corresponding to the healthy state where the response is much more rapid.

The testing for electromagnetic hypersensitivity can be done merely by having the patient in the same room as an ordinary laboratory oscillator tuned to the required frequency; sufficient signal for this purpose usually leaks from the oscillator, just as there are enough signals leaking out of a television set to be found by a detector van, or from a computer enabling it to be read by remote surveillance systems. The senior writer uses a level of ELF alternating magnetic field strength of the order of 10–30 nT to commence testing patients for electromagnetic hypersensitivity. This level of magnetic field would be generated 1 m away from a long wire carrying a current of $\frac{1}{10}$ amp.

It was found, perforce necessity, that a tube of water or saline exposed to a magnetic field at the patient's neutralising frequency has a clinical effect as if it were a homoeopathically potentised remedy of the patient's neutralising dilution of allergen. Dr Monro has compared diluted allergens with the same substance homoeopathically 'potentised' and finds them clinically equivalent. It is possible to trigger allergic responses either chemically or electrically and to neutralise them either electrically or chemically, whichever way the allergic response was triggered initially. This emphasises the involvement of the patient's own regulatory systems in this condition.

Both electronic equipment and other nearby patients may need protection from allergic subjects. When in a reacting condition, they may also emit electromagnetic signals. The case histories of the more than 100 patients tested include many such instances. The emission of coherent electromagnetic radiation by living systems is widespread, thus, the allergic status of any clinician, or any person handling live biological materials, is as important as any source of electromagnetic field exposure to laboratory water. These matters should be well documented in records of experiments.

There is evidence that information can be electromagnetically 'written' into environmental water, particularly that retained in the stone or brick of a building. Effects corresponding to the frequencies of electromagnetic fields can be precisely retained by water for extended periods and a reacting allergic subject should be able to 'read-out' this information at a later time by electromagnetically 'zapping' the environment.

At the moment of death, the component organs of the body do not also all die at the same instant; otherwise, organ transplantation would not work. But, when a person dies, the acquisition of sense information ceases; the information storage locations in the brain cease to function and decomposition sets in. If this information acquired throughout a life-time is not to be lost for ever, it must be 'accessed' and 'dumped' elsewhere, preferably as pure, immaterial, information; perhaps it passes through the necrotic electromagnetic radiation and in some circumstances becoming structured into environmental water or stone.

If each cell of the living body is able coherently to convert the energy from a reservoir corresponding to its thermal environment at 310 K into electromagnetic radiation, then man would be capable of emitting 100 watts/m^2 of radiation – about the strength of sunlight in temperate latitudes in a different approach, Professor Pethig has estimated the total electron transport along each metabolic pathway in the body to be about 200 amps. Since the energy band gap of proteins is about 5 eV, this represents an electrical power of about 1 kW, comparable, as it must be, to metabolic outputs. If all this power could be briefly converted into coherent radiation, then two reacting allergic subjects should be able to communicate line-of-sight on most frequencies. If a person could generate this power at frequencies below 30 MHz, where the ionosphere behaves as a reflecting layer or mirror, there is potentially enough power available for communication, albeit with very limited bandwidth, between hypersensitive subjects beyond the horizon and half-way round the world.

This leads to the final question, 'What level of electromagnetic radiation is safe?' In a world in which the only certain thing in 'life', is 'death', and in which road traffic accidents are running at epidemic proportions, the reply must be, 'How *safe* do you want *safe* to be? One cannot eliminate hayfever by stopping farmers from growing grass, it grows without assistance, and many people spend all their lives in the country without ever getting hayfever. One cannot eliminate headaches by legislating that there shall be no more thunderstorms; there are about 2000 occurring somewhere in the world at any given time.'

The present US and UK guidelines of 100 W/m^2 (10 mW/cm^2) limiting exposure to microwave radiation represents a fraction of the power density of tropical sunlight. But it is only reasonable from the point of view of avoiding widespread thermal injury, and represents enforceable legislation. The level of non-ionising radiation which will produce no effects of any kind in any person could not be lived with from an engineering stand-point in view of the expectations society has from modern electronics. It is even below the level of non-ionising radiation which people can themselves emit and which can affect other hypersensitive persons in their vicinity. It is also below the level of geomagnetic disturbances and environmental factors like the weather.

The UK, as yet, has no guidelines on ELF but there is now coming together for the first time some indication as to what the threshold might be for an increased statistical risk of cancers, behavioural effects and suicides following long-term low-level exposures to coherent, alternating, power frequency magnetic fields. Most biological systems and populations are characterised by a sigmoidal (s-shaped) response to stress, and there will be some individuals right out on the tail of high sensitivity. The ultimate 'safe' level for a given individual probably also depends upon his or her genetic, nutritional, environmental and hormonal status. One would not wish to have people involved in litigation against their parents because they are dissatisfied with their genetic or allergic inheritance.

There is no simple ready-made solution to the environmental problems other than to clean up the environment. On present running, Sweden and New Zealand will probably come up with the most practical solution in terms of a 'No Fault' compensation scheme, which currently pays from taxation, compensation at an agreed scale for injuries, disability and even death to victims of medical accidents. The compensation can be paid within months, instead of the five or six years that it takes in Britain to obtain compensation by suing through the courts. The British Medical Association and the Law Society have been again discussing these possibilities for Britain. There are real worries that Britain is moving in the direction of the American style of medical litigation. 'No Fault' legislation would need to include environmentally induced disease. It should be remembered that it is more difficult and expensive to take legal action in the UK than in the USA. Recalling the old adage that 'a government is not an "honest man"', it is quite possible that in environmental matters governments may not allow themselves to be sued. Even the EEC has its difficulties. If a moratorium were instituted in respect of environmental illnesses, the sufferers from effects due to power-lines, for example, might get compensation without the CEGB having to accept liability; but, if the electricity undertakings were privatised, the CEGB might disappear, the purchasers might deny liability, and there would be nothing tangible left to sue. The only recourse would be the ballot box. Fortunately, all the 1988 political party conferences seem to have seen the 'green light', although their commitment to correcting and preventing 'electropollution' remains to be seen.

Once the dirty environment is clearly seen to be costing governments and polluters money, there will be a real incentive to clean it up. In Scandinavia, a whole house has been transported to a site away from overhead power-lines, but the Baltic is biologically dead. In Texas, a very substantial punitive award of about $25 million was made against a utility for siting power-lines over a school. The judgement was upheld at appeal, although the punitive damages were removed, while the utility had spent $8 million in resiting the lines. In Florida, juries have awarded $1 million to owners of land next to high-voltage power-lines. In parts of California, health warnings, like those on cigarette packets, are being issued to potential buyers of properties near power-lines.

The risk of a flood of litigation must be one of the factors which prevents the USA from officially admitting that there may be effects due to non-ionising radiation at non-thermal levels, even though the military in both the USA and the USSR have long accepted this 'Catch-22' situation as the price to be paid for having unrestricted use of any and every part of the electromagnetic spectrum.

As mentioned already, the National Research Council (USA) accepted, in July 1986, that non-thermal effects of non-ionising electromagnetic radiation can occur but stopped short of admitting the possibility that there might be harmful effects. The situation changed even as this book was being written for, on 1 July 1987, the New York State Power Lines Project published its Final Report. Six years previously, it had been constituted to spend $5 million to investigate ELF health effects as ordered by the State's Public Service Commission in its ruling on a ten-year-old dispute over planning for a power-line to import cheap and clean hydro-electricity from Canada. Overall, the conclusion is that funded studies have indicated a 'variety of effects' not 'previously appreciated' and that 'several areas of potential concern for public health have been identified' (*Microwave News*, July/August 1987).

A cleaner environment is in the interests of all on planet Earth. Yet, it is difficult to get funding for environmental research because it is not seen as being 'important'. A speaker on American television once said that it is irresponsible for researchers to do environmental research which might result in higher costs for industry! Dr Bill Rea is most emphatic that a dirty environment costs far more through illness and lost efficiency in the work force than would be the cost of cleaning it up. However, this assumes that work people in industry are not just 'expendible hands', who are expected to pay for their own health care anyway. Fortunately for the United States, they now have a Federal Law (FIDAL) which 'has teeth'; this requires employers to inform their employees of any hazards in the work place and it is not sufficient for them to be told in a meaningless form of words.

In Britain, the Environmental Medicine Foundation have collected enough resources to be able to establish a Chair of Environmental Medicine at the Robens Institute of the University of Surrey. The proposals in the recently published (UK) Education Bill lend themselves to being so interpreted as to allow the dismissal of any incumbent whose championing of a healthy environment conflicts with government policy. The Bill does not even enshrine academic freedom as sought by the Committee of Vice-Chancellors and Principals to protect from dismissal staff holding controversial or unpopular views (*Guardian*, 21 November 1987). If retaining an academic post in the UK only becomes possible for a 'Vicar of Bray', it will be a sad day for the World Environment.

Since the UK spends 30 per cent of its research budget on defence work, almost any environmental research involving electromagnetic field effects and man is bound to have implications affecting costs of defence projects and procurement. Since there is no 'Freedom of Information Act' and a catch-all 'Official Secrets Act' (currently under review), such pressure as may be applied to universities will be very difficult for them to withstand. It is not unknown in academic circles to hear that someone in a university has been 'pressured' by vested interests.

Chernobyl emphasised once and for all that environmental pollution does not recognise the boundaries of states or power blocs. The environment, like the weather (and taxation) reaches to the poorer countries which do not have the health, nutrition and material resources to mitigate the effects of environmentally induced disease. Environmental protection must include the removal of pollutants, or the provision of adequate safe-havens to protect the hypersensitive from all the contaminants, chemical and electromagnetic which 'foul the nest' of Planet Earth.

In 1964, the magazine *Time* remarked that the annual turnover of General Motors exceeded the Gross National Product of India. But ideas are more powerful than money or multi-nationals. In Europe, the year 1987 was designated 'European Year of the Environment'. This was much overdue in view of the fact that throughout recorded history, armies have fought for the possession of some or other small patch of Europe. It indicates that 'all the armies of the world are not as powerful as an idea whose time has come'. Electromagnetic fields have changed the course of history. This century, for the first time since the city-states of ancient Greece, one man can through radio and television speak to the nation; more recently through satellite transmissions, and for the first time since the beginning of the human race, one person can be seen to address all humankind. The time has come for these ideas. Will Electromagnetic Man speak words of love or hate, good or evil?

Let those who eat the bread and watch the circuses made possible by high technology, be mindful of those fellow humans who have barely two pieces of alternative technology to rub together but who still retain the gift of life and who seek justice and fulfillment according to their status as members of the human race. The more one sees patients, the more one realises that illness is the great leveller of persons from all walks of life to what is basic and common to their humanity.

> Whatever can be useful to starving millions is beautiful to my mind. Let us give today the first vital things of life, all the graces and ornaments of life will follow.
>
> Mahatma Gandhi

Postscript

During the course of writing this book, it became clear that whenever we finished it, it would not still be up-to-date by the time it was published. Research and debate are accelerating in the area of environmental electromagnetic effects and everything is beginning to snow-ball. Before radio and television made their impact on the news telling, all the papers carried a 'STOP PRESS' column. Written at the last possible moment, this Postscript is our Stop Press. After we have stopped writing, the American publications *Microwave News* and *VDT News* under their Editor, Dr Louis Slesin (PO Box 1799, Grand Central Station, New York, NY 10163, USA), must be recommended as the best informed source of material for keeping up-to-date on non-ionising radiation effects. We have restricted ourselves so far as possible to the discussion of non-ionising radiation, but this is inevitably some overlap. Alpha and beta radiations carry electric charge and interact with electromagnetic fields. Gamma-rays, like X-rays, are electromagnetic radiation. With the recent publicity being given to radon gas in the environment, these properties of ionising radiation should not be forgotten. The effects of free radicals in the body and the possibility of biological transmutations considered by Kervran (1972) are also relevant.

For further reading on coherence, Professor Fröhlich has edited a book entitled *Biological Coherence and Response to External Stimuli* (Fröhlich, 1988), which presents an extensive treatment of the introduction of modern physical concepts into biology. In particular, the concept of coherence finds wide application and yields novel results in connection with long-range cellular effects and resonant interactions of biological tissues with low-intensity electromagnetic radiation.

Another book, *Modern Bioelectricity*, edited by Andrew A. Marino

(1988), who has doctorates in both biophysics and law, assembles contributions covering the development of bioelectricity during the past 20 years. Initially, people had said that physiological effects of electromagnetic fields did not exist, or if they did, they were 'classical'. That is, they were non-quantum effects, thermal in nature and the magnitude of the effect produced was directly proportional to the stimulus. Hence, they presented no threat to the scientific 'status quo'. But, as is remarked, it is the duty of each citizen to contribute to the collective judgment of how scientific facts are to be incorporated into the fabric of their society. This book represents a major contribution to that scientific and social dialogue; it includes sections covering the regulation of life processes, the electrical properties of tissue, the biological effects of electromagnetic fields, the therapeutic applications of electromagnetic energy, and finally, the health hazards of electromagnetic energy.

Dr Fritz Popp (Popp *et al.*, 1988) has edited a second and enlarged edition of his book *Electromagnetic Bioinformation*. This deals specifically with the ways in which living systems can emit and show spectral responses throughout the whole spectral range, from the extremely slow fluctuations below 1 Hz up to the ultraviolet region and possibly above, and use such waves for regulatory processes or, more generally, for communication within living systems.

The proceedings (mostly in French) of the transdisciplinary seminars on synergism and coherence in biological systems which have been held since 1983 in Paris, and have been edited by Dr Zbigniew William Wolkowski (1988), are a salutary reminder that not everything of importance happens in English. In the third series of the Proceedings, there is a paper *Man and Milligauss* by Professor Yves Rocard (the father of the present Prime Minister of France) in which one finds that, although his last resume in English appeared in Barnothy (1964), much work has been done since then.

The senior author has had another paper accepted by the journal *Clinical Ecology* in which he reports that the logarithms of the neutralising frequencies (see Chapter 6) appear to be proportional to the logarithms of the natural numbers. This means that when the first two have been found, the remaining provocation and neutralisation frequencies should be predictable.

There have been several recent theoretical developments relating to electromagnetic man, these include an important paper by Del Giudice, Preparata and Vitiello (1988) in which they show that the usually neglected interaction between the electric dipole of the water molecule and the quantised electromagnetic radiation can be treated in the context of a recent quantum field theory formulation of collective dynamics. The result is the possibility that coherent interactions between water electric dipoles and the radiation field can generate ordered structure in macroscopic domains of the order of a hundred microns in size. Such domains could be the basis of the memory properties of water described in this book. In a further paper, Del Giudice and Preparata (to be published) consider the consequences of a laser mechanism acting in liquid water which is predicted to behave as a physical system far from equilibrium. A consequence of highly coherent structuring is that within the structured region, as in the electron beam laser, the relation – frequency times wavelength equals the constant velocity of propagation of the electromagnetic wave, does not apply. Rather, the wavelength is the constant and there are many velocities and proportional frequencies.

If the dimensions of regions of coherence in water correspond to a 100 μm wavelength, then the critical magnetic field for one flux quantum to link each of them is of the order of 100 nanotesla. This implies that the threshold for any effects, whether harmful or not, associated with structured water in a living system will be of the order of 100 nanotesla. The senior writer tests patients for electrical hypersensitivity at about 30 nT. The extrapolations of the suicides data of Perry, the leukaemia data of Wertheimer and Leeper, and Savitz, the threshold of magnetic field perception by dowsing, the warning threshold chosen for the Kombi-Test environment field monitor, and geomagnetic disturbances, all come in this region. Maxey (1975) reported preliminary results of experiments using alternating magnetic fields (0.6–30 Hz, 30–1800 nT) at the heads of subjects during routine EEG recording in a hospital. In some of the patients, coupling occurred at 30 nT between the ELF and the rhythmic brain activity similar to the photic driving by a flashing light. Coupling at low frequencies increased the amplitude of the brain waves, coupling at higher frequencies reduced them. Spontaneous bursts of theta brain waves (4–7 Hz) were liable to cause decoupling. An interesting possibility is that communications to submerged submarines could be read or interfered with by sensitive persons.

All this is taking place at considerably greater field strengths than predicted for cooperative effects involving the whole man, based on energy considerations. However, it does suggest that magnetic fields which are able to influence macroscopic domains in water need to be taken seriously as possible biological stressors. Unfortunately, most of the fields generated by the activities of modern technology must therefore be classed as possible biological stressors.

Synthesis from the latest work enables one to begin to appreciate in a simplistic manner how water can remember frequencies and chemical structures to which it has been exposed and thence affect living systems. The senior writer has proposed that water must have a helical structure to be able to interact with a magnetic field. The coherent structures predicted for water (Del Giudice, *et al.*, 1988) of the order of 100 μm, and the constancy of wavelength within a highly coherent region makes the frequency proportional to the velocity; this, in turn, will be proportional to the charge hopping rate, where the maximum rate is 10^{11} hops per second. A feature essential for a liquid is that length will not define a resonant frequency, only the precision with which frequency can be specified. Dilution and succussion will therefore only increase the precision of the frequency determined by coherence and hopping rate. Thus, there should be a limiting frequency resolution of the order of tens of milliHertz; resonant frequencies of about 6 kHz in highly potentised preparations and 30 kHz in lower potencies. Dr Wolfgang Ludwig (1988) has observed such frequency spectra in homoeopathic and similar preparations. He has presented preliminary results at a number of seminars, including those of the Brügemann Institute.

The apparatus needed is a state-of-the-art Rockwell Signal Analyser. A bandwidth of 0.25 Hz can be used over the frequency range up to 50 kHz. With careful electromagnetic screening, the detection of water signal levels of the order of a microvolt across the 20 megohm input impedance of a specially constructed pre-amplifier is possible. The upper bounds of the so-called 'Ultra-Fine Bio-Energy Region' can thus be defined. This term was coined to describe the weak field effects being measured by the MORA apparatus. It must be noted that although such electro-diagnosis and therapy instruments are basically low frequency amplifiers and bridges, high frequency signals from patients and testers can be guided efficiently along their open wires especially as they are covered with insulation (Goudau, 1950) and can be detected through the amplifier non-linearities. Such surface wave propagation applies generally and with equal force to overhead transmission lines and electrical wiring in general.

The bond angles of the water molecule lead naturally to a basic pentagonal structure for their simplest planar arrangement. These should form naturally into a dodecahedron (a 12-sided, near-spherical cavity) at the interface of collapsing bubbles formed by the succession of a homoeopathic potency. This is strangely consistent with Benveniste's findings that only those dilution ratios which correspond to the planes of symmetry of a dodecahedron produced effects at his homoeopathic levels of dilution. A pearl-chain of dodecahedrons would also provide a helical structure and this would make the fundamental 'bit' for information storage the relative dynamic positions of the hydrogen bond and the covalent bond between the oxygen atoms of water molecules around a dodecahedron.

The senior writer sees the fundamental action of homoeopathic potencies on a living organism as being the seeding of the frequencies of specific resonant modes in the multi-mode, multi-frequency dielectric resonator which is constituted by the organism's morphology. Just as light travels down a glass rod or a fibre optics light guide, any block of dielectric whatever its refractive index (i.e. any organism) always has at least one propagating electromagnetic mode and without any need for the bounding metal walls of the cavity resonator. There is an external field to a dielectric resonator which is not radiated but which will induce currents in nearby objects (i.e. other organisms) and receive power from them (Whitmer, 1948; Hondors and Debye, 1910). This is just the right sort of resonator to account for the observed properties of metabolically pumped coherent oscillations in living systems.

Over the past 30 years, Burkhard Heim, of Northeim near Göttingen, in West Germany has developed a new logic, a new system of mathematics and a universal quantum field theory, which overcomes the difficulties encountered by Einstein, Heisenberg, Leibnitz and Newton in trying to formulate a theory which would unite the macrocosmos and the microcosmos.

Heim's Theory (1980, 1984) can give the precise values of the constants of elementary particles. It predicts a 6 – dimensioned cosmos, which includes the 3 – dimensions of space we already use, the dimension of time, and two further dimensions which are considered to be outside physical experience, namely the psychic and the spiritual. It appears that photons, the energy components of the electromagnetic field, have components in the fifth and sixth dimensions too. The fundamental noise limitation in electronic amplifiers arises from electron-phonon scattering; electromagnetic waves are perturbed in the time dimension by this interaction and hence they become noisy with consequent corruption of the information they are carrying. But they should remain noise-free and the information carried remain uncorrupted if they can be intercepted in Heim's fifth and sixth dimensions. In effect, this possibility was considered in relation to necrotic radiation in Chapter 12.

Operator-related anomalies in the performance of a wide range of engineering devices, systems and processes have been investigated by Robert Jahn, Dean Emeritus of the School of Engineering and Applied Sciences, Princeton University (Jahn and Dunne, 1987). The primary effect in psychokinesis experiments is only a very marginal effect, but it has been replicable in over two million experiments and occurs at a probability level that would be unacceptable in space technology. A theoretical model based on quantum mechanical metaphors has been worked out by them.

Professor Jacques Benveniste, in Paris, observed the biological activity of high dilutions in the course of his work on mode of action of homoeopathic remedies. He had published this work in the European Journal of Pharmacology (Davenas, Poitevin and Benveniste, 1987) and in the British Journal of Pharmacology (Poitevin, Davenas and Benveniste, 1988) but its significance had still not been noticed by the scientific community at large. Parallel experiments had been made in the laboratory of Professor Z.Bentwich at the Kaplan Hospital in Rehovot, Israel, and in Milan and Toronto. These were by no means the first attempts to investigate homoeopathic potencies by classical scientific experiments (Reilly, 1988).

Benveniste had by then been trying for two years to get the journal, *Nature* (London), to check the data and publish it. On the 30 June 1988, their paper, now with 13 co-authors from five different laboratories, appeared in *Nature*. Then, an inquisitorial team comprising the Editor of *Nature*, an American specialist in the subject of misconduct in science and a well known American professional magician visited just one of the participating laboratories, that of Professor Benveniste at INSERM, Clamart near Paris, the following week. In the issue of *Nature* dated 28 July 1988, they reported on the basis of this visit that the 'High Dilution' experiments were a delusion (Maddox et al., 1988), to which Benveniste (1988) gave a spirited reply.

Fifteen weeks later, Cyril Smith visited Professor Benveniste's laboratory and found strong signals coming from the cold store room, one of the benches and a nearby incubator. Inside the cold store, the source was a brown paper package containing the tubes handled by the inquisitors and the bench and incubator showing stress regions were those used by them. For such effects to remain for this period of time, at least one of the inquisitors must have been radiating very strongly, strongly enough to overwrite the high dilutions of antigen with his own signals while handling the tubes or pipetting. The onus is therefore on these people to demonstrate that they did not influence the course of the experiments that they were there for the purpose of validating.

It is well known that tubes of neutralising allergy dilutions should not be handled by other persons, as they often are rendered useless thereby. If this appears too far-fetched, Dr Leonhard Hochenegg's trick of lighting a fluorescent tube held in his hand (Playfair, 1988) should emphasise the electrical 'potentiality' of certain persons. Further, a Granada television report made some years ago showed a lady, who features in Shallis (1988), generating 1600 volts while holding the leads of an electrostatic voltmeter. The senior writer was not involved in this demonstration, but from seeing a video-recording it is clear that this is not a simple electrostatic phenomenon, rather, it is a high voltage being generated by a reacting allergic subject. It emphasises that electrical appliances should be designed to tolerate operator applied electrical stresses at least equivalent to the application of a high-voltage 'Megger' insulation tester without electrical breakdown or other failure.

A recent demonstration test carried out by the senior writer and Werner Kropp at the laboratories of Wekroma AG (Wekroma AG, Via Storta 78, CH-6645 Brione S/M., Switzerland) further shows the possibility of interactions between an experimenter and water. The apparatus used was a Perkin Elmer differential spectrometer (Model Lambda 3 UV/VIS) covering the range 190 nm to 900 nm. Two 10 cm path-length quartz cuvettes were used for the reference and sample beams. The instrument was set to record differences in absorbance of ±0.03 full scale. In Figure P.1, the zero tracing is for pure water in both beams. When Cyril Smith held the water in a beaker in the palm of the left hand for a minute and then returned it to the cuvette, the smaller of the deflections on the tracing was recorded. When this was repeated with fresh water and the beaker this time was held while standing on a strong geophysical anomaly within the laboratory, which was cut into the granite of the hillside, the even larger deflections were obtained. The tracings are very non-linear, not characteristic of thermal effects on the water spectrum such as might have been generated by the heat of the hand. Furthermore, the tracings are different in the two adjacent locations, with identical thermal conditions. However produced, such changes must be considered as possible perturbers of bio-photon communication systems, and thus as another example of possible experimenter interaction with living systems.

Werner Kropp has gone further than the work described by the senior author in Chapter 6 of this book in that he has determined the electromagnetic conditions necessary for a number of remedies which can be produced on a commercial basis within sealed ampoules of saline and which are not dependent on the neutralisation frequencies of a particular patient. Kropp too, is well aware of the ability of the electrical environment to influence his preparations. He takes anti-static precautions like those taken by workers with field effect transistors. He also has had a thin gold metallic coating applied to the outside of the bottles for his preparations, to serve as a light and electrical shield.

There are a number of pieces of evidence showing interesting left/right differences in man's electromagnetic interactions. The blood sedimentation rate (ESR) appears to be different depending on whether the blood is taken from the left or right side of the body as reported by Dr Bodo Kohler of Freiburg at a recent Brügemann Institute Seminar. The difference varies periodically in time. There is apparatus made in West Germany that records the capillary blood flow (plethysography) simultaneously from the left and right fingers. This is said to show differences under the same environmental conditions that dowsers obtain responses.

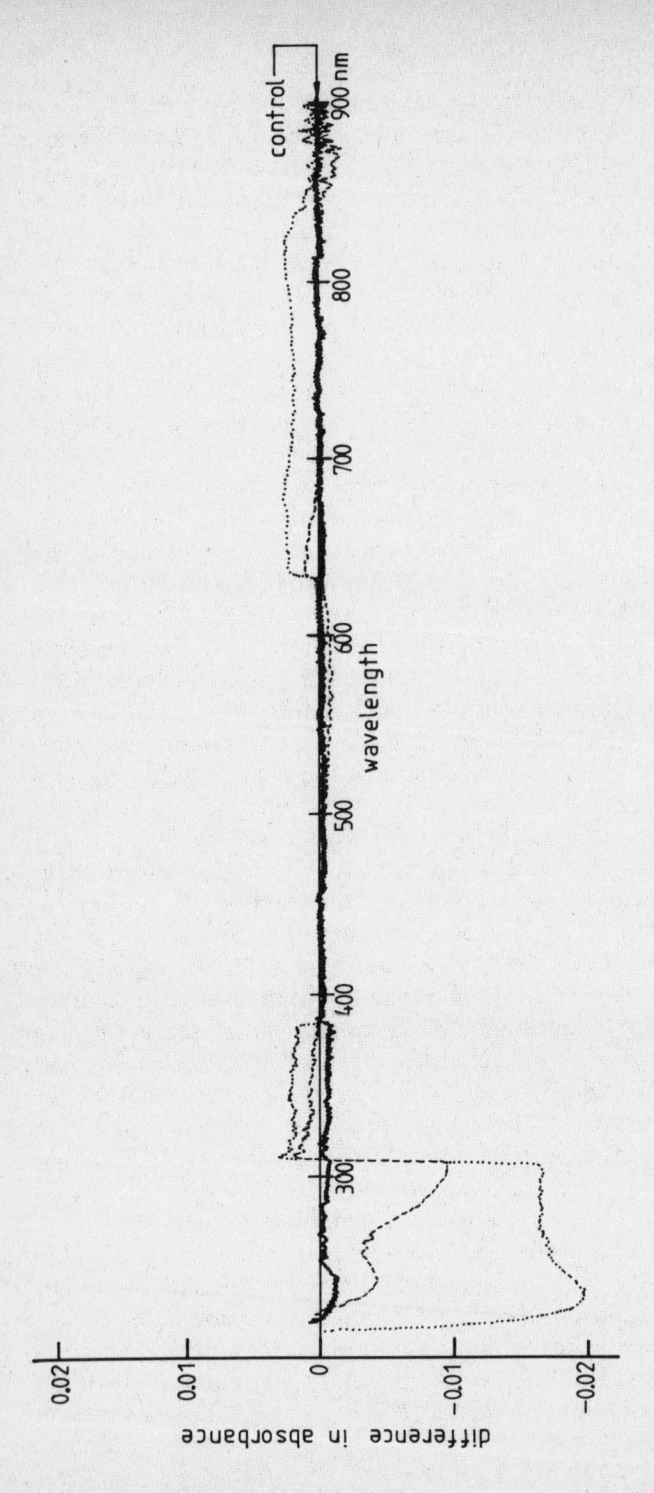

Fig. P.1 The change in the optical spectrum of water produced by the senior writer holding a beaker of water in the left hand for one minute. The traces were recorded using a Perkin Elmer differential spectrometer (Model: Lambda 3, UV/VIS) covering the range 190 to 900 nm, with 10 cm path length quartz cuvettes in the sample and reference beams.

The continuous trace was taken with pure water in each cuvette. The dashed trace was taken with an aliquot of the same water in the sample cell after holding it in a beaker for one minute. The dotted trace was taken similarly, except that it was held for one minute while standing over a known geophysical anomaly within the laboratory. The changes around 700 nm may be due to solvated electrons.

Roger Coghill (1988, 1989) has developed the hypothesis that there exists a cerebral morphogenetic radiation (CMR) system in the brain which makes use of polarity differences between the left and right hemispheres to convert steady potentials into a wide range of electromagnetic signals for regulation purposes, particularly for the initiation of protein synthesis. If this is correct, is must involve the Josephson effect. Electrical insulation is assumed to be provided by the myeling sheathing.

The purpose of paradoxical sleep, it appears, is to shut down motor and sensory activities at the thalamus-hypothalamus interface so that the CMR signals enjoy optimal conditions.

He notes that in cases of Sudden Infant Death Syndrome (SIDS) these children have nearly always been chronically exposed to some factor, perhaps electromagnetic radiation, which shows up as a demyelination of the corpus callosum. Likewise, recent outbreaks of meningococcal meningitis have all occurred near powerful sources of electromagnetic radiation.

The CMR signals are given downward directivity by the lateral brain ventricles. If this CMR system is interfered with by extraneous electromagnetic fields the cerebral control of cellular activity is disturbed, possibly leading to neoplasms.

Coghill notes that circulatory lymphocytes are the most sensitive of all body tissues to radiation, and suggests that AIDS itself may not have a viral aetiology, but may be the result of damage to the CMR system during infancy which shows up eventually as an immune deficiency. He points out that in the brain, the cortical array concerned with the genitalia (a signal important for survival of the species) are found deep in the central longitudinal fissure, and predicts that the immune control system lies between that region and the corpus callosum itself. Both of these are damaged when the corpus callosum is stressed and thermally damaged. Hence the associations of AIDS with sexual deviancy is simply because both immune defence and procreative drive mechanisms have been damaged.

As Adams (1989) points out, AIDS-like diseases have been described from at least the sixteenth century. Arguments against HIV causing AIDS are also based on the alleged finding of HIV patients having no trace of the virus, and of healthy people with HIV but no signs of AIDS. Thus, some contend AIDS is a mutant strain of syphilis.

Wilson (1988) has shown that chronic exposure to ELF electric or magnetic fields can disrupt normal circadian rhythms in rat pineal seratonin-N-acetyl-transferase activity as well as in seratonin and melatonin concentrations. Such disruptions in the circadian rhymicity of pineal melatonin secretion have been associated with certain depressive disorders in humans which Perry *et al.*, 1989, have again recently linked to power frequency exposure.

A vivid demonstration of the power of geopathic stress was provided by a photograph, shown at a recent Symposium of the Brügemann Institute, depicting identical quadruplet boys at about the age of seven, two of which were almost a head shorter and appeared stunted in growth compared with their siblings. They had always all slept in the same bedroom, but there were geopathic stress lines running through the beds of the two stunted in growth which missed the beds of those showing normal development. Geopathic stress zones have been followed through all 15 storeys of a tower block through persistant damp patches precisely aligned on all the floors and which cleared as soon as the geopathic stress had been cured. Research on geopathic stress has been taken seriously and been funded at the level of DM400,000 by the West German Government. It is being carried out by Professor Hildebert Wagner at the Institute of Pharmaceutical Biology in the University of Munich and a report is due early in 1989 (Best, 1988). Geopathic stress research is also being carried out at Szczecin, in Poland.

Work done in the senior writer's laboratory (M.Britton, to be published) showed that plants left over the weekend in a geopathic stress zone in which the magnetic field gradient was about $100 nT/metre$ were almost dead by the Monday and recordings showed a steady drop in activity throughout the weekend. The plants also seemed able to sense the small geomagnetic changes which originate in the ionosphere when sun illuminates it at dawn. Thus, they prepare themselves for photosynthesis as soon as daylight breaks at ground level.

In Chapter 11, we emphasised the dual role of light and water presented in the two Biblical accounts of the Creation. All the recent developments have reinforced the sense of wonder at the phenomenon of Man in an Electromagnetic Environment. The recently reported dating of the Turin Shroud fabric to a definite post-Christ era may still not be the final word. Remembering the work of Kervran (1972), living systems seem to be able to rearrange nucleons, including radioactive isotopes. Thus, the radio-isotope dating of any object closely involved with life must remain suspect so long as it is based on the assumption that there has been no change in the radioisotope content since, in this case, the material from which the fabric was originally woven had died.

The practical politics of life may be improved if the victims of medical and environmental accidents are compensated on a Scandinavian-system where fault does not have to be proved. This was discussed at a recent 'no fault legislation' conference in London (Times, 1988). What can be done for those of the 80,000 persons in the UK and many more throughout the world living under power lines who are being excessively stressed? To move the lines will give someone else the stress and NIMBY (not-in-my-backyard) will be invoked. Power line frequencies are the most difficult to shield, but a system of active compensation is possible (Malmivuo *et al.*, 1987) at least for the sleeping area. Radio and microwave frequencies are easier to shield with metal foil wallpaper.

There is yet another question of 'whose fault' which still needs to be addressed. In the nineteenth century, Bechamp and Pasteur (Hume, 1947) clashed over the possibility of pleomorphism (the occurrence of multiple forms of an organism in a single life cycle). Bechamp went even further, maintaining that bacteria could devolve into smaller invisible forms. In the 1930s Kendall, Rosenow and Rife (Lynes, 1987) demonstrated, with the Rife microscope, that the tubercule bacillus went through many changes including a form which passed through a bacterial filter. In 1948 there was proof that a cancer virus was actually a pleomorphic bacterium. In 1987, Lynes (1987) has described why 'The Cancer Cure That Worked' has never come to pass. As we have said in Chapter 1, the 'zeitgeist' and its prophets still wield great power over ideas. However, the Rife microscope and Rife oscillator are again being built; it has also been said that similar results have been obtained with a high quality optical microscope and two lasers.

At the 1988 round of UK Party Political Conferences, it was notable that all Parties seemed to have seen the 'Green Light'. In the context of Electromagnetic Man, the environmental problems are part scientific, part medical, part technological, part legal, and part political. When in 1986, *Save British Science* put an advertisement in *The Times* (13/1/1986) the Government was completely taken by surprise. Science does not enter the minds of Members of Parliament very much unless their constituents write about it. The then Treasury view was still that science was not of any benefit to the economy; this was based on a paper written some 20 years earlier. It will be very interesting to see, in 20 years' time, what actions governments have taken to clean up the electromagnetic environment. 1989 is European year for cancer; hopefully UK cancer charities will follow the lead of the American National Cancer Institute in funding major research projects into the link between cancer and EMF exposure.

If this book is to have a message, it is that we must now focus on the fundamental electromagnetic aspects of man's structure and function (long range coherence) and not be inhibited by the contemporary zeitgeist, or vested interests, into seeking exclusively chemical (short range coherence) explanations if we are to reach the limits of the possible and break through towards understanding, or at least accepting, the psychic and spiritual components of that Phenomenon we call Man.

Glossary

Airy disc: when a lens forms an image of a point of light, such as a star, the image is a bright spot of finite size, called the Airy Disc (named after the astronomer) surrounded by a halo of rings. The larger the diameter of the optical system, the smaller this resolution limiting image will be.

Allergy: the term allergy was coined by the Austrian paediatrician, von Pirquet (1905), from the Greek words 'ALLOS' = change and 'ERGON' = action. It describes a state of altered reactivity on exposure to a specific environmental factor. It is often used in the more restricted sense to refer to the subset of allergic patients who have abnormal immunoglobulin-E antibody effects.

Alpha-helix: the polymerised peptide groups of atoms which form proteins take on a helical configuration forming a hollow cylinder from which the side-groups radiate outwards.

Anaerobe: Anaerobic bacteria: organisms that do not need air or free oxygen molecules to be able to live and reproduce.

Anisotropy: this is used in the physics sense whereby specific properties have different values in different spatial directions.

Anti-oxidant: a chemical which prevents or inhibits molecular oxygen from acting as an unwanted oxidising agent (e.g. vitamin C).

Assay: the qualitative or quantitative determination of the atomic or molecular composition of a substance.

ATP: this is short for 'adenosine triphosphate' which is a co-enzyme assisting other enzymes in effecting the biochemical reactions necessary for metabolism.

Avogadro's number: this is the number of molecules needed to make up one gram-molecular weight of any substance, it has the value 6.02×10^{23} molecules (in German speaking countries, this is usually called Loschmidt's number).

Bandwidth: this is a measure of the sharpness of a resonance (see Figure 2.3) or wave filter, it is the frequency difference measured between the points at which the power has fallen to one half of its value at the peak.

Bioelectromagnetics: is the study of the interactions between biological systems and electromagnetic fields.

Boltzmann's constant: is the GAS CONSTANT divided by AVOGADRO'S NUMBER, it relates to the energy per degree absolute of temperature.

Boson: Bose condensation: bosons are particles that behave according to Bose-Einstein statistics. The wave function describing a pair of bosons is symmetrical and two such particles can be in the same state. This includes quanta of electromagnetic radiation, or photons. Under certain conditions, all the bosons in a system may condense in a single energy state to give an extremely intense and coherent oscillation.

Carcinogen: any agent which incites carcinoma or other malignant condition.

Catalyst: a substance which in small amounts can increase the rate at which a chemical reaction proceeds without itself being used up.

Coherence: the existence of definite fixed relationships between the phases of otherwise separate waves makes them coherent. It is a measure of the degree of precision of the velocity, frequency and wavelength. Coherence makes interference effects between waves possible.

Cytokinesis: this term is used in respect of certain biological cells to denote the division of the cell contents, cytoplasm, which may follow division of the cell nucleus and precede the formation of a new cell wall.

Dielectric: in general, every substance which is not a metal is a dielectric. However, it usually refers to an electrical insulator or near insulator which can sustain an electric field without thermal damage. The Dielectric Constant is the ratio of the electric field strength in vacuum to that in the material, for the same distribution of electric charge.

Dielectrophoresis: small objects including biological cells, experience appreciable forces due to alternating electric fields because of natural or induced dipoles. The magnitude and direction of these forces depend on the difference in dielectric constant between the particle and its surroundings and the square of the electric field.

Dipole: a system having two distinct and spatially separated poles, e.g. the North and South poles of a magnet, or electric + and − charges.

DNA: (deoxyribonucleic acid) is a polymer present in the chromosomes and some viruses which carries the genetic information encoded in the sequence of base groups attached to a sugar and phosphate polymer chain most being in the form of a two stranded helix kept together by hydrogen bonds.

Electric charge: is a basic property of fundamental particles which occurs in (positive, negative or zero) integer multiples of the proton charge. It is detected by the mechanical force existing between charges. An electrostatic field is a property of electric charge at rest, a magnetic field is a property of electric charge in steady motion, radiation is a property of electric charge being accelerated, or decelerated.

Electric field: this is a fundamental field of force in nature measured as the mechanical force per unit charge, or the gradient of the electrical potential.

Electromagnetic field (EMF): is a combination of an electric field and a magnetic field which may propagate as a wave, when it becomes Electromagnetic Radiation (EMR).

Energy (joule): a basic quantity in physics is the capacity of a system for doing work or absorbing work. In electricity, it is the work associated with moving an electric charge in the presence of an electric field.

Entropy: a measure of the disorder in a system, it is expressed at the energy which can be absorbed by a system divided by its absolute temperature. It is also equal to Boltzmann's Constant multiplied by the natural logarithm of the number of energy states of the system.

Enzyme: living cells produce these proteins which catalyse the various chemical processes essential to life without themselves being used up.

Enzyme-substrate complex: in enzymology texts a reaction intermediate, the term substrate is not to be confused with the physical and technological term 'substrate' meaning a lower layer usually providing mechanical support.

Free radicals: these are molecules which have the surplus spin of at least one un-paired electron. They are detected by electron spin resonance and may be highly reactive.

Frequency (Hertz): the number of cycles of an oscillation per second.

Gas constant: is the constant of proportionality relating the pressure, volume and absolute temperature of a so-called 'Perfect Gas'.

Hall effect: is the deflection of an electric current by a magnetic field and its importance is that it gives the sign and number of charge carriers per unit volume of the conductor or semiconductor.

Hydrogen: the simplest chemical element, comprising a single proton and electron. Water is an oxide of hydrogen comprising two hydrogen atoms for each oxygen atom. In water, (and certain other molecules) each hydrogen has a closer covalent bond to one oxygen atom than that at the other end of the linkage which is a HYDROGEN BOND.

Hydrophilic: water seeking or liking.

Hydrophobic: water avoiding or repelling.

Hydrolase: an enzyme that catalyses the hydrolysis of proteins, nucleic acids, starch, fats and macromolecular substances.

Hydrolysis: is chemical decomposition by water.

Inertia: resistance to a change in momentum.

Ion: an isolated electron or positron, or an atom or molecule (in a solid, liquid or gas) which has acquired a net electric charge by the gain or loss of one or more electrons.

Ionising and non-ionising radiation (NIR): electromagnetic radiation may be sufficiently energetic (high enough in frequency) to ionise an atom or molecule absorbing it. The boundary between ionising and non-ionising radiation is in the ultraviolet part of the spectrum, about 3×10^{15} Hz.

Josephson effect: occurs at a weak-link junction between two superconductors and is associated with quantised magnetic flux. It provides an interconversion between frequency and voltage.

Joule: the physical unit of energy or work. A force acting through a distance in the direction of the force does work and energy is expended. The unit is named after James Prescott Joule (son of a Salford brewer) who first measured and published the relation between heat and work in 1847.

Kilo-: prefix denoting one thousand times the basic unit, e.g. 1 kilovolt or 1 kV, equals 1000 volts.

Linearity (linear response): the output being in direct proportion to the input.

Lysozyme: a defence enzyme which hydrolyses the walls of certain types of invading cells.

Lyse: lysis: the dissolving of cells or tissues.

Magnetism: a phenomenon in the space around electric charge in uniform motion in a closed circuit, wire or coil (electromagnet), or an interacting domain of charge orbiting or spinning in an atom or molecule (permanent magnet).

Magnetic Field: the spatial distribution of the force between magnets.

Mega-: a prefix denoting one million times the basic unit, e.g. 1 MV = 1,000,000 V.

Micro-: a prefix denoting a one millionth fraction of the basic unit, e.g. 1 micrometre, 1 micron, $1 \mu m = 10^{-6}$ m.

Microwave: electromagnetic radiation decimetres, centimetres or millimetres in wavelength; it is used for cooking by energy absorption, also for radar and telecommunications as it can be formed into narrow beams.

Milli-: a prefix denoting a one thousandth fraction of the basic unit, e.g. 1 millimetre, $1 mm = 10^{-3}$ m.

Mitosis: In the asexual reproduction of cells, division of the cell nucleus takes place in such a way that the daughter cells receive identical copies of the genetic information from the parent cell. The sequence of events by which this takes place is conventionally divided into a number of arbitrary stages.

Newton's Laws: In his *Principia* written between 1684 and 1697, Newton postulated definitions of quantity of matter, inertia, force, and stated the three fundamental laws of motion, which are of general validity except at velocities close to the velocity of light when Einstein's Relativity modifications must be applied. Newton's Laws may be summarised:

I: Every body perseveres in its state of rest, or uniform motion in a straight line, except in so far as forces act upon it.

    II: Change of motion is proportional to the force and takes place in that direction.
    III: An action is always opposed by a equal and opposite reaction.

Newton also discovered the law of gravitational attraction which states that, any two particles attract with forces proportional to the masses and inversely proportional to the square of the distance separating them. This was verified by Kepler's Laws of Planetary Motion.

Nucleus:
    I: in the context of the cell, it is the major membrane encased compartment containing the chromosomes and RNA synthesis structures of the eukaryotic cell.
    II: in the context of atomic structure, it is the massive part of the atom containing the protons and neutrons within a sphere of about 10^{-15} m radius, compared with the 10^{-10} m radius of the surrounding cloud of electrons.

Oscillation: a periodic variation in e.g. a voltage or current or mechanical displacement.

Oxidation-reduction (REDOX): Chemical reactions involving electron movements are fundamental to all living systems. Some atoms (such as oxygen) have a greater affinity for electrons than others. In a chemical or electrochemical reaction, the atom which loses an electron is said to be oxidised, the atom which acquires an electron is said to be reduced.

Peek and Poke: are computer instructions, the former reads the contents of a specific memory location, the latter allows data to be inserted there.

Photoelectric effect: is the direct conversion of light into the mechanical energy of an electron emitted from surface into a vacuum. Each electron is the result of a light quantum (PHOTON) interaction, its energy depends on the frequency of the light and Planck's Constant.

Piezoelectric: certain anisotropic crystals (e.g. quartz) generate a voltage between faces when deformed mechanically and vice-versa. The effect is used in pick-up sensors for electromechanical recordings and in oscillators to give a stable frequency.

Polynucleotide: the structural units of DNA and RNA are called nucleotides, they combine a phosphate group, a sugar group and one of four different base groups. The sequence of units in the polymer provides the molecular mechanism for storing and transmitting genetic information.

Protein: is a polypeptide having a molecular weight above about 10,000 and a definite three-dimensional structure. Various proteins form much of the fabric of the animal body.

Provocation – neutralisation: This describes a clinical technique for the diagnosis and treatment of food allergy. It was first discovered by Dr Carleton Lee of St Joseph, Missouri. Subsequently, Dr Joseph Miller (1972) of Mobile, Alabama studied it and organised it into a comprehensive procedure for clinical testing, through the recording and interpretation of wheals following the

Glossary

pricking of the patient's skin with an allergen, and various other symptoms which might occur. It was found that if the allergen is serially diluted, certain dilutions produced symptoms while certain other dilutions nullified those symptoms; these results repeated in a cyclical pattern as the dilution proceeded. With very sensitive allergy patients it is not practicable to skin-prick or inject with allergen or vaccine hundreds or even thousands of times. For such patients, Dr Jean Monro has developed the technique of 'SURFACE APPLICATION' for which the drop of serially diluted allergen need only remain on the surface of the intact skin long enough to test for a reaction, after which it can be wiped away and replaced by a drop of a different dilution.

Quantum, (pl. Quanta): In 1900, Planck postulated that the emission and absorption of radiation takes place in discrete, finite sized QUANTA of energy each equal to Planck's Constant multiplied by the frequency.

Rectification: The conversion of an alternating voltage or current into a steady, unidirectional source.

RNA (Ribonucleic acid): a polynucleotide involved in cell protein synthesis. It is de-polymerised by the enzyme – ribonuclease.

Schumann radiation: ELF electromagnetic radiation between 1Hz and 30Hz originating in the resonator formed between the conducting Earth and the conducting ionosphere; the resonance is stimulated by distant thunderstorms.

Semiconductor: non-metallic materials (e.g. silicon) which have an energy band structure to their electrical conduction processes; they are used in many electronic devices.

Sonication: a process of cleaning by immersion in a bath agitated by high power ultrasonics.

Spectroscopy: Measurement of the frequencies contained in EMR, which are usually displayed as intensity vs. frequency.

Sync:
  I: short for synchronisation in electronics parlance, e.g. the (sync or synch) pulses ensure a stable television picture by providing the necessary synchronisation with the waveforms in the camera.
  II: a mathematical function written as $\sin x/x$, which relates for example to the spectrum of a pulse.

Talmud: the fundamental code of Jewish Civil and Canon Law comprising: the Mishnah which is the oral law finally redacted in AD 220, and the Gemara which is commentary and complement.

Thermodynamics: a theoretical technique for the derivation of physical properties involving changes of temperature and energy conversion.

Uncertainty principle (Heisenberg's): quantifies the absolute limit to the precision with which the position and momentum (or instant and energy) of a particle can be measured as equal to Planck's Constant.

Ultrasonic: acoustic oscillations at frequencies too high to be heard (usually

METRE-KILOGRAM-SECOND

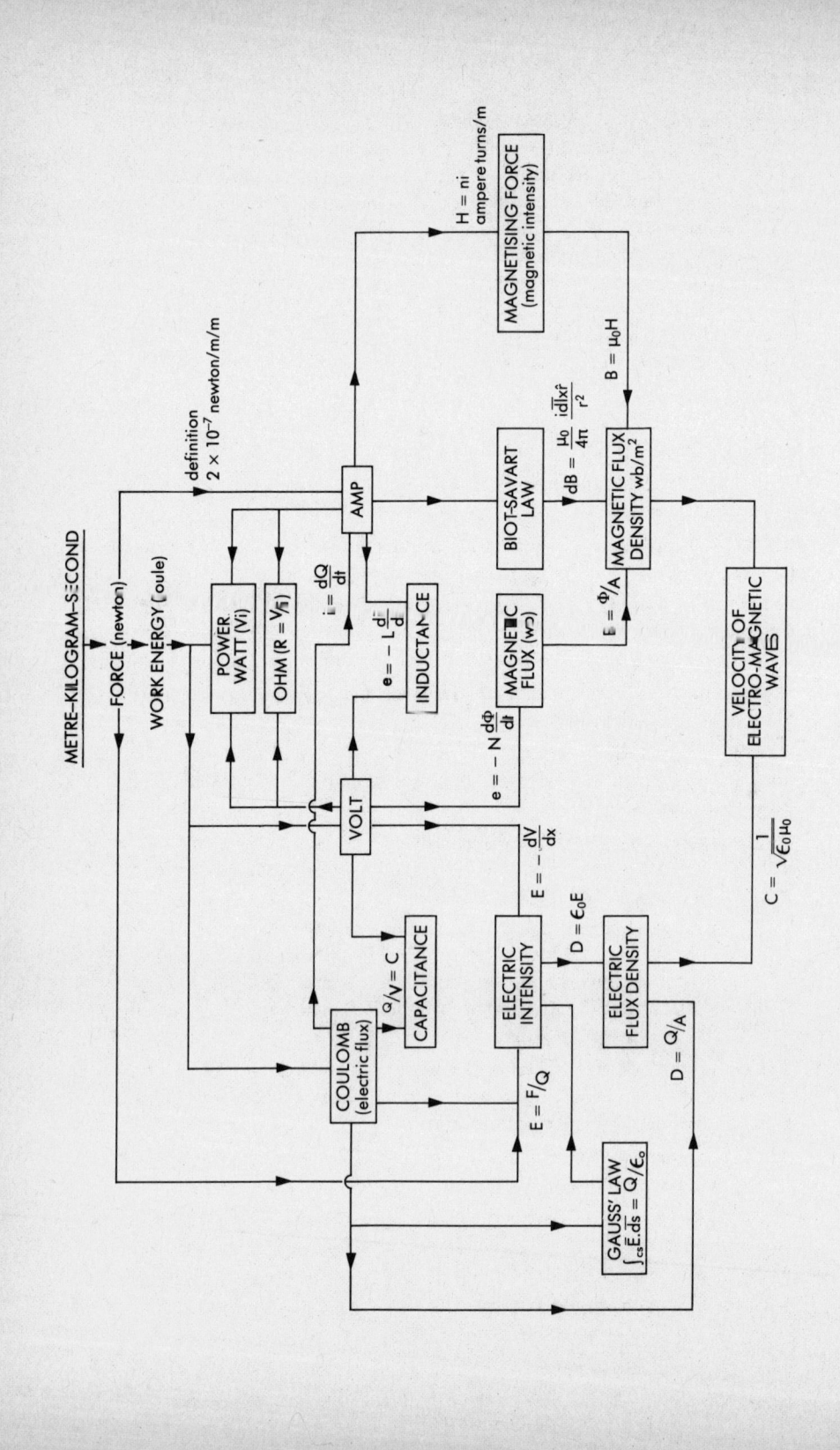

FORCE (newton) — definition 2×10^{-7} newton/m/m

WORK ENERGY (joule)

POWER WATT (Vi)

OHM ($R = V/i$)

$i = \dfrac{dQ}{dt}$

$e = -L\dfrac{di}{dt}$

INDUCTANCE

AMP

BIOT-SAVART LAW

$dB = \dfrac{\mu_0}{4\pi} \dfrac{i\,\overline{dl} \times \hat{r}}{r^2}$

MAGNETIC FLUX DENSITY wb/m²

$B = \mu_0 H$

MAGNETISING FORCE (magnetic intensity)

$H = ni$ ampere turns/m

MAGNETIC FLUX ($w\phi$)

$e = -N\dfrac{d\Phi}{dt}$

$E = \Phi/A$

VOLT

$E = -\dfrac{dV}{dx}$

COULOMB (electric flux)

$Q/V = C$

CAPACITANCE

ELECTRIC INTENSITY

$E = F/Q$

$D = \epsilon_0 E$

ELECTRIC FLUX DENSITY

$D = Q/A$

GAUSS' LAW

$\int_{cs} \overline{E} \cdot \overline{ds} = Q/\epsilon_0$

VELOCITY OF ELECTRO-MAGNETIC WAVE

$C = \dfrac{1}{\sqrt{\epsilon_0 \mu_0}}$

above 20 kHz). Most ultrasonic devices use piezoelectric transducers and frequencies between 100 kHz and 5 MHz.

Units: physical quantities need to be specified in terms of both magnitude and a physical unit of measurement which can be related back to the fundamentals of mass, length, time, and electric charge. Figure G.1 shows the interrelationships between the various electric, magnetic and electromagnetic units used.

Velocity: is usually used for speed in a specified direction.

Wavelength: the distance between two successive peaks of a wave. The wavelength (metres per wave) multiplied by the frequency (waves per second) gives the velocity of propagation of the wave (metres per second).

Wave number: the number of wavelengths per centimetre, this is used for convenience particularly by spectroscopists.

Wave-particle duality: the particles of matter can only be adequately described by assuming they have both particle and wave properties. The (de Broglie) wave amplitude may be considered to represent the probability of finding the particles at a given position and instant.

X-ray crystallography: is the technique of using photographically recorded patterns of spots produced by the diffraction of a beam of monochromatic X-rays passing through a single crystal, to determine the three dimensional arrangement of atoms within the crystal and thus the molecules forming it.

References

Introduction

Best, S. T. (1984), 'Laying it on the power line', *Guardian*, 24 October.
Fröhlich, H. (1950), 'Theory of the superconducting state', *Phys. Rev.*, 79, 845–56.
Hyland, G. J. (1987), 'From theoretical physics to biology: the forward path of theory with Herbert Fröhlich', in *Energy Transfer Dynamics*, eds Barrett, T. W. and Pohl, H. A., Heidelberg: Springer-Verlag, 146–63.
Panorama (1988), *Electricity – A Shock in Store?* BBC1 Television, 21 March.
Smith, C. W. and Aarholt, E. (1982), 'Possible effects of environmentally stimulated, endogenous opiates', *Health Physics*, 43, 929–30.

Chapter 1   History of a phenomenon

Aschoff, D. von (1986), 'Geopathische Zonen – physikalische Grundlage der Krebsentstehung', presented. at Intl. Cong. Z.D.N. Essen, 19 October 1985. Dusseldorf: Mehr Wisen Buch-Deinst.
Becker R. O. and Marino, A. A. (1982), *Electromagnetism and Life*, Albany: SUNY Press.
Becker, R. O. and Selden, G. (1985), *The Body Electric*, New York: Morrow.
Bernal, Prof. J. D. (1939), *The Social Function of Science*, London: Routledge.
Brillouin, L. (1934), 'Fluctuations of current in a conductor', *Helv. Phys. Acta*, 7, (Suppl. 2), 47–67 (in French).
Didot, F. (ed.) (1861), *Nouvelle biographie générale*, Paris: Firmin Didot, 'Mesmer' – Col. 147–62 (in French).
Dubos, R. (1973), *Man Adapting*, New Haven, London: Yale.
Geddes, L. A. and Hoff, H. E. (1971), 'The discovery of bioelectricity and current electricity – the Galvani–Volta controversy', *IEEE Spectrum*, 8(12), 38–46.
Gilbert, W. (1600/trs. 1958), *De Magnete*, New York: Dover.

Lakhovsky, G. (1939), *The Secret of Life*, trs. Clement, M., London: Heinemann.
O'Neill, J. J. (1968), *The Life of Nikola Tesla: Prodigal Genius*, London: Neville Spearman; (paperback ed. 1980), Frogmore: Granada.
Stillings, D. and Roth, N. (1978), 'When electroquackery thrived', *IEEE Spectrum*, 15(11), 56–61.
Taylor, A. J. P. (1967), *Europe: Grandeur and Decline*, Harmondsworth: Penguin (Pelican).

Chapter 2 Basic concepts
Bronowski J. (1973), *The Ascent of Man*, London: BBC.
Chiabrera, A.(1986), Lecture given at BRAGS Conference, Utrecht, Netherlands, 19–22 October 1986.
Del Giudice, E., Doglia, S., Milani, M. and Vitiello, G. (1986), 'Electromagnetic field and spontaneous symmetry breaking in biological matter', *Nuclear Physics B275 [FS 17]*, 185–99.
Del Giudice, E., Preparata, G. and Vitiello, G. (1988), 'Water as a free electric dipole laser', *Phys. Rev. Lett.*, 61(9), 1085–8.
Levine, S. A. and Kidd, P. M. (1985), *Antioxidant Adaptation, Its Role in Free Radical Pathology*, San Leandro, CA: Allergy Research Group, ISBN 0-9614630-0-7.
Mott, N. F. (1972), *Elementary Quantum Mechanics*, London: Wykeham.
Pappas, P. T. and Obolensky, A. G. (1988), 'Thirty-six nanoseconds faster than light', *Electronics and Wireless World*, December, 1162–5.
Popp, F.-A. (1979), 'Photon storage in biological systems', in *Electromagnetic Bioinformation*, eds Popp, F.-A. and Becker, B., Munich: Urban & Schwarzenberg, pp. 123–49 (2nd edn, 1988).

Chapter 3 The cosmic connection
Adderley, E. and Bowen, E. (1962), 'Lunar component in precipitation data', *Science*, 137, 748.
Ahmed, N. A. G., Calderwood, J. H., Fröhlich, H. and Smith, C. W. (1975), 'Evidence for collective magnetic effects in an enzyme: likelihood of room temperature superconductive regions', *Phys. Lett. 53A*, 129–30.
Andrews, E. A. (1961), 'Moon talk: the cyclic periodicity of postoperative hemorrhage', *J. Florida Medical Assoc.*, 46, 362–6.
Arendt, J. (1986), 'Assay of melatonin and its metabolites: results in normal and unusual environments', *J. Neurotransmission, 21(Supp)*, 11–13.
Baker, R. and Smith, C. W. (1985), 'Comment on the paper, "Growth of yeast cultures in an *in-vitro* model for investigating homoeopathic remedies"', *Brit. Hom. J.*, 74(2), 93–6.
Baker, R. R. (1984), 'Signal magnetite and direction finding', *Phys. Technol.*, 15, 30–6.
Baker, R. R. (1985a), 'Magnetoreception in man and other primates', in (eds) Kirschvink, J. L., Jones, D. S. and McFadden, B. J., *Magnetite*

Biomineralisation and Magnetoreception in Organisms: A New Magnetism, New York: Plenum. Chap. 26.

Baker, R. R. (1985b), 'Human navigation: a summary of American data and interpretations', in (eds) Kirschvink, J. L., Jones, D. S. and McFadden, B. J., *Magnetite Biomineralisation and Magnetoreception in Organisms: A New Magnetism*, New York: Plenum. Chap. 34.

Barr, M. L. (1979), *The Human Nervous System*, Hagerstown: Harper & Row.

Bell, B. and Defouw, R. J. (1966), 'Dependence of the lunar modulation of geomagnetic activity on the celestial latitude of the Moon', *J. Geophysical Res.*, 71(3), 951–7.

Bigg, E. A. (1963), 'Lunar and planetary influences on geomagnetic disturbances', *J. Geophysical Res.*, 68, 4099–104.

Bradley, D. A., Woodbury, M. A. and Brier, G. W. (1962), 'Lunar synodical period and widespread precipitation', *Science*, 137, 748–9.

Brown, F. A. (1954), 'Persistent activity rhythms in the oyster', *American Scientist*, 178, 510.

Brown, F. A. (1962), *Biological Clocks*, Boston: Heath.

Brown, F. A. (1972), 'Some orientational influences of non-visual, terrestrial electromagnetic fields', *Ann. N.Y. Acad. Sci.*, 188, 221–41.

Brown, F. A. (1983), 'The biological clock phenomenon: exogenous timing hypothesis', *J. Interdiscipl. Cycle Res.*, 14(2), 137–62.

Brown, F. A. and Chow, C. S. (1973), 'Lunar-correlated variations in water uptake by bean seeds', *Biol. Bull*, 45, 265–78.

Bunning, E. (1964), *The Physiological Clock*, Berlin: Springer.

Burr, H. S. (1945), 'Diurnal potentials in the maple tree', *J. Biol. and Med.*, 17, 727–34.

Burr, H. S. (1972), *Blueprint for Immortality, The Electric Patterns of Life*, London: Neville Spearman.

Burr, H. S. and Northrop, F. S. (1935), 'The electromagnetic field theory', *Quarterly Rev. Biol.*, 10, 322–33.

Chizhevsky, A. L. (1934), 'Effets de l'activite periodique solaire sur les phenomenes sociaux', in Piery, M. (ed.), *Traite de Climatologie Biologique et Medicale*, Paris: Masson, vol. 1: 576–86.

Chizhevsky, A. L. (1971), 'Physical factors of the historical process', *Cycles*, January, 11–23.

Cope, F. W. (1971), 'Evidence from activation energies for superconductive tunnelling in biological systems at physiological temperatures', *Physiol. Chem. Phys.*, 3, 403–10.

Cope, F. W. (1978), 'Discontinuous magnetic field effects (Barkhausen Noise) in nucleic acids as evidence for room temperature organic superconduction', *Physiol. Chem. Phys.*, 10, 233–46.

Cremer-Bartels, G., Krause, K. and Kuchle, H. J. (1983), 'Influence of low magnetic field strength variations on the retina and pineal gland of quails and humans', *Graefe's Arch. Klin. Exper. Ophthal.*, 220, 248–32.

Currie, R. (1988), 'Lunar tides and the wealth of nations', *New Scientist*, 5 November, 52–5.

References

Downer, J. (1988), *Supersense*, London: BBC Publications.

Dewey, E. R. with Mandino, O. (1972), *Cycles: The Mysterious Forces that Trigger Events*, New York: Manor Books.

Dubrov, A. P. (1978), *The Geomagnetic Field and Life: Geomagnetobiology*, New York: Plenum.

Farmer, C. B. et al. (1987), *Nature*, 329, 126–30.

Friedman, H., Becker, R. O. and Bachman, C. H. (1965), 'Psychiatric ward behaviour and geophysical parameters', *Nature*, 205, 1050–2.

Fröhlich, H. (1984), Discussions at Workshop on 'Collective Behaviour of Biological Systems', Vulcane, Sicily, 25–27 June 1984.

Fröhlich, H. (1985), Discussions at Colloquium on 'Bioelectronics and Biosensors', UCNW, Bangor, 17–19 April 1985.

Ganong, W. F. (1969), *Review of Medical Physiology*, Los Altos, CA: Lange Medical Publ.

Gauquelin, M. (1982), *The Cosmic Clocks: from Astrology to a Modern Science*, San Diego, CA: Astro Computing Services (Updated edition of 1973 original Paladin Books).

Gendrin, R. and Stefant, R. (1964), 'Magnetic records between 0.2–30 c/s', in (ed.) Blackman, W. T., *Propagation of Radio Waves at Frequencies below 300 kc/s*, London: Pergamon.

Jacobi, E. (1979), *Pathopsysiologie der Thrombozytenadhasivität*, Bern: Verlag Hans Huber.

Jacobi, E. and Kruskemper, G. (1975), 'Wirkungen simulierter sferics (wetterbedingte, elektromagnetische Strahlungen) auf die Thrombozytenadhasivität', *Inn. Med.*, 2, 73–81.

Kauffman, G. B. and Beck, M. T. (1987), 'Self-deception in science: the curious case of Giorgio Piccardi', *Spec. Sci.*, 10(2), 113–22.

Kauffman, G. B. and Belloni, L. (1989), 'Giorgio Piccardi (1895–1972), Italian Physical Chemist and Master of the Sun', *J. Chem. Education*, (to be published).

Klinowska, M. (1972), 'A comparison of the lunar and solar activity rhythms of the golden hamster', *J. Interdiscipl. Cycle Res.*, 3, 145–50.

Keeton, W. T. (1979), 'Avian orientation and navigation', *Brit. Birds*, 72, 451–70.

Kirschrink, J. L., Jones, D. S. and MacFadden, B. J. (eds) (1985), *Magnetite Biomineralization and Magnetoreception in Organisms. A New Biomagnetism*, New York: Plenum.

Kollerstrom, N. (1980), 'Plant response to the lunar synodic cycle', *Cycles*, 31(3), 61–3.

König, H. L. (1979), 'Bioinformation – electrophysical aspects', in (eds) Popp, F.-A. and Becker, G. *Electromagnetic Bio-information*. Munich: Urban and Schwarzenberg, 25–54.

Lieber, A. L. (1979), *The Lunar Effect*, London: Corgi.

Luette, J. P., Park, C. G. and Helliwell, R. A. (1979), *J. Geophysical Res.*, 84, 2657–68.

Ravitz, L. J. (1951), 'Comparative clinical and electrocyclical observations of twin brothers concordant as to schizophrenia', *J. Nerv. and Mental Diseases*, 121, 72–87.

Ravitz, L. J. (1962), 'History, measurement and applicability of periodic changes in the electromagnetic field in health and disease', *Ann. N.Y. Acad. Sci.*, 98(4), 1144–201.

Rotton, J. and Kelly, I. W. (1985), Much ado about the full moon: a meta-analysis of lunar-lunacy research', *Psychological Bull.*, 97, 286–306.

Rounds, H. D. (1975), 'A lunar rhythm in the occurrence of blood-borne factors in cockroaches, mice and man', *Comp. Biochem. Physiol.*, 50C, 193–7.

Piccardi, G. (1962), *The Chemical Basis of Medical Climatology*, Springfield, Ill.: C. C. Thomas.

Playfair, G. L. and Hill, S. (1978), *The Cycles of Heaven*, London: Souvenir.

Semm, P., Schnieder, T. and Vollrath, L. (1980), 'Effects of an earth-strength magnetic field on electrical activity of pineal cells', *Nature*, 288, 607–8.

Smith, C. W. and Baker, R. D. (1982), 'Comments on the paper, "Environmental power-frequency magnetic fields and suicide"', *Health Physics*, 43(3), 439–41.

Smith, C. W. (1985), 'Superconducting areas in living systems', in (ed.) Mishra, R. K., *The Living State II*, Singapore: World Scientific, 404–20.

Smith, C. W. (1986), 'High sensitivity biosensors and weak environmental stimuli', *Proc. Colloq. Bioelectronics and Biosensors*, UCNW Bangor, 17–19 April 1985, in *Industrial Biotechnology Wales*, Apr./May, 1986, Art. 4: 2–85.

Sweeney, B. M. (1969), *Rhythmic Phenomena in Plants*, London: Academic Press.

Tromp, S. W. (1949), *Psychical Physics*, Amsterdam: Elsevier.

Tromp, S. W. (1963), *Medical Biometeorology*, Amsterdam: Elsevier.

Tromp, S. W. 1967), 'Blood sedimentation rate patterns in The Netherlands during the period 1955–1965', *Int. J. Biometeor.*, 11, 105–17.

Tromp, S. W. (1973), 'Short and long periodical fluctuations in blood sedimentation rate, haemoglobin and diastolic blood pressure, observed in healthy male donors in 18 bloodbanks in the northern and southern hemisphere', *J. Interdiscipl. Cycle Res.*, 4(3), 207–20.

Tromp, S. W. (1975a), 'Possible extra-terrestrial triggers of interdisciplinary cycles on earth. A review', *J. Interdiscipl. Res.*, 6(3), 303–15.

Tromp, S. W. (1975b), 'Possible geophysical causes of long-term fluctuations in blood sedimentation rate patterns in the world', *J. Interdiscipl. Cycle Res.*, 6(1), 71–2.

Tromp, S. W. (1979), *Biometeorological Survey. Vol. 1, 1973–1978*, London: Heyden & Sons.

Voss, K. (1964/5), 'Weitere Folgerungen aus Steigversuchen', *Neue Aspeckte*, 15, 1–11.

Wever, R. A. (1973), 'Human circadian rhythms under the influence of weak electric fields and the different aspects of these studies', *Int. J. Biometerol.*, 17(3), 227–32.

Wever, R. A. (1985), 'The electromagnetic environment and the circadian rhythms of human subjects', in (eds) Grandolfo, M., Michaelson, S. M. and Rindi, A., *Static and ELF Electromagnetic Fields: Biological Effects and Dosimetry*, New York: Plenum.

Wever, R. A. (1987), Personal communication (verbal) to Cyril Smith.

Wilson, B. (1988), 'Chronic exposure to ELF fields may induce depression', *Bioelectromagnetics*, 9, 195–205.

Wiseman, A. (1987), 'Soviets link magnetic body fields to health', *Times*, March 23.

Chapter 4 Human biology and electromagnetic fields

Aarholt, E., Jaberansari, M., Jaffary-Asl, A. H., Marsh, P. N. and Smith, C. W. (1988), 'NMR conditions and biological systems', in *Modern Bioelectricity*, (ed.) A. A. Marino, New York: Marcel Dekker, Ch. 4, 75–104.

Barker, A. T., Jaffe, L. F. and Vonable, J. W. (1981), 'Lateral voltage gradients near mammalian skin wounds', *A.M. Zoolog.*, 21(4), 998–1007.

Barker, A. T. and Foulds, I. S. (1983), 'Human skin battery potentials, their variation with site, age and sex', *Clin. Phys. P.*, 4(1), 101–2.

Becker, R. O. and Selden, G. (1985), *The Body Electric*, New York: Morrow.

Bell, D. A. (1960), *Electrical Noise: Fundamentals and Physical Mechanism*. London: Van Nostrand.

Bullock, T. H. (1977), 'Electromagnetic sensing in fish', *Neurosci. Res. Program Bull.*, 15(1), 17–22.

Faraday, M. (1855/reprint 1965), *Experimental Researches in Electricity*, London: Taylor and Francis, New York: Dover (reprint).

Freeston, I. L., Barker, A. T. and Jalinous, R. (1984), 'Nerve stimulation using magnetic fields', in 'Frontiers of Engineering and Computing in Health Care', *Proc. 6th Ann. Conf. IEEE Eng. in Med. & Biol. Soc.* (Cat. No. 84CH2058-6). Los Angeles, CA: 15–17 Sept. '84. New York: IEEE, 557–61.

Fröhlich, H. (1969), *Theoretical Physics and Biology*, (ed.) Marois, M., Amsterdam NL: North Holland.

Fröhlich, H. (1975), 'The extraordinary dielectric properties of biological molecules and the action of enzymes', *Proc. Nat. Acad. Sci. USA*, 72, 4211–15.

Fröhlich, H. (1978), 'Coherent electric vibrations in biological systems', *IEEE Trans., MTT*, 26, 613–17.

Gamow, R. I. and Harris, J. F. (1972), 'What engineers can learn from nature', *IEEE Spectrum*, 9(8), 36–42.

Grundler, W. (1985), 'Frequency-dependent biological effects of low intensity microwaves', in *Interactions between Electromagnetic Fields and Cells*, (eds) Chiabrera, A., Nicolini, C. and Schwan, H. P., NATO ASI Series 97A, New York: Plenum.

Grundler, W., Keilmann, F., Putterlik, V., Santo, L., Strube, D. and Zimmermann, I. (1983), in *Coherent Excitations in Biological Systems*, (eds) Fröhlich, H. and Kremer, F., Berlin: Springer-Verlag, 21.

Illingworth, C. M. (1974), 'Trapped fingers and amputated fingertips in children', *J. Pediatr. Surg.*, 9(6), 853–8.

Jafary-Asl, A. H. and Smith, C. W. (1983), *Ann. Rep. Conf. Electrical Insulation & Dielectric Phenomena*, IEEE Publ. 83 CH 1902–6, 350–5.

Jaffe, L. F. (1977), 'Electrophoresis along cell membranes', *Nature*, 265, 600–2.

Kelly, J. A., Sielecki, A. R., Sykes, B. D., James, M. N. G. and Phillips, D. C. (1979), 'X-ray crystallography of the binding of the bacterial cell wall trisaccharide NAM-NAG-NAM to lysozyme', *Nature* (London), 282, 875–8.

Molyneux, D. H., Wallbanks, K. R. and Ingram, G. A. (1987), 'Trypanosomatid-vector interfaces – in vitro studies on parasite substrate interactions', in (eds) Chang, K-P., and Snary, D., *Host-Parasite Cellular and Molecular Interactions*, Heidelberg: Springer-Verlag, 387–96.

Nordenström, B. E. W. (1983), *Biologically Closed Electrical Circuits: Clinical, Experimental and Theoretical Evidence for an Additional Circulatory System*, Stockholm: Nordic Medical.

Nordenström, B. E. W. (1985), 'Biokinetic impacts on structure and imaging of the lung: the concept of biologically closed electric circuits', *Am. J. Roentgenol.*, 145, 447–67.

Overall, R. and Jaffe, L. F. (1985), 'Patterns of ionic current through *Drosophila* follicles and eggs', *Dev. Biol.*, 108(1), 102–19.

Pohl, H. (1978), *Dielectrophoresis: The Behaviour of Neutral Matter in Nonuniform Electric Fields*, Cambridge, UK: Cambridge University Press.

Pohl, H. (1983), 'Natural oscillating fields of cells', in *Coherent Excitations in Biological Systems*, (eds) Fröhlich, H and Kremer, F., Heidelberg: Springer-Verlag, 199–210.

Rosen, D. (1963), 'Dielectric properties of protein powders with absorbed water', *Trans. Farad. Soc.*, 59, 2178–91.

Shaw, T. M. (1942), 'The elimination of errors due to electrode polarization in measurements of the dielectric constants of electrolytes', *J., Chem. Phys.*, 10, 609–17.

Smith, C. U. M. (1971), *Molecular Biology, A Structural Approach*, London: Faber & Faber.

Smith, C. W. (1985), 'Superconducting areas in living systems', in *The Living State II*, (ed.) Mishra R. K. Singapore: World Scientific, 404–20.

Smith C. W. (1986), 'High sensitivity biosensors and weak environmental stimuli', *Proc. Colloq. Bioelectronics and Biosensors, UCNW. Bangor, 17–19 April, 1985, in International Industrial Biotechnology*, 6(3), (April/May, 1986), Article: 4:2:85.

Smith, C. W., Jafary-Asl, A. H., Choy, R. Y. S. and Monro, J. A. (1987), 'The emission of low intensity electromagnetic radiation from multiple allergy patients and other biological systems', in *Proc. 1st. Intl. Symp. on Photon Emission from Biological Systems*, Wroclaw, Poland, January 24–26, 1986, (eds) Jezowska-Trzebiatowska, B., Kochel, B., Slawinski, J. and Strek, W., 110–26.

Taubes, G. (1986), 'An electrifying possibility', *Discover*, April, 23–37.

Chapter 5 Electromagnetic fields in medicine

Baker, R. R. (1984), 'Sinal magnetite and direction finding', *Phys. Technol.*, 15, 30–6.

Baker, R. R. (1985), 'Magnetoreception by man and other primates', in *Magnetite Biomineralisation and Magnetoreception in Organisms: A New Magnetism*, (eds) Kirschvink, J. L., Jones, D. S. and McFadden, B. J., New York: Plenum, Ch. 26.

Barr M. L. (1979), *The Human Nervous System*. Hagerstown, MD: Harper & Row.

Becker, R. O. and Selden, G. (1985), *The Body Electric*, New York: Morrow.

Brown, E. and Behrens, K. (1985), *Your Body's Responses*, Dallas: Madison Avenue.

British Standards Institute (B.S.I.) (1979, amended 1982, 1985), *Medical Electrical Equipment*, B.S. 5724, Pt. I – *General Safety Requirements*, Pt. II – *Particular Requirements for Safety*, London: British Standards Institute.

Bydder et al. (1982). 'Clinical NMR imaging of the brain: 140 cases', *Am. J. Roentgenology*, 139, 215–36.

Cameron, J. R. and Skofronick, J. G. (1978), *Medical Physics*, Chichester: Wiley-Interscience.

Clayton, E. B. (1958), *Electrotherapy and Actinotherapy*, London: Balliere, Tindall & Cox, 3rd. edn.

Clegg, J. S. (1984), 'Properties and metabolism of the aqueous cytoplasm and its boundaries', *Am. J. Physiol.*, 246, (*Regulatory Integrative Comp. Physiol.*, 15); R133–51.

Fishman, S. N. (1985), 'Movement of charges in excitable membranes', *Speculations in Science and Technology*, 8(3), 163–9.

Green, J. H. (1968), *An Introduction to Human Physiology*, London: Oxford Univ. Press.

Hahnemann, S. (1982), *Organon of Medicine*. Los Angeles: Tarcher.

Hill, D. and Parr, G. (eds) (1963), *Electroencephalography*, London: Macdonald.

Jafary-Asl, A. H., Solanki, S. N., Aarholt, E. and Smith, C. W. (1982) 'Dielectric measurements on live biological materials under magnetic resonance conditions', *J. Biol. Phys.*, 11, 15–22.

Johns, H. E. and Cunningham, J. R. (1969), *The Physics of Radiology*, Springfield, Ill: C. C. Thomas.

Keeton, W. T. (1979), 'Avian orientation and navigation', *Brit. Birds*, 72(10), 451–70.

Kenyon, J. (1982, 1983), *Modern Techniques of Acupuncture*, Wellingborough: Thorsons. Vols I & II, 1982; Vol. III, 1983.

Lakhovsky, G. (1939), *The Secret of Life*, trs. Clement, M., London: Heinemann.

Mayer-Gross, W., Slater E. and Roth, M. (1969), *Clinical Psychiatry*, 3rd. edn., London: Bailliere, Tindall & Cassell.

Patterson, M. A. (1978), 'The significance of current frequency in Neuroelectric Therapy (NET) for drug and alcohol addictions', in Wageneder, F. M. &

Germann, R. H. (eds), *Electrotherapeutic Sleep and Electroanaesthesia*, Graz: R. M. Verlag.

Patterson, M. A. (1986), *Hooked? NET: The New Approach to Drug Cure*. London: Faber & Faber.

Reid, K. H. (1974), 'Mechanism of action of dental electro-anaesthesia', *Nature*, 247, 150–1.

Röntgen, W. C. (1896), 'On a new kind of ray', *Nature*, (London), 53, 274 (English translation of the original German paper).

Rutherford, E. (1905), *Radio-activity*, Cambridge: University Press.

Sances, A., Jr. and Larson, S. L. (1970), 'Electroanesthesia research', in Clynes, M. and Milsum, J. H. (eds), *Biomedical Engineering Systems*, New York: McGraw-Hill, Ch. 8.

Semm, P., Schneider, T. and Vollrath, L. (1980), 'Effects of an earth-strength magnetic field on electrical activity of pineal cells', *Nature*, (London), 288, 607–8.

Smith, C. W., Choy, R. and Monrop, J. A. (1985), 'Water – friend or foe?', *Laboratory Practice*, 34(10), 29–34.

Smith C. W. (1986), 'High sensitivity biosensors and weak environmental stimuli', *Proc. Colloq. Bioelectronics and Biosensors*, UCNW. Bangor, 17–19 April, 1985, In *International Industrial Biotechnology*, 6(3), (April/May, 1986), Article: 4:2:85.

Stead, G., Reynolds, R. J., Finzi, N. S., Andrews, C., Lacassagne, A. and Case, J. T. (1956), 'Sixty years of radiology', *Brit. J. Radiol.*, 29, 234–55.

Strong, P. (1970), *Biophysical Measurements*, Beaverton, Oregon: Tektronix Inc.

Taubes, G. (1986), 'An electrifying possibility', *Discover*, April, 23–37.

Welkowitz, W. and Deutsch, S. (1976), *Biomedical Instruments: Theory and Design*, London: Academic Press.

Wever, R., (1985), 'Circadian rhythms of human subjects', in *Static and ELF Electromagnetic Fields: Biological Effects and Dosimetry*, (eds) Grandolfo, M. Michaelson, S. M. Rindi, A., New York: Plenum, 477–523.

Young, I. R., et al. (1982), Initial clinical evaluation of a whole body nuclear magnetic resonance (NMR) tomograph', *J. of Computer Assisted Tomography*, 6(1), 1–18.

Chapter 6 Electrical sensitivity and allergy

Aschoff, D. von (1986), 'Geopathische Zonen – physikalische Grundlage der Krebsentstehung', presented at: Intl. Cong. Z.D.N. Essen, 19 October, 1985. Dusseldorf: Mehr Wisen Buch-Deinst.

Brown, E. and Behrens, K. (1985), *Your Body's Response*, Dallas, Tx: Madison Avenue.

British Society for Clinical Nutrition (1985), 'Hazards in Dentistry: The Mercury Debate'. Cambridge, 15–16 July.

Hayashi, H. (1988), 'Clinical experiences obtained from the use of electrically reformed water'. Paper presented at 6th. Intl. Symp. on Man and His Environment in Health and Disease, Dallas, Texas, February 25–28.

Jhon, M. S (1987), 'Physico-chemical approaches to the role of water in modern diseases such as cancer, diabetes and AIDS'. *Speculations in Science and Technology*, 10(3), 179–85.

Kervran, L. C. (1972), *Biological Transmutations*, Crosby: Lockwood.

Li, K. H. (1987), 'Physical basis of coherent radiations from biomolecules', in: Proc. 1st. Intl. Symp. on Photon Emission from Biological Systems, Wroclaw, Poland, January 24–26, 1986, eds Jezowska-Trzebiatowska, B., Kochel, B., Slawinski, J. and Strek, W., pp. 63–95.

Miller, J. B. (1972), *Food Allergy: Provocative Testing and Injection Therapy*, Springfield (Ill.): C. C. Thomas.

Miller, J. B. (1987), *Relief at Last*, Springfield, Ill: C. C. Thomas.

Monro, J., Carini, C. and Brostoff, J. (1984), 'Migraine is a food-allergic disease', *Lancet*, 2, 719–21.

Moon, M. J. and Jhon, M. S. (1986), 'The studies on the hydration energy and water structures in dilute aqueous solution'. *Bull. Chem. Soc. Jpn.* 59, 1215–22.

Patterson, M. A. (1978), 'The significance of current frequency in Neuroelectric therapy (NET) for drug and alcohol addictions', in: Wagender, F. M. and Germann, R. H. (eds), *Electrotherapeutic Sleep and Electroanaesthesia*, Graz: R. M. Verlag.

Patterson, M. A. (1986), *Hooked? NET: The New Approach to Drug Cure*, London: Faber & Faber.

Persinger, M. A. (1974), *ELF and VLF Electromagnetic Field Effects*, New York: Plenum.

Pohl, G. F. von (1987), *Earth Currents – Causative Factor of Cancer and other Diseases*, Stuttgart: French Verlag (English translation of 1932 German original).

Popp, F.-A. (1986), *Bericht an Bonn*, Essen: Verlag fur Ganzheitsmedizin.

Rea, W. J. (1987), 'Electromagnetic assessment under environmentally controlled conditions'. 5th. Ann. Intl. Symp. on: 'Man and his Environment in Health and Disease', Dallas, Texas, February 26 – March 1.

Smith, C. W. and Aarholt, E. (1982), 'Possible effects of environmentally stimulated endogenous opiates', *Health Physics*, 43(6), 929–30.

Smith, C. W., Choy, R. Y. S. and Monro, J. A. (1985), 'Water – friend or foe?', *Laboratory Practice*, 34(10), 29–34.

Smith, C. W., Al-Hashmi, S. A. R., Kushelevsky, A., Slifkin, M. A., Choy, R. Y. S., Monro, J. A., Clulow, E. E. and Hewson, M. J. C. (1986), 'Preliminary investigations into the acceptability of fabrics by allergy patients', *Clinical Ecology*, 4(1), 7–10.

Smoker, P. (ed) (1988), *The Risk of Nuclear War*, Richardson Institute for Peace Studies, Lancaster University.

Ziff, S. (1984) *Silver Dental Fillings: The Toxic Time Bomb*, Sante Fe: Aurora Press.

Chapter 7 Alternative medicine – the potential breakthrough

British Medical Association (1986), *Report of the BMA Board of Science*

Working Party on Alternative Therapy, London: BMA. (Comment in: *The Guardian*, 13 May, and *The Observer*, 18 May).

Brown, E. and Behrens, K. (1985), *Your body's Response*, Dallas, TX: Madison Avenue.

Brucato, and Stephenson, (1966), 'Dielectric strength testing of homoeopathic dilutions of HgCl. *J. Amer. Inst. Hom.*, 59, 281–6.

Callinan, P. (1985). 'The mechanism of action of homoeopathic remedies', *Complementary Med. 3(1)*, 35–36.

Callinan, P. (1986), 'Vibratory energy in water: a model for homoeopathic action', *Complementary Medicine*, 2, February, 34–53.

Celan, E., Gradinaru, D. and Celan, B. (1986), 'The evidence of selective radiation emitted by a cell culture which destructively affects some tumoral cell lines', in *Photon Emission from Biological Systems*, Jezowska-Trzebiatowska, B., Kochel, B., Slawinski, J. and Strek, W., Singapore: World Scientific, 219–25.

Chemical Rubber Company (CRC) (1976), *Handbook of Chemistry and Physics*, ed. Weast, R. C., Cleveland: CRC Press.

Collier, R. J. and Donarski, R. J. (1987), 'Non-invasive method of measuring resonant frequency of a human tibia *in vivo*, Part 1 and 2', *J. Biomed. Eng.*, 9, October, 321–8 and 329–31.

Consumers Association (1986) 'Magic or Medicine?'. *Which?* October, 443–7.

Cox, H. J. E. (1985), Letter re. cost-effectiveness of clinical ecology, in Thomson, G. M., *Report of the ad hoc Committee on Environmental Hypersensitivity Disorders*, Appendix 2, Toronto, Ontario: Provincial Court (Family Division).

Davenas, E., *et al.* (including Benveniste, J.) (1988), 'Human basophil degranulation triggered by very dilute antiserum against IgE', *Nature, 333*, 30 June, 816–18.

Day, L. and De La Warr, G. (1957), *New Worlds Beyond the Atom*, London: Vincent Stuart.

Egely, G. (1986), 'Experimental investigation of biologically induced energy transfer anomalies'. Proc. 6th. Intl. Conf. on Psychotronic Research. Zagreb: Society for Natural Sciences, 29–30.

Fidler, J. Havelock (1983), *Ley Lines, their Nature and Properties. A Dowser's Investigation*, Wellingborough: Turnstone.

Gordon, R. (1988), *Are You Sleeping in a Safe Place*? Dulwich Health Society, 130 Gipsy Hill, London SE 19.

Gutfreund, H. (1977), *Enzymes: Physical Principles*, London: Wiley.

Hawkins, L. H. (1981), *'Air ionisation and office health'*, *Building Services and Environmental Engineer*, April.

Hodges, H. (1970), *Technology in the Ancient World*, London: Allen Lane, Penguin Press.

Jussal, R. L., Meera, S., Dua, R. D. and Mishra, R. K. (1982), 'Physical effects on the suspending medium by compounds in asymptotically infinite dilutions', *Hahnemannian Gleanings, 49(3)*, 114–20.

Jussal, R. L., Meera, S., Dua, R. D. and Mishra, R. K. (1984), 'Effect of ultra-

dilutions on neurotransmitter enzyme', *Hahnemannian Glean*, 51, 143–6.
Kenyon, J. (1982a and b, 1983), *Modern Techniques of Acupuncture*, Wellingborough: Thorsons, Vols I & II 1982, Vol. III 1983.
Kervran, L. C. (1972), *Biological Transmutations*, Crosby: Lockwood.
Kirlian, S. D. and Kirlian, V Kh. (1961), 'Photography and visual observation by means of high frequency currents', *Journal of Scientific and Applied Photography*, 6, 397–403.
Ludwig, W. (1986, 1988), Papers presented at seminars of the Brügemann Institute, Postfach 1262, Pippinstrasse 10, D-8035 Gauting, W. Germany.
Manners, P. G. (1986), *Proc. World Research Foundation Congress of Bio-Energetic Medicine*, Los Angeles, November, 7–9. World Research Foundation, 15300 Ventura Blvd., Ste. 405, Sherman Oaks, CA 91403, USA.
Mandel, P. (1986), *Beitrage zur Theorie-Diagnose-Therapie*, Internationale Gesellschaft für Kirlianfotografie und bioelektronische Diagnose und Therapie e.V., Hildastrasse 8, D, D-7520 Bruchsal, W. Germany.
Miller, J. B. (1972), *Food Allergy: Provocative Testing and Injection Therapy*, Springfield (Ill.): C. C. Thomas.
Miller, J. B. (1987), *Relief at Last*, Springfield, Ill: C.C.Thomas.
Oldfield, H. and Coghill, R. (1988), *The Dark Side of the Brain*. Shaftesbury: Element Books.
Ostrander, S. and Schroeder, L. (1970), *PSI, Psychic Discoveries behind the Iron Curtain*. London: Abacus, Sphere Books.
Reilly, D. T., Taylor, M. A., McSharry, C. and Aitchison, T. (1986), 'Is homoeopathy a placebo response? Controlled trial of homeopathic potency with pollen in hayfever as model'. *Lancet*, October 18, 881–6.
Sacks, A. D. (1985), 'Nuclear magnetic resonance spectroscopy of homoeopathic remedies', *Journal of Holistic Medicine*, 5(2), 172–7.
Slawinska, D. and Slawinski, J. (1986), 'Biophoton emission from cucumber seedlings perturbed by formaldehyde as a possible indicator of the effectiveness of homoeopathic drugs' in: *Bericht an Bonn*, ed. Popp, F.-A., Essen: Verlag für Ganzheitsmedizin.
Stanway, A. (1979), *Alternative Medicine, A Guide to Natural Therapies*. Harmondsworth: Penguin.
Watterson, J. G. (1982), 'Model for a cooperative structure wave', in: *Biophysics of Water*, eds Franks, F. and Mathias, S. F., London: Wiley.
Wever, R. A. (1985), 'The electromagnetic environment and the circadian rhythms of human subjects', in *Static and ELF Electromagnetic Fields: Biological Effects and Dosimetry*, eds Grandolfo, M., Michaelson, S. M. and Rindi, A. New York: Plenum.

Chapter 8 Electromagnetic environmental pollution
Aarholt, E., Flinn, E. A. and Smith, C. W. (1980), 'Biological effects of extremely low-frequency non-ionizing radiation'. *Intl. Symp. URSI/CNFRS*, Electromagnetic Waves and Biology, Jouy-en-Josas, Paris.
Aarholt, E., Flinn, E. A. and Smith, C. W. (1981), 'Effects of low frequency magnetic fields on bacterial growth rate', *Phys. Med. Biol.*, 26, 613–21.

Adey, W. R. and Sheppard, A. R. (1983), Report to Montana Department of National Resources and Conservation, Montana, USA.

Ahmed N. A. G. and Smith, C. W. (1981), 'The application of Rutherford Backscattering Technique to dental hard tissue', in *Recent Developments in Condensed Matter Physics*, eds Devreeses, J. T., Lemmens, L. F., Van Doren, V. E. and Van Royen, J. New York: Plenum, Vol. 4: 321–8.

Ahmed, N. A. G., Calderwood, J. H., Fröhlich, H. and Smith, C. W. (1975), 'Evidence for collective magnetic effects in an enzyme: likelihood of room temperature superconductive regions', *Phys. Lett.*, 53A, 129–30.

Asanova, T. P. and Rakov, A. I. (1975), 'The state of health of persons working in electrical fields of outdoor 400 and 500kV switchyards', in Knickerbocker, G. (Translation): *Hygiene of Labor and Professional Diseases*, Vol. 5, Special Publication no. 10, Piscataway NJ: IEEE Power Engineering Society, p. 1966.

Bacon, H. (1986), 'The hazards of high-voltage power lines', in Goldsmith, E. and Hildyard, N., *Green Britain or Industrial Wasteland?* Oxford: Polity Press/Basil Blackwell.

Banks, M. J. J., Keitley, R. and Stringfellow, G. C. (1968), 'Radio noise and corona loss studies at 275/400 and 750 kV on test and operational power lines', in IEE Conf. Publ. No. 44, *Progress in Overhead Lines and Cables for 220 kV and Above*, 306–13.

Becker, R. O. (1977), 'Testimony before the State of New York Public Service Commission: Cases 26529, 26559 – Common Record Hearings on Health and Safety of 765 kV Transmission Lines'.

Becker, R. O. and Marino, A. A. (1982), *Electromagnetism and Life*, Albany: SUNY Press, p. 21.

Becker, R. O. and Selden, G. (1985), *The Body Electric*, New York: Morrow.

Best, S. T. (1981), 'Pylon power', *Doctor*, March 19.

Best, S. T. (1982), 'Scots farmers fight health-risk pylons', *Observer*, April 18.

Bloch, F. (1968), 'Simple interpretation of the Josephson effect', *Phys. Rev. Lett.*, 21, 1241–3.

Boericke, W. (1927), *Homeopathic Materia Medica*. Philadelphia: Boericke & Runyon.

Box, W. R. and Symes, R. F. (1968), '400 kV tower design and testing progress', IEE Conf. Publ. No. 44. *Progress in Overhead Lines and Cables for 220 kV and Above*, pp. 168–73.

Braganza, L. F., Blott, B. H., Coe, T. J. and Melville, D. (1983), *Biochim. Biophys. Acta*, 731, 137–44.

Coleman, M., Bell, J. and Skeet, R., 'Leukemia incidence in electrical workers', *Lancet*, 2, 982–3.

Currently at Risk, (1984), Channel Four TV, London, September.

Danilin, V. A., Veronin, A. K., and Maderakij, V. A. (1969), 'Labour, hygiene and occupational diseases', Abst. MIOT 135, translated by CIS Intern. Occ. Safety and Health Info. Center, USA; Institute of Occ. Health and Safety, London, May, 2293.

Delgado, J. M. R., Leal, J., Monteagudo, J. L. and Gracia, M. G. (1982),

'Embryological changes induced by weak, extremely low frequency electromagnetic fields', *J. of Anatomy*, 134(3), 533–51.
Goldberg, D. P. (1972), *The Detection of Psychiatric Illness by Questionnaire*. London: Oxford University Press. (see also: Goldberg, D. (1986), 'Use of the General Health Questionnaire in clinical work', *British Medical Journal*, 293, 1188–9).
Golding, E. (1987), Letter to Simon Best.
Hawkins, L. H. (1981), 'Air ionisation and office health', *Building Services and Environmental Engineer*, April.
Hildyard, N. (1983), *Cover Up*, London: New English Library, 67–97.
Jafary-Asl, A. H., Solanki, S. N., Aarholt, E. and Smith, C. W. (1982), 'Dielectric measurements on live biological materials under magnetic resonance conditions', *J.Biol. Phys. II*, 15–22.
McAuliffe, K. (1985), 'The mind fields', *OMNI*, February, 7(5), 41–4, 96–104.
McDowall, M. E. (1983), 'Leukaemia mortality in electrical workers in England and Wales', *Lancet*, January 29, 246.
Marino, A. A. and Ray, J. (1986), *The Electric Wilderness*, San Francisco: San Francisco Press.
Meda, E., Carrescia, V., and Cappa, S. (1969), Abstr. held at Institute for Occupational Health and Safety, London.
Milham, S. Jr. (1982), 'Mortality from leukaemia in workers exposed to electrical and magnetic fields', *New England J. Med.* 307, 249.
Nordstrom, S., Birke, E., and Gustavsson, L. (1983), 'Reproductive hazards among workers at high voltage substations.' *Bioelectromagnetics*, 4, 91–101.
Perry, F. S., Reichmanis, M., Marino, A. A., and Becker, R. O. (1981) 'Environmental power-frequency magnetic fields and suicide', *Health Physics*, 41, 267–77.
Pethig, R. (1973), 'Electronic conduction in biological systems', *Electronics & Power*, 19, 445–9.
Phillips, R. D. (1986), 'Health effects of ELF fields: research and communications regulation', *Intl. Utilities Symp.*, Toronto, September, 1986.
'Picture Week', *Time-Life* (1985), 23 December.
Popp, F-A., Becker, G., Konig, H. L. and Peschka, W. (1979), *Electromagnetic Bio-information*, Munich: Urban & Schwarzenberg.
Rocard, Y. (1964), 'Actions of a very weak magnetic gradient: the reflex of the dowser', in *Biological Effects of Magnetic Fields*, ed. Barnothy, M. F., New York: Plenum.
Savitz, D. A. (1987), 'Childhood cancer and electromagnetic field exposure', in *Biological Effects of Power Line Fields*, eds Ahlbom, A. *et al.*, New York State Power Lines Project, Scientific Advisory Panel Final Report, July 1.
Science News (1984), 'DNA helix found to oscillate in resonance with microwaves', 125, 21 April, 248.
Seba, D. B. (1987), 'Man and his environment: an unhealthy relationship', *5th. Ann. Intl. Symp. on Man and his Environment in Health and Disease*, Dallas TX, February 26 – March 1.
Seba, D. B. (1988), 'Environmental and health '88: Part I, A chronic cancer;

Part II, Healing the wound'. *6th. Ann. Intl. Symp. on Man and his Environment in Health and Disease*, Dallas TX, February 25–28.

Smith, C. W. and Aarholt, E. (1982), 'Possible effects of environmentally stimulated endogenous opiates', *Health Physics*, 43, 929–30.

Smith, C. W. and Baker, R. D. (1982), 'Comments on the paper "Environmental power-frequency magnetic fields and suicide"', *Health Physics*, 43(3), 439–41.

Smith, C. W., Choy, R. Y. S. and Monro, J. A. (1985), 'Water – friend or foe?', *Laboratory Practice*, 34(10), 29–34.

Smith, C. W., Choy, R. and Monro, Jean A. (1985a), 'Environmental, allergenic and therapeutic effects of electromagnetic fields', presented at 3rd. Ann. Intl. Symp. 'Man and his Environment in Health and Disease', Dallas, Texas.

Smith, C. W., Jafary-Asl, A. H., Choy, R. Y. S and Monro, J. A. (1987) 'The emission of low intensity electromagnetic radiation from multiple allergy patients and other biological systems', *Proc. Intl. Symp. on Photon Emission from Biological Systems, Wroclaw, Poland, January 24–26, 1986*, eds Jezowska-Trzebiatowska, B., Kochel, B., Slawinski, J. and Strek, W., Singapore: World Scientific, 110–126.

Stead, G., Reynolds, R. J., Finzi, N. S., Andrews, C., Lacassagne, A., and Case, J. T. (1956), 'Sixty years of radiology', *Brit. J. Radiol.*, 29, 234–55.

Stewart, A., Webb, J., Giles, D. and Hewitt, D. (1956), 'Preliminary communication: malignant disease in childhood and diagnostic irradiation *in utero*', *Lancet*, 2, 447–55.

Stewart, A., Webb, J. and Hewitt, D. (1958), 'A survey of childhood malignancies', *Brit. Med. J.*, 1, 1495–1508.

Strumza, M. V. (1970), 'Influence sur la santé humaine de la proiximité des conducteurs d'électricité à haute tension', *Archives de Maladies Professionelles de Médecine du Travail et de Securité Sociale*, 31,(b), 269–76.

Swicord, M. L. and Davis, C. C. (1983), *Bioelectromagnetics*, 4(1), 21–42.

Szent-Gyorgyi, A. von (1978), *The Living State and Cancer*. New York: Marcel Dekker.

The Times (1986), Obituary: Walter Stoessel. 12 December.

Tomenius, L. (1982), 'Electrical constructions and 50 Hz magnetic fields at the dwellings of tumour cases (0–18 years) in the county of Stockholm', International Symposium, Prague, 1982.

US Navy (1973), *Project Sanguine*, Report to the White House, Washington, DC.

US Navy (1974), *Project Sanguine*, Report to the White House, Washington, DC.

Waibel, R. (1975), *Der Einfluss niederfrequenter elektrischer Felder auf Lebewesen*, PhD Dissertation, University of Graz, Austria.

Wellenstein, G. (1973), 'The influence of high tension lines on honey bee colonies', *Zeitschrift für Angewandte Entomologie*, 74, 86–94.

Wertheimer, N. and Leeper, E. (1979), 'Electrical wiring configurations and childhood cancer', *Am. J. Epidem.*, 109, 273–84.

Wertheimer, N. and Leeper, E. (1982), 'Adult cancer related to electrical wires near the home', *Int. J. Epidemiol.*, 345–55.

Wever, R. A. (1967), 'Uber die Beeinflussung der circadian Periodik des

Menschen durch schwach elektromagnetische Felder', *Z. vergl. Physiol.*, 56, 111–28.

Wever, R. A. (1973), 'Human circadian rhythms under the influence of weak electric fields and the different aspects of these studies, *Intl. J. Biometeorology, 17(3)*, 227–32.

Wright, W. E., Peters, J. M. and Mack, T. M. (1982), 'Leukaemia in workers exposed to electrical and magnetic fields', *Lancet*, ii, January 29, 1160–1.

Young, L. (1973), *Power over People*, Oxford: OUP.

Young, L. (1974), 'Pollution by electrical transmission', *Bull. of the Atomic Scientists*, December.

Zaret M. M., Cleary, S. F. Pasternack, B., Eisenbud, M. and Schmidt, H. (1963), *A Study of Lenticular Imperfections in the Eyes of a Sample of Microwave Workers and a Control Population*, Final Report RADC-TDR-63-125. Rome Air Development Center: United States Air Force.

Zaret M. M. (1977), 'Potential hazards of hertzian radiation and tumors', *New York State J. Med.*, 77(1), 146–7.

Zaret, M. M. (1988), 'Electromagnetic energy and cataracts', in *Modern Bioelectricity*, ed. Marino, A. A., New York: Marcel Dekker, Ch. 24.

Chapter 9 Chronic electromagnetic field exposure, health risks and safety regulations

Adey, W. R. (1980), 'Frequency and power windowing in tissue interactions with weak electromagnetic fields', *Proc. IEEE.*, 68(1), 119–25.

Adey, W. R., Bawin, F. M. and Lawrence, A. F. (1982), 'Effects of weak, amplitude-modulated fields on calcium efflux from awake cat cerebral cortex', *Bioelectromagnetics*, 3, 295–308.

Ahlbom, A., *et al.* (1987), *Biological Effects of Power Line Fields*. New York State Power Lines Project Scientific Advisory Panel Final Report. New York, NY: NYS Dept of Health, Corning Tower, Empire State Plaza, Albany, NY 12237.

Bawin, S. M. and Adey, W. R. (1976), 'Sensitivity of calcium binding in cerebral tissue to weak environmental electric fields oscillating at low frequency', *Ann. NY Acad. Sci.*, 247, 74.

Becker, R. O. and Marino, A. (1982), *Electromagnetism and Life*. Albany: State University of New York Press.

Becker, R. O. (1986), *The Body Electric*. New York: Morrow.

Bellamy, D., *et al.* (1979), 'Inhibition of the development of Walker 256 carcinoma with a simple metal-plastic implant', *Europ. J. Cancer*, 15, 223–32.

Best, S. T. (1984), 'Laying it on the power line', *Guardian*, October 24.

Best, S. T. (1988), 'The electropollution effect', *J. Alternative & Complementary Med.*, May, pp. 17, 18, 26, 30, 34, 43.

Blackman, C. F., *et al.* (1977), 'Two parameters affecting radiation-induced calcium efflux from tissue', *URSI Symp.*, Airlie, Virginia.

Blackman, C. F., *et al.* (1989), 'Calcium efflux from brain tissue: power density versus internal field intensity dependencies at 50 MHz RF radiation', *Bioelectromagnetics*, 1, 277–83.

Blackman, C. F., et al. (1985), 'Effects of ELF (1–120 Hz and modulated (50 Hz) —RF fields on the efflux of calcium ions from brain tissue in vitro', *Bioelectromagnetics*, 6, 1–11.
Bonnell, J. A. (1979), Letter to Mrs Stella Ross, of Innsworth, Gloucestershire. January 12.
Bonnell, J. A. (1982), 'Effects of electric fields near power-transmission plant', *J. Roy. Soc. Med.*, 75, 933–41.
Bonnell, J. A., et al. (1983), 'Environmental power frequency magnetic fields and suicide – Comment', *Health Physics*, 44(6), 697–8.
Bouchat, J. and Marsol, C. (1967), 'Cataracte capsulaire bilaterale et radar', *Arch. Ophthalmol.* (Paris), 27, 593.
Bowman, J. D., et al. (1988), 'Exposures to extremely low frequency electromagnetic fields in occupations with elevated leukemia rates', *Appl. Ind. Hygiene*, 3, 189–94.
Braganza, L. F., et al. (1984), 'The superdiamagnetic effect of magnetic fields on one and two component multilamellar liposomes', *Biochemica et Biophysica Acta*, 801, 66–77.
Brennock, M. (1986), 'ESB pylons plan opposed by Bord Failte', *Irish Times*, 5 September.
Broadbent, D. E. and M. et al. (1985), 'Health of workers exposed to electric fields', *Br. J. Ind. Med.*, 42, 75–84.
Brown, H. and Chattopadhyay, S. (1988), 'Electromagnetic field exposure and cancer', *Can. Biochem. Biophys.*, 9, 295–342.
Butrous, G. S., et al. (1982), 'Effects of high-intensity power-frequency electric fields on implanted, modern, multiprogrammable, cardiac pacemakers', *J. Roy. Soc. Med.*, 75, 327–31.
Byus, C. V., Pieper, S. E., and Adey, W. R. (1987), 'The effects of low energy 60 Hz environmental electromagnetic fields upon the growth-related enzyme ornithine decarboxylase', *Carcinogenesis*, 8, 1385–9.
Byus, C. V., Pieper, S. E., and Adey, W. R. (1988), 'Increased ornithine decarboxylase activity in cultured cells exposed to low energy modulated microwave fields and phorebol ester tumor promoters', *Cancer Research*, 48, 4222–6.
Carpenter, R. L. and Donaldson, D. D. (1970), 'Bilateral cataracts following miocrowave diathermy treatments: a case study', *5th Intern. Symp.* International Microwave Power Institute, Scheveningen, The Netherlands.
Cartensen, E. L. (1987), *Biological Effects of Transmission Line Fields*, New York: Elsevier.
CEGB (1988), '£500,000 new magnetic field study', *Press release*. London: CEGB.
CEGB (1988a), *Power Points. Electric and magnetic fields – your questions answered*, (Pamplet). London: CEGB.
Choy, R., Monro, J. A. and Smith, C. W. (1987), 'Electrical sensitivities in allergy patients', *Clin. Ecol.*, 4, 93–102.
Clarke, J. (1983), *Multiple Sclerosis: A New Theory Concerning Cause and Cure*, Sheffield: New Age Science Press.

Coggon, D. et al. (1986), 'A survey of cancer and occupation in young and middle-aged men. II. Non-respiratory cancers', *Br. J. Ind. Med.*, 43, 381–6.

Coleman, M., Bell, J. and Skeet, R. (1983), 'Leukemia incidence in electrical workers', *Lancet*, 1, 982–3.

Coleman, M., Beral, V. (1988), 'A review of epidemiological studies of the health effects of living near or working with electricity generation and transmission equipment', *Intern. J. Epidemiol.*, 17(1), 1–13.

COMARE (1986), *First Report: The Implications of the New Data on the Release from Sellafield in the 1950s for the Conclusions of the Report on the Investigations of the Possible Increased Incidence of Cancer in West Cumbria.* London: HMSO.

COMARE (1988), *Second Report: Investigation of the possible Increased Incidence of Leukemia in Young People near the Dounreay Nuclear Establishment, Caithness, Scotland.* London: HMSO.

Cox, R. (1987), Phone conversation with Simon Best, October 27.

Cook-Mozaffari, P. J. et al. (1987), Cancer Incidence and Mortality in the Vicinity of Nuclear Installations, England and Wales 1959–1980. London: OPCS/HMSO. No 51.

Dixey, R. and Rein, G. (1982), '^{3}H-noradrenaline release potentiated in a clonal nerve cell line by low-intensity pulsed magnetic fields', *Nature*, 296, 253–6.

Dixon, B. (1988), 'Scientifically speaking', *BMJ*, March 26; 296, 940.

Dowson, D., et al. (1988), 'Overhead high voltage cables and recurrent headache and depressions', *The Practitioner*, April 22, 435–6.

Dutta, S. K. and Millis, R. M. (eds) (1986), *Biological Effects of Electropollution: Brain Tumors and Experimental Models*, Philadelphia: Information Ventures Inc.

Environmental Protection Agency (EPA) (1986a), *An Investigation of Microwave and Radiofrequency Radiation Levels in Vernon Township, New Jersey, November 10–16, 1985.* Trenton, NJ: Bureau of Radiation Protection.

EPA (1986b), *The Radiofrequency Radiation Environment: Environmental Exposure Levels and RF Radiation Emitting Sources*, Hankin, N. (ed.), Washington, DC: EPA.

Florig, H. K. (1986), *Population Exposure to Power-Frequency Fields: Concepts, Components and Control.* (PhD thesis). Ann Arbor, MI., Dissertation Information Service, University Microfilms.

Fröhlich, H. (ed.) (1988), *Biological Coherence and Response to External Stimuli*, Heidelberg: Springer.

Fulton, J. P., Cobb, S. and Preble, L. (1980), 'Electrical wiring configurations and childhood leukemia in Rhode Island', *Am. J. Epidemiol.*, 111, 292.

Goodman, N. (1988), 'Medicine and the media', *BMJ*, April 9; 296, 1059.

Goldhaber, G., Polen, M. and Hiatt, R. (1988), 'Risk of miscarriage and birth defects among women who use video display terminals during pregnancy', *Am. J. Ind. Med.*, 13, 695–706.

Hawkins, L. and D'Auria, D. (1987), 'Leukemia risks near nuclear sites', Points. *BMJ*, December 5, 295, 1488.

References

Hicks, N., et al. (1984), 'Childhood cancer and occupational radiation exposure in parents', *Cancer*; 53(8), 1637–43.

Hollows, F. C. and Douglas, J. B. (1984), 'Microwave cataract in radiolinemen and controls', *Lancet*, 2, 406–7.

Industrial Injuries Advisory Council (IIAC) (1987), *Non-Ionising Radiation*. Cm 253, London: HMSO.

Irish Press (1986), 'ESB defends Wicklow scheme', 6 September.

IRPA/INIRC (1988), 'Alleged radiation risks from visual display units', *Health Physics*, 54(2), 231–2.

Leeper, E. (1988), *Possible Inexpensive Modifications of Waterbed Heaters to Reduce AC Magnetic Field Production*, Salina Star Route, Boulder, CO 80302, USA.

Lester, J. R. and Moore, D. F. (1982), 'Cancer incidence and electromagnetic radiation', *J. Bioelectricity*, 1, 59–76.

Lester, J. R. and Moore, D. F. (1982a), 'Cancer mortality and air force bases', *J. Bioelectricity*, 1, 77–82.

Lester, J. R. and Moore, D. F. (1985), 'Reply to "Cancer mortality and air force bases: a re-evaluation"', *J. Bioelectricity*, 4, 129–32.

London Hazards Centre (1987), *VDU Hazards Handbook*, Huws, U. (ed.).

London Hazards Centre (1987a), *Fluorescent Lighting – A Health Hazard Overhead*, London: LHC.

Lin, R. S., et al. (1985), 'Occupational exposure to electromagnetic fields and the occurrence of brain tumors', *J. Occ. Med.*, 27, 413–19.

Lunt, M. J. and Watson, B. W. (1982), 'A system for investigating the in vitro effects of low-frequency pulsed magnetic fields', *Clin. Phys. and Physiol. Measurement*, 3, 221–5.

Macmillan, I. S. (1986), *Electromagnetic Fields, Electric Power and Public Health. A community resource document based on the Victorian experience, 1985–86*. Collingwood Community Health Centre, Collingwood, Victoria 3066, Australia.

Mansfield, P. and Monro, J. (1987), *Chemical Children*, London: Century.

Marino, A. A. (ed.) (1988), *Modern Bioelectricity*. New York: Marcel Dekker.

Marino, A. A. and Ray, J. (1986), *The Electric Wilderness*. San Francisco: San Francisco Press.

Marriott, I. A. and Stuchly, M. A. 1986), 'Health aspects of work with visual display units', *J. Occ. Med.*, 28(9), 833–48.

McAuliffe, K. (1985), 'The mind fields', *Omni*, February, 41 ff.

McDonald, F. (1987), 'Power line fears growing', *Irish Times*, October 10.

McDowall, M. E. (1983), 'Leukemia mortality in electrical workers in England and Wales', *Lancet*, 1, 246.

McManus, T. (1988), *EMFs and HV Transmission Lines*, Dublin: Govt Publ. Sale Office.

Meecham, W. and Shaw, N. (1979), 'Effects of jet noise on mortality rate', *Br. J. Audiology*, 13, 77–90.

Microwave News (1981), February.

Microwave News (1983), September, p. 5.

Microwave News (1985), November/December, p. 1.

Microwave News (1986), January/February, p. 2.
Microwave News (1986), March/April, p. 4.
Microwave News (1986), May/June, p. 3; p. 5; p. 6.
Microwave News (1986), July/August, p. 2; p. 4; p. 8; p. 9.
Microwave News (1986), September/October, p. 5; p. 14.
Microwave News (1986), November/December, p. 4; p. 6; p. 12.
Microwave News (1987), January/February, p. 7.
Microwave News (1987), March/April, p. 7; p. 9.
Microwave News (1987), July/August, p. 1; p. 6; p. 11.
Microwave News (1987), November/December, p. 10.
Microwave News (1988), March/April, p. 9.
Microwave News (1988) May/June, p. 3.
Microwave News (1988), July/August, p. 9.
Microwave News (1988), September/October, p. 1; p. 7.
Milham, S. (1982), 'Mortality from leukemia in workers exposed to electrical and magnetic fields', *New Engl. J. Med.*, 307, 249.
Milham, S. (1985), 'Silent keys: leukemia mortality in amateur radio operators', *Lancet*, 6 April, 812.
Milham, S. (1988), 'Increased mortality in amateur radio operators due to lymphatic and hematopoietic malignancies', *Am. J. Epidemiol.*, 127(1), 50–4.
Mirakian, R. *et al.* (1986), 'Protracted diarrhoea of infancy: evidence in support of an autoimmune variant', *BMJ*, 293, 1132–6.
Myers, A. *et al.* (1985), 'Overhead powerlines and childhood cancer', in *Proc. Intern. Conf. on Electric and Magnetic Fields in Medicine and Biology, London, December, 1985*. London IEE Conf. Publ. no. 257, 126–30.
New Scientist (1988), 'ECC wants safer screens', 9 June, 37.
Nordenström, B. (1983), *Biologically Closed Electric Circuits; Clinical, experimental, and theoretical evidence for an additional circulatory system*. Stockholm: Nordic Medical.
Nordenström, B. (1984), 'Biologically closed electric circuits: activation of vascular, interstitial, closed, electric circuits for treatment of inoperable cancers', *J. Bioelectricity*, 3(162), 137–53.
Norris, W. T. *et al.* (1985), 'People in alternating electric and magnetic fields near electric power equipment', *Electronics and Power*, February, 137–41.
NCRP (1986), *Biological Effects and Exposure Criteria for Radiofrequency Electromagnetic Fields*, (No. 86), Bethesda, MD: NCRP Publications.
NRC (1986), *Non-Thermal Effects of Non-Ionizing Radiation*. Washington, DC: National Research Council.
NRPB (1986), *Advice on the Protection of Workers and Members of the Public from the Possible Hazards of Electric and Magnetic Fields with Frequencies below 300 GHz. A Consultative Document*. May. Didcot, Oxon: NRPB. Final Document, 1989. ISBN 0–859–51–314–9. London: HMSO.
NRPB (1987), *Corporate Plan 1987/88 to 1990/91*. Didcot, Oxon: NRPB.
NRPB (1989), Radiation Exposure in the UK Population. 1988 Review. London: HMSO.
Olsen, R. G. (1985), 'The magnetic field environment of electric power lines',

in *Panel Session on Biological Effects of Power Frequency Electric and Magnetic Fields*, Feero, W. E. (ed.), Piscataway, NJ: IEEE.

Paz, J. et al. (1987), 'Potential ocular damage from microwave exposure during electrosurgery: dosimetric survey', *J. Occ. Med.*, 29(7), 581–3.

Pearce, N. E. et al. (1985), 'Leukemia in electrical workers in New Zealand', *Lancet*, 6 April, 811–12.

Pearce, N. E. (1988), 'Leukemia in electrical workers: a correction', *Lancet*, 2 July, 48.

Perry, F. S.et al. (1981), 'Environmental power-frequency magnetic fields and suicide', *Health Physics*, 41, 267–77.

Perry, F. S. and Pearl, L. (1988), 'Health effects of ELF fields and illness in multistorey blocks', *Public Health*, 102, 11–18.

Phillips, J. L. et al. (1986a), 'In vitro exposure to electromagnetic fields: changes in tumor cell properties', *Intern. J. Rad. Biol.*, 49, 463–9.

Phillips, J. L. et al. (1986), 'Transferrin binding to two human colon carcinoma cell lines: characterization and effect of 60 Hz fields', *Cancer Research*, 46, 239–44.

Pienaar, J. (1988), 'Labour claim on electricity dismissed by Parkinson', *Independent*, March 29.

Polk, C. and Postow, E. (1986), *CRC Handbook of Biological Effects of Electromagnetic Fields*. Boca Raton, FL: CRC Press.

Polson, P. and Merritt, J. H. (1985), 'Cancer mortality and air force bases: a reevaluation', *J. Bioelectricity*, 4(1), 121–7.

Prentice, T. (1986), 'Childhood cancer research to check radiation', *Times*, 17 May.

Rea, W. (1987), Lecture at 5th Intern. Symp. on Man and his Environment in Health and Disease, Dallas, TX.

Ross, S. (1987), Private communication to Simon Best.

Sadcikova, M. N. (1974), 'Clinical manifestations of reactions to microwave irradiation in various occupational groups', in *Biologic Effects and Health Hazards of Microwave Radiation*, Warsaw: Polish Medical Publishers.

Salzinger, K. (1987), 'Behavioral effects of ELF', *NYSPLP, Appendix 10*. New York, NY: State of NY Dept of Health, July 1.

Samoilenko, I. I. et al. (1984), Prikl. Biokhim. Mikiobiol. 20(2), 230–44 (English summary).

Savitz, D. A. (1986/7), 'Childhood cancer and electromagnetic field exposure', *NYSPLP, Appendix 15*. New York, NY: State of NY Dept of Health, July 1.

Savitz, D. A. (1988), 'Childhood cancer and electromagnetic field exposure', *Am. J. Epidemiol.*, 128, 21–38.

Savitz, D. A. and Calle, E. E. (1987), 'Leukemia and occupational exposure to electromagnetic fields: review of epidemiological surveys', *J. Occ. Med.*, 29, 47–51.

Sigler, A. T. et al. (1965), 'Radiation exposure in parents of children with Down's syndrome', *John Hopkins Med. J.*, 117, 374–99.

Smith, C. W. (1984), 'Electromagnetic phenomena in living systems', in *Proc. 6th Ann. Conf. IEEE. Eng. in Med. and Biol. Soc., London*, IEEE Publ. No. CH2058-6/84/0000–0176, 176–80.

Smith, C. W. and Baker, R. D. (1982), 'Comments on the paper "Environmental power-frequency magnetic fields and suicide"', *Health Physics*, 43(3), 439–41.

Smith, C. W., Marsh, P. N. and Croft, L. R. (1985), 'Microwaves', University of Salford, *Venture and Enterprise Fund Supplement*, September, 8–9.

Smith, C. W. *et al.* (1986), 'The emission of low-intensity electromagnetic radiation from multiple allergy patients and other biological systems', *Proc. Intern. Symp. on Photon Emission from* Biological Systems, Wroclaw, Poland, January 24–26, 1986.

Smith, N. (1982), 'Claims that ESB lines are "Grave Danger"', *Irish Independent*, 2 November.

Standard Association of Australia (1985), *Maximum Exposure Levels – Radiofrequency Radiation – 300 kHz to 300 GHz*, AS 2772-1985. SAA, PO Box 458, North Sydney 2060, Australia.

Speers, M. *et al.* (1988), 'Occupational exposures and brain cancer mortality: a preliminary study of East Texas residents', *Am. J. Ind. Med.*, 13, 629–38.

Spitz, M. R. and Johnson, C. C. (1985), 'Neuroblastoma and paternal occupation in electric and electronic industries', in *Biological Effects of Electropollution: Brain Tumors and Experimental Models*, Dutta, S. K. and Millis, R. M. (eds), Philadelphia, PA: Information Ventures Inc.

Stern, F. B. *et al.* (1986), 'A case-control study of leukemia at a naval nuclear shipyard', *Am. J. Epidemiol.*, 123, 980–92.

Stewart, A. *et al.* (1956), 'Preliminary communication: malignant disease in childhood and diagnostic irradiation in utero', *Lancet*, 2, 447.

Stevens, R. G. (1987), 'Epidemiological studies of cancer and residential exposure to EMFs', *NYSPLP, Appendix 16*. New York, NY: State of NY Dept of Health, July 1.

Stevens, R. G. (1987a), 'Electric power use and breast cancer: a hypothesis', *Am. J. Epidemiol.*, 125(4), 556–61.

Swerdlow, A. J. (1983), 'Epidemiology of eye cancer in adults in England and Wales, 1962–1977', *Am. J. Epidemiol.*, 118, 294–300.

Sykes, J. M. (1988), *Sick Building Syndrome: A Review*, Bootle, Health and Safety Executive.

Tell, R. and O'Brien, P. J. (1977), *An Investigation of Broadcast Radiation Intensities at Mount Wilson, California*, ORP/EAD-77-2. Las Vegas, Nevada: EPA.

Thatcher, M. (1986), Letter to Mrs Elizabeth Scott, February 24.

Tomenius, L. (1986), '50 Hz electromagnetic environment and the incidence of childhood tumours in Stockholm county', *Bioelectromagnetics*, 7, 191–207.

Tornquist, S. *et al.* (1986), 'Cancer in the electric power industry', *Br. J. Ind. Med.*, 43, 212–13.

Trevithick, J. *et al.* (1985), 'In vitro studies of microwave-induced cataract: reciprocity between exposure duration and dose rate for pulsed microwaves', *Experimental Eye Research*, 40, 1–13.

Tumanyan, M. A. and Samoilenko, I. I. (1983), *Radiobiology*, 23, 415–19.

VDT News (1988), July/August, p. 1.

Walsh, C. (1985) 'In the paths of the pylons' march', *Irish Times*, 31 August.
Watson, B. (1986), *Medical Electronics and Physics at Bart's, 1964–1986*. London: Dept of Med. Electronics, St Bartholomew's Hospital.
Wertheimer, N. and Leeper, E. (1979), 'Electrical wiring configuration and childhood cancer', *Am. J. Epidemiol.*, 109, 273–84.
Wertheimer, N. and Leeper, E. (1980), Reply to Fulton *et al.* (1980). *Am. J. Epidemiol.*, 111(4), 461–2.
Wertheimer, N. and Leeper, E. (1982), 'Adult cancer related to electrical wires near the home', *Intern. J. Epidemiol.*, 11(4), 345–55.
Wertheimer, N. and Leeper, E. (1986), 'Possible effects of electric blankets and heated waterbeds on fetal development', *Bioelectromagnetics*, 7, 13–22.
Wertheimer, N. and Leeper, E. (1987), 'Magnetic field exposure related to cancer subtypes', *Ann. NY. Acad. Sci.*, 502, 43–54.
Wertheimer, N. and Leeper, E. (1988), *Microwave News*, January/February.
Wertheimer, N. and Leeper, E. (1988a), 'Some supplementary analyses of data from the Two Epidemiological Studies in the New York Power Lines Project, March 31. Dept of Preventive Medicine and Biometrics, University of Colorado Medical Center, Denver, Colorado 80262, USA.
Wertheimer, N. and Leeper, E. (1989), *Am. J. Epidemiol.*, 120, 18–25.
WHO (1982), *Non-Ionizing Radiation Protection*. Suess, M. J. (ed.), WHO Regional Publ. European Series No. 10, Geneva: WHO.
WHO (1984), *Extremely Low Frequency Fields*. Environmental Health Criteria Series No. 35, Geneva: WHO.
WHO (1987), *Magnetic Fields*. EHC Series No. 69, Geneva: WHO/IRPA.
Wilson, B. *et al.*, (1988) 'Chronic exposure to ELF fields may induce depression', *Bioelectromagnetics*, 9, 195–205.
Wrixon, A. *et al.* (1988), *Radon*. London: Inst. Environmental Health Officers.
Yousef, G. *et al.* (1988), 'Chronic enterovirus infection in patients with postviral fatigue syndrome', *Lancet*, 1, 146–50.
Zaret, M. (1964), 'An exploratory study of the cataractogenic effects of microwave radiation', *RADC Tech. Doc. Rpt. No. 64–273*.
Zaret, M. (1969), 'Ophthalmic hazards of microwave and laser environments', *Proc. Aero. Med. Assoc. Ann. Meeting*, 29.
Zaret, M. (1973), *Testimony before Senate Committee on Commerce, Science and Transport Hearings on Radiation Control for Safety and Health*. Washington: US Senate, No. 93–24, 104.
Zaret, M. (1979), 'Air safety', *NY State J. Med.*, 79, 1964.
Zaret, M. (1980), 'Cataracts following use of cathode ray tube displays', *Proc. Intern. Symp. on Electromanetic Waves and Biology*, Jovey-en-Josas, France.
Zaret, M. (1984), 'Cataracts and visual display units', in *Health Hazards of VDTs?* Pearce, R. G. (ed.), Chicester: Wiley.
Zaret, M. *et al.* (1963), *Final Report: A Study of a Sample of Microwave Workers and a Control Population*. RADC Tech. Doc. Rpt., 63–125.
Zaret, M. and Synder, W. Z. (1977), 'Cataracts and avionic radiations', *Br. J. Ophthalm.*, 61, 380.

Ziff, S. (1984), *Silver Dental Fillings: The Toxic Timebomb*, Santa Fe, NM: Aurora Press; also (UK), Wellingborough: Thorsons, 1985.

Chapter 10   Beware: military at work

Becker, R. O. (1987), Private letter to Dr Louis Slesin, Editor: *Microwave News*, 3 January.

Becker, R. O. and Selden, G. (1985), *The Body Electric*, New York: Morrow.

Beischer, D. E., Grissett, J. D. and Mitchell, R. E. (1973), *Exposure of Man to Magnetic Fields Alternating at Extremely Low Frequency*, 30 July. Bureau of Medicine and Surgery, Project No. MF 51.524.015-0013BEOX, Naval Aerospace Medical Research Laboratory, Pensacola, Florida, USA.

Bertell, R. (1986), 'Personal Testimony re: Greenham Common Peace Camp', Toronto, Canada, 7 July, reproduced in Besly, K. (1986).

Besly, K. (1986), *Microwave/Electromagnetic Pollution: A little known health hazard; A means of control?*, October, Southbourne, Emsworth, Hants: Inlands House.

Best, S. T. (1987), Letter to Sir Russell Johnston, MP, 14 November.

Birge, R. *et al.* (1987), *J. Amer. Chem. Soc.*, 109, 2090–101.

Boffey, P. M. (1976), 'Project Seafarer: Critics attack National Academy's review group', *Science*, 18 June, 192, 1213–4.

Brodeur, P. (1977), *The Zapping of America. Microwaves, Their Deadly Risk and the Cover-up*, New York: Norton.

Brown, P. (1985), 'Highlands to get 30-mile aerial for nuclear submarine control', *Guardian*, 12 March.

Burrows, W. (1987), *Deep Black, The Secrets of Space Espionage*, New York: Bantam.

CAMROC (Campaign Against Military Research On Campus) (1988), *Military Research in London's Universities and Polytechnics*, May, c/o 190 Burdett Road, Bow, London E3.

Central TV (1984), *Opening Pandora's Box*, Part 3 of *The Good, the Bad and the Indefensible*, Channel 4, 8 September.

Chomet, J. (1986), 'Wave of concern', *The Times*, 12 January.

Danielsson, B. and M.-T. (1986), *Poisoned Reign*, London: Penguin.

Dawe, T. (1988), 'Car phone owners given bug warning', *The Times*, 13 February.

Drori, J. (1985), 'Springing a leak in the system', *Guardian*, 28 February.

Electronics Today (1985), '"Electronic weapons being used against us", Greenham women claim', 23 December.

Evans, M. (1987), 'The spies that never sleep', *The Times*, 28 December.

Fox, B. (1988), 'Electronic smog fouls the ether', *New Scientist*, 7 April, 34–8.

Fitzgerald, P. and Leopold, M. (1987), *Stranger on the Line. The Secret History of Phone Tapping*, London: Bodley Head.

Freeman, R. (1988), Letter to Sir Russell Johnston, MP, 27 April.

Graham Smith, F. and Lovell, B. (1987), 'Soviet space aims may be harmful', Letter to the Editor, *The Times*, 20 August.

Grant, E. *et al.* (1987), *Nature*, 9 July, 328, 145–6.

Green, D. (1985), 'Fibre optics move into the office', *The Times*, 2 July.

Grissett, J. D. (1980), 'Biological effects of electric and magnetic fields associated with ELF communications systems', *Proc. IEEE*, January, *68(1)*, 98–104.

Hamblin, T. J. (1987), 'A shocking American report with lessons for us all', *BMJ*, 11 July, *295*, 73.

Hamilton, A. (1987), Reply to Sir Russell Johnston, MP, 5 January.

Hanson, C. (1986), 'The "virus" threat to defence secrets', *The Times*, 12 August.

Hughes, C. (1985), 'Sites explored for improving radio links to submarines', *The Times*, 22 April.

Hyder, K. (1988), 'Government taps 30,000 phone lines', *Observer*, 30 October. See also Sweeney, J. (1989), 'Confessions of a hi-tech eavesdropper', Observer, 2 April.

ITV/Television New Zealand (1987), *Tahiti Witness*, Independent Television, 24 November.

Lacoste, B. (1987), 'Spot, the spy in the sky', *The Times*, 20 October.

Lester, J. R. and Moore, D. F. (1982), 'Cancer mortality and Air Force bases', *J. Bioelectricity*, *1*, 121–7.

Lester, J. R. and Moore, D. F. (1985), 'Reply to "Cancer mortality and Air Force bases: A reevaluation"', *J. Bioelectricity*, *4*, 129–31.

Lowther, W. (1986), 'Here's looking at you, Sid, Elmer, Hans, Ivan, Pierre, Jose, Gino, Bruce, Chang', *Mail on Sunday YOU Magazine*, 9 March.

McAuliffe, K. (1985), 'The mind fields', *OMNI*. February, *7(5)*, 41–4, 96–104.

Manchester City Council Police Monitoring Unit Document (1986), Extracted in Besly, K. (1986), January.

Marino, A. (ed.) (1988), *Modern Bioelectricity*, New York: Marcel Dekker.

Matthews, R. (1988), 'Nuclear war "More likely by accident than design"', *The Times*, 1 June.

Microwave News (1986), January/February, 'Air Force recommends 50 V/m safety level for VLF from GWEN', p. 5.

Microwave News (1986), May/June, 'Gearing up for Star Wars', p. 13; 'Naval EMC: Incompatibility sinks ship', p. 2.

Microwave News (1986), July/August, 'DoD's TEMPEST program badly run. GAO reports', p. 7.

Microwave News (1986), November/December, 'Microwave Weapons', p. 4.

Microwave News (1987), January/February, 'New support for cancer risk from MW/RF exposure', pp. 1, 13; 'Swedish Academy of Engineering: ELF fields may not be risk free...', p. 7; 'ZAP!', p. 5; 'Woodpecker Project', p. 9; 'Will EMPRESS II close down Baltimore harbour?', p. 2; 'EMPRESS II EMI to nuclear power plant and ship electronics', p. 3.

Microwave News (1987), May/June, 'Project ELF', p. 7; 'TEMPEST market strong and growing', p. 11; 'GWEN DEIS', p. 6.

Microwave News (1987), July/August, 'DNA MW absorption contested', p. 5.

Microwave News (1987), September/October, 'Suit seeks more protection against HERO and ESD risks', p. 2; 'Vision, stealth and mechanisms', pp. 1, 15.

Microwave News (1988), March/April, 'Microwaves in Moscow', p. 7.

Microwave News (1988), May/June, 'Burning a hole in the atmosphere', p. 11; 'DoD shuts down EMP simulators', p. 7.

Ministry of Defence (1989), *Guide to the Practical Safety Aspects of the Use of Radio Frequency Energy*. Defence Standard, 05–74. Glasgow.

National Radiological Protection Board (NRPB) (1986), *Advice on the Protection of Workers and Members of the Public from the Possible Hazards of Electric and Magnetic Fields with Frequencies below 300 GHz: A Consultative Document*, May, Chilton, Didcot, Oxfordshire.

New Scientist (1984), 'Radio beams damage electronic components', 30 August, 24.

Norton-Taylor, R. (1985), 'US aerials for station', *Guardian*, 6 March.

Parry, G. (1986), 'Peace women fear electronic zapping at base', *Guardian*, 10 March.

Sainsbury, T. (1987), Letter to Sir Russell Johnston, MP, 30 June.

Schiefelbein, S. (1979), 'The invisible threat. The stifled story of electric waves', *Saturday review* (US journal, now defunct), 15 September, 16–20.

Smith, C. (1986), 'Comments on the Consultative Document: NRPB (1986)', Dept. of Electronic and Electrical Engineering, University of Salford.

Smoker, P. (ed.) (1988), *The Risk of Nuclear War*, Richardson Institute for Peace Studies, Lancaster University.

Szmigielski, S. *et al.* (1988), 'Immunologic and cancer-related aspects of exposure to low-level microwave and radiofrequency fields', in Marino, A. (ed.), *Modern Bioelectricity*, New York: Marcel Dekker, 861–925.

The Times (1986), Obituary, Mr Walter Stoessel, 12 December.

The Times (1988), 'Lecturers worried by secret research projects', 5 April.

Tumanyan, M. A. and Samoilenko, I. I. (1983), 'Influence of alternating magnetic field on the bacteriocidal effect of ionizing radiation', *Radiobiology*, 23(3), 415–19.

US Senate (1979), *Microwave Irradiation of the US Embassy in Moscow*, US Committee on Commerce, Science and Transportation, Washington, DC.

US House of Representatives Subcommittee (1986), *American Nuclear Guinea Pigs: three decades of radiation experiments on US citizens*, Committee on Energy and Commerce, Washington, DC.

Webb, C. (1987), 'Searching out an electronic menace', *The Times*, 7 Feb.

White, M. (1985), 'Russians bug typewriters in US Embassy', *Guardian*, 27 March.

Williams, I. (1985), 'Saving volts from jolts', *Sunday Times*, 12 May.

Williams, P. and Wallace, P. (1989), Unit 731, London: Hodder and Stoughton.

Witherow, J. (1986), 'Loose talk and hi-tech hotlines', *Sunday Times*, 9 March.

Witherow, J. (1987), 'Computer bugs that threaten nuclear war', *Sunday Times*, 10 May.

Wright, P. with Greengrass, P. (1987), *Spycatcher*, New York: Viking Penguin.

Zaret, M. M. and Snyder, W. Z. (1977), 'Cataracts and avionic radiations', *Brit. J. Ophthalmol.*, 61, 380.

Chapter 11 Old wisdom, new understanding

Abell, G., Kurtz, P., Zelen, M. (1983), 'The Abell–Kurtz–Zelen "Mars Effect" experiments: a reappraisal', *Skeptical Inquirer*, 7(3), 77–82.

Aschoff, D. von (1986), 'Geopathische Zonen – physikalische Grundlage der Krebsentstehung', presented at Intl. Cong. Z.D.N. Essen, 19 October 1985. Dusseldorf: Mehr Wisen Buch-Deinst.

Barnothy, M. F. (1964), *Biological Effects of Magnetic Fields*, New York: Plenum. Vol. I.

Barnothy, M. F. (1969), *Biological Effects of Magnetic Fields*, New York: Plenum. Vol II.

Beadon, C. V. (1980), 'Ley lines and black streams – facts and fancies', *J. Brit. Soc. of Dowsers*, 27(189), 242–50.

Best, S. T. (1988), 'What we don't know about Earth radiation', *J. Alternative and Complementary Med.*, November, 17–18 and 30.

Brooker, C. (1983), 'Magnetism and the standing stones', *New Scientist*, 13 January, 105.

Brooker, C. (1988), 'The Earth's magnetic field and its effect on the animal nervous system', in *Energy Medicine around the World*, ed. Srinivasan, T. M., Phoenix, AZ: Gabriel Press, 271–86.

Brown, E. and Behrens, K. (1985), *Your Body's Response*, Dallas, TX: Madison Avenue.

Brügemann Institute for ultra-fine Bio-cybernetics (1984), *Research and Teaching for Therapeutic and Diagnostic Methods in the Ultra-fine Energy Region*. Postfach 1262, Pippinstrasse 10, D-8035 Gauting, W. Germany.

Carlson, S. (1985), 'A double-blind test of astrology', *Nature*, 318, 419–25.

Charpentier, L. (1983), *The Mysteries of Chartres Cathedral*. Trans. Sir R. Fraser, 1st edn 1972. Research Into Lost Knowledge Organisation. Distributor, Thorsons: Wellingborough.

Comité Para (1976), 'Considerations critiques sur une recherche faite par M. M. Gauquelin dans le domaine des influences planétaires', *Nouvelles Brèves*, September, 43, 327–33.

Curry, P. (1982), 'Research on the Mars Effect', *Zetetic Scholar*, 9, 34–53.

Dean, G. (1977), *Recent Advances in Natal Astrology*, Subiaco, Western Australia: Analogic.

Dean, D. (1986), 'A note on the "healing?" infra-red twin peaks', *J. of the Society for Psychical Research*, 53(805), 456–8.

Evans, M. W. (1984), 'Barrier crossing theory for ultra-fine far infrared structure in the liquid state', *Physica Scripta*, 30, 222–4.

Edwards, G. S. *et al.* (1985), 'Microwave-field-driven acoustic modes in DNA', *Biophys. J.*, 47, 799–807.

Eysenck, H. J. (1975), 'Planets, stars and personality', *New Behaviour*, 246–9.

Eysenck, H. J. (1986), 'A double-blind test of astrology', Letter to the Editor, *Correlation*, 6(1), 15–16.

Eysenck, H. J. (1987), 'The Committee for Objective Research in Astrology', *Astro-Psychological Problems*, 5(1), 4.

References

Eysenck, H. J. and Nias, D. B. (1982), *Astrology: Science or Superstition?*, London: Temple Smith.

Faraday, M. (1855/reprint 1965), *Experimental Researches in Electricity*, London: Taylor and Francis; New York: Dover (reprint).

Fidler, J. Havelock (1983) *Ley Lines, Their Nature and Properties. A Dowser's Investigation*, Wellingborough: Turnstone.

Field, J. W. (1984), 'A Lutheran astrology: Johannes Kepler', *Archive for History of the Exact Sciences*, 31(3), 189–292.

Gauquelin, F. (1982), *The Personality of the Planets*, San Diego, CA: Astro Computing Services.

Gauquelin, M. (1955), *L'Influence des Astres*, Paris: Dauphin (see 1988a).

Gauquelin, M. (1960), *Les Hommes et les Astres*, Paris: Denoel (see 1988b).

Gauquelin, M. (1966), *L'Heredité Planetaire*, Paris: Planète.

Gauquelin, M. (1976), *Cosmic Influences on Human Behaviour*, London: Futura.

Gauquelin, M. (1982), *The Cosmic Clocks*, San Diego, CA: Astra-Computing Services.

Gauquelin, M. (1983), *The Truth about Astrology*, London: J. M. Dent.

Gauquelin, M. (1984), 'Professional and heredity experiments: computer re-analysis and investigations on the same material', *Correlation, J. of Research into Astrology*, 4(1), 8–24. (PO Box 39, North P. D. O., Nottingham NG5 5PD, UK.)

Gauquelin, M. (1986), 'Bibliographical chronology of Michel Gauquelin's planetary hereditary research', Letter to the Editor, *Correlation*, 6(1), 16–17.

Gauquelin, M. (1988a), *Written in the Stars*. Wellingborough: Thorsons.

Gauquelin, M. (1988b), *Planetary Heredity*. Updated trans. of 1966 original. San Diego, CA: Astro Computing Services.

Gauquelin, M. et al. (1979), 'Personality and the positions of the planets at birth', *Brit. J. of Soc. and Clin. Psychol.*, 18, 71–5.

Gauquelin, M. et al. (1981), 'Eysenck's personality analysis and the positions of the planets at birth: a replication on American subjects', *Personality and Individual Differences*, 2, 346–50.

Geller, U. and Playfair, G. L. (1986), *The Geller Effect*, London: Cape.

Genzel, L., Edwards, G. S. and Powell, J. W. (1986), 'Microwave-driven LAM and intrinsic A-tract bending in DNA', *Biopolymers Res. Comm.*

Gordon, R. *Are You Sleeping in a Safe Place?*, London: Dulwich Health Society.

Graves, T. (1978), *Needles of Stone*, London: Turnstone.

Graves, T. (1986), *Needles of Stone Revisited*, Glastonbury: Gothic Image Publications.

Grundler, W. (1985), 'Frequency-dependent biological effects of low intensity microwaves', in *Interactions between Electromagnetic Fields and Cells*, eds Chiabrera, A., Nicolini, C. and Schwan, H. P., NATO ASI Series A, Life Sciences; V.97, New York: Plenum, 459–81.

Hahnemann, S. (1982), *Organon of Medicine*, Los Angeles: Tarcher.

Hodges, H. (1970), *Technology in the Ancient World*, London: Allen Lane, Penguin Press.

Kollerstrom, N. (1984), *Astrochemistry*, Frome: Urania Trust.
Lakhovsky, G. (1939), *The Secret of Life*, trs. Clement, M., London: Heinemann.
Landscheidt, T. (1989), *Sun, Earth, Man: A Mesh of Cosmic Oscillations*, Frome: Urania Trust.
Le Lorrain, SJ. (1693), *Occult Physics or a Treatise on the Divining Rod*, Paris.
Lerner, E. J. (1984), 'Biological effects of electromagnetic fields', *IEEE Spectrum*, 21(5), 57–69.
McGillion, F. (1980), *The Opening Eye*, London: Coventure.
Maddox, J. (1986), 'Physicists about to hi-jack DNA?, *Nature* (London), 324, 6 November, 11.
Newman, Cardinal J. H. (1883), *The Pillar of the Cloud: Lead Kindly Light*, (early editions include: London: Nelson (1887), cited in Oxford Dictionary of Quotations).
Patrovsky, V. (1986) Proc. 6th Intern. Conf. on l'sychotronic Res., Zagreb, Nov. 13–16: 244–5.
Pethig, R. (1973), 'Electronic conduction in biological systems', *Electronics & Power*, 19, 445–9.
Pohl, G. F. von (1987), *Earth Currents: Causative Factor of Cancer and other Diseases*, trans. of 1932 original by Ingrid Lang, Stuttgart: Frech-Verlag.
Pohl, H. A. (1985), 'AC field effects of and by living cells', in *Interactions between Electromagnetic Fields and Cells*, eds Chiabrera, A., Nicolini, C. and Schwan, H. P., NATO ASI Series A, Life Sciences; V.97, New York: Plenum, pp. 437–457.
Popp, F.-A., Becker, G. König, H. L. and Peschka, W. (eds) (1979), *Electromagnetic Bio-information*, Munich: Urban and Schwarzenberg.
Preuss, J. (1978), *Biblical and Talmudic Medicine*, Brooklyn, NY: Hebrew Publ.
Rawlins, D. (1981), 'sTarbaby', *Fate*, October.
Rea, W. J., Schamhart, D. and Smith, C. W. (1986), Seminar (Item C86-26 (audio tape), C86-27 (video tape)), World Research Foundation Congress of Bio-energetic Medicine, 15300 Ventura Blvd. Suite 405, Sherman Oaks, CA 91403, USA.
Rochard, Y. (1964), 'Actions of a very weak magnetic gradient: the reflex of the dowser', in *Biological Effects of Magnetic Fields*, ed. Barnothy, M. F., New York: Plenum.
Schwenck, T. (1973), 'Experiment at the laboratory of the Swiss Weleda Company', in *The Secrets of Metals*, Pelikan, W., New York: Anthroposophical Press.
Searle, S. (1974), 'The Church points the way', *New Scientist*, 3 January, 10–13.
Seymour, P. A. H. (1986), *Cosmic Magnetism*, Bristol: Adam Hilger.
Seymour, P. A. H. (1988), *Astrology: The Evidence of Science*, Luton: Lennard Publishing.
Slawinska, D. and Slawinski, J. (1986), 'Biophoton emission from cucumber seedlings perturbed by formaldehyde as a possible indicator of the effectiveness of homoeopathic drugs', in *Bericht an Bonn*, ed. Popp, F.-A., Essen: Verlag fur Ganzheitsmedizin.

Slawinski, J. (1987), 'Electromagnetic radiation and the afterlife', *J. Near Death Studies*, 6(2), 79–94.
Smith, C. W. (1984), 'Electromagnetic phenomena in living biomedical systems', *Proc. 6th Ann. Conf. IEEE in Med. & Biol. Soc.*, IEEE Publ. CH2058, 176–80.
Smith, C. W. (1988), 'Electromagnetic and geomagnetic fields in hypersensitivity, energy medicine and bio-navigation', in *Energy Medicine around the World*, ed. Srinivasan, T. M., Phoenix AZ: Gabriel Press, 219–38.
Smith, C. W., Al-Hashmi, S. A. R., Kushelevsky, A., Slifkin, M. A., Choy, R. Y. S., Monro, J. A., Clulow, E. E. and Hewson, M. J. C. (1986), 'Preliminary investigations into the acceptability of fabrics by allergy patients', *Clinical Ecology*, 4(1), 7–10.
Smith, C. W., Jafary-Asl, A. H., Choy, R. Y. S. and Monro, J. A. (1987), 'The emission of low intensity electromagnetic radiation from multiple allergy patients and other biological systems', *Proc. Intl. Symp. on Photon Emission from Biological Systems, Wroclow, Poland, January 24–26, 1986*, eds Jezowska-Trzebiatowska, B., Kochel, B., Slawinski, J. and Strek, W., Singapore: World Scientific, 110–26.
Stanway, A. (1982), *Alternative Medicine*, Harmondsworth: Penguin.
Stark, F. (1986), 'How strong is the Gauquelin planetary effect really?', *Astro-Psychological Problems*, 4(3), 12–17.
Stark, F. (1987), 'Replication of the "Gauquelin Effect" with ordinary people', *Astro-Psychological Problems*, 5(2), 15–22.
Startup, M. (1984a), 'The validity of astrological theory as applied to personality, with special reference to the angular separation between planets', PhD thesis (Psychology), Goldsmiths' College, London University.
Startup, M. (1984), 'Planets, personality and ordinary people: a reappraisal', *Correlation*, 4(1), 5–7.
Taylor, A. J. P. (1967), *Europe: Grandeur and Decline*, Harmondsworth: Penguin (Pelican).
Tucker, R. D. and Schmitt, O. H. (1978), 'Tests for human perception of 60 Hz moderate strength magnetic fields', *IEEE Trans. BME-25(6)*, 509–18.

Chapter 12 The last frontiers
Burr, H. S. (1972), *Blueprint for Immortality*, London: Neville Spearman.
Debes, J. and Morris, R. (1982), 'Comparison of striving and non-striving instructional sets in a PK study', *J. of Parapsychology*, 46(4), 297–312.
Fidler, J. Havelock (1983), *Ley Lines, Their Nature and Properties. A Dowser's Investigation*, Wellingborough: Turnstone.
Hieronymus, T. G. (1968), *Tracking the astronauts in Apollo 8: A quantitative evaluation of the well-being of the three men through the period from two days before lift off until two days after splash down*. Preliminary Report from Advanced Sciences Research and Development Corporation, Lakemont, Georgia, 30552, USA.
Morris, R. L. (1986), 'PSI and human factors: the role of PSI in human-

equipment interactions', *Proc. Intl. Conf. on Current Trends in PSI Research*, 1984, eds Shapin, B. and Coly, L., Parapsychology Foundation Inc., NY.

O'Keefe, J. and Nadel, L. (1978), *The Hippocampus as a Cognitive Map*, Oxford: Clarendon Press.

Ostrander, S. and Schroeder, L. (1970), *PSI, Psychic Discoveries behind the Iron Curtain*, London: Abacus, Sphere Books.

Pethig, R. (1973), 'Electronic conduction in biological systems', *Electronics & Power, 19*, 445–9.

Popp, F-A., Becker, G., König, H. L. and Peschka, W. (eds) (1979), *Electromagnetic Bio-information*, Munich: Urban and Schwarzenberg.

Puharich, A. (1962), *Beyond Telepathy*, London: Souvenir Press.

Puharich, A. (1986), 'A common scientific allopathic, homeopathic, surgical, herbal and healing form of medical practice based on a new general theory of healing dynamics', *Proc. 6th Intl. Conf. on Psychotronic Research*, Zagreb: Society for Natural Sciences, 204–8.

Shallis, M. (1988), *The Electric Shock Book*, London: Souvenir.

Slawinski, J. (1987), 'Electromagnetic radiation and the afterlife', *J. Near Death Studies, 6(2),* 79–94.

Smith, C. W., Choy, R. Y. S. and Monro, J. A. (1985), 'Water – friend or foe?', *Laboratory Practice, 34(10),* 29–34.

Smith, C. W. (1987), 'Comments on "Electromagnetic radiation and the afterlife"', *J. Near Death Studies, 6(2),* 109–12.

Thomson, Judge G. M. (1985), *Report of the ad hoc Committee on Environmental Hypersensitivity Disorders*, Toronto, Ontario: Provincial Court (Family Divison).

Vonier, Abbot A. (1953), *The Collected Works of Abbot Vonier*, vol. 3, London: Burns Oates.

Conclusion

Davenas, E. *et al.* (1988), *Nature, 333,* 30 June, 816–18.

Benveniste, J. (1988), *Nature,* 28 July, *334,* 291.

Smith, C. W., Jafary-Asl, A. H., Choy, R. Y. S. and Monro, J. A. (1987), 'The emission of low intensity electromagnetic radiation from multiple allergy patients and other biological systems', *Proc. Intl. Symp. on Photon Emission from Biological Systems, Wróclow, Poland, January 24–26, 1986,* eds Jezowska-Trzebiatowska, B., Kochel, B., Slawinski, J. and Strek, W., Singapore: World Scientific, 110–26.

Postscript

Adams, J. (1989), *Aids: The HIV Myth*, London: Macmillan.

Barnothy, M. F. (1964), *Biological Effects of Magnetic Fields*, New York: Plenum.

Benveniste, J. (1988), 'Dr. Jacques Benveniste replies:', *Nature 334,* 291.

Best, S. T. (1988), 'What we don't know about Earth radiation', *J. Alternative & Complementary Medicine*, November, 17–18 and 30.

References

Coghill, R. (1988), 'The real missing link?', *J. Alternative & Complementary Medicine*, October, 19–21.

Coghill, R. (1989), 'An hypothesis of cerebral morphogenetic radiation with implications for morphology and immunology', *Medical Hypotheses*, in press.

Davenas, E. *et al.* (1988), 'Human basophil degranulation triggered by very dilute antiserum against IgE', *Nature* (London), 333, 30 June, 816–18.

Davenas, E., Poitevin, B. and Benveniste, J. (1987), 'Effect on mouse peritoneal macrophages of orally administered very high dilutions of silica', *European J. Pharmacol.*, 135, 313–19.

Del Giudice, E., Preparata, G. and Vitiello, G. (1988), 'Water as a free electric dipole laser', *Phys. Rev. Lett.*, 61, 1085–8.

Fröhlich, H. ed. (1988), *Biological Coherence and Response to External Stimuli*, Heidelberg: Springer-Verlag.

Goubau, G. (1950), 'Surface waves and their application to transmission lines', *J. Appl. Phys.*, 21, 1119–28.

Heim, B. (1980), *Elementarstrukturen der Materie*, vol. 1, Innsbruck: Resch-Verlag.

Heim, B. (1984), *Elementarstrukturen der Materie*, vol. 2, Innsbruck: Resch-Verlag.

Hondors, D. and Debye, P. (1910), 'Elektromagnetische Wellen an dielektrischen Drahten', *Ann. der Phys.*, 32, 465–76.

Hume, E. D. (1947), *Bechamp or Pasteur*, Essex: C. W. Daniel.

Jahn, R. G. and Dunne, B. J. (1987), *Margins of Reality: The Role of Consciousness in the Physical World*, San Diego, New York, London: Harcourt Brace Jovanovich.

Kervran, C. L. (1972), *Biological Transmutations*, (English translation), Crosby: Lockwood.

Ludwig, W. (1988), Seminar Proceedings of the Hans Brügemann Institute, Postfach 1262, D-8035 Gauting, West Germany.

Lynes, B. (1987), *The Cancer Cure that Worked*, Wash., D.C. 200/6: Box 5564.

Maddox, J., Randi, J. and Stewart, W. W. (1988), '"High Dilution" experiments a delusion', *Nature* (London), 334, 287–90.

Malmivuo, J., Lekkala, J., Kontro, P., Suomaa, L. and Vihinen, H. (1987), 'Improvement of the properties of an eddy current magnetic shield with active compensation', *J. Phys. E: Sci. Instrum.*, 20, 151–64.

Marino, A. A. ed. (1988), *Modern Bioelectricity*, New York: Marcel Dekker.

Maxey, E. S. (1975), 'Critical aspects of human versus terrestrial electromagnetic symbiosis', presented at the US National Committee/International Union of Radio Science 1975 Meeting, Boulder CO: October 20–23.

Perry, F. S., Pearl, L. and Binns, R. (1989), 'Power frequency magnetic field; depressive illness and myocardial infarction', *J. Public Health*, May.

Playfair, G. L. (1988), 'The "Wonder Healer" of the Tyrol', *J. of Alternative & Complementary Medicine*, November, 19.

Poitevin, B., Davenas, E. and Benveniste, J. (1988), '*In vitro* immuniological degranulation of human basophils is modulated by lung histamine and *apis mellifica*', *Brit. J. Clin. Pharmacol.*, 25, 439–44.

Popp, F-A. *et al.*, eds (1988), *Electromagnetic Bio-Information*, (2nd edn), Munich: Urban & Schwarzenberg.

Reilly, D. T. (1988), Letter to Nature, *Nature* (London), 28 July, 334, 285.

Reppert, S., Weaver, D. R., Rivkees, S. A. and Stopper, E. G. (1988), 'Putative melatonin receptors in a human biological clock', *Science*, 242, 78.

Save British Science Society, Suite 208 Grosvenor Gardens House, Grosvenor Gardens, London SW1W 0BS.

Times (1988), 'Clash on no-fault medical compensation', September 3, 16.

Whitmer, R. M. (1948), 'Fields in nonmetallic waveguides', *Proc. IRE*, 36, 1105–9.

Wilson, B. W. (1988), 'Chronic exposure to ELF Fields may induce depression', *Bioelectromagnetics*, 9, 195–205.

Wolkowski, Z. W. (1988), *Synergie et Cohérence dans les Systèmes Biologiques*, (Troisième serie, 1985–6), Paris: Université Pierre et Marie Curie.

Glossary

Miller, J. B. (1972), *Food Allergy: Provocative Testing and Injection Therapy*, Springfield (Ill.): C. C. Thomas.

Miller, J. B. (1987), *Relief at Last*, Springfield, Ill: C. C. Thomas.

von Pirquet, C. F. and Schick, B. (1905), *Die Serumkrankheit*, Leipzig, Vienna: Deuticke.

Name index

Aarholt, E.: Fishpond test, 151–2; on *E. coli*, 149; on NMR conditions, 59; on stimulation of endogenous opiates, 3, 86, 145, 156
Abell, G., 253
Abrams, Albert, 122–3
Acheson, Donald, 188, 198
Adams, J., 287
Adderley, E., 37
Adey, Ross: on calcium efflux, 182; on EM bio-effects, 172; on power line hazards, 143–4; on pulse modulation, 228; rejects Graves report, 174; testimony, 165, 171, 207–8
Agricola, 238
Ahlbom, A., 169, 171
Ahmed, Nadir A. G., 52, 153
Aldini, Giovanni, 11
Alexander the Great, 11
Andreev, 106
Andrews, E. A., 41
Arendt, Josephine, 49
Aristotle, 10
Arsonval, Arsène d', 15, 75
Aschoff, D., 16, 94, 245
Ash, Michael, 141
Avogadro, Amedeo, 111
Axelrod, Patricia, 230

Bach, Edward, 108
Bachman, C. H., 41
Bacon, Hiliary: after Fishpond, 160; before Fishpond, 161–2; Fishpond campaign, 4, 6, 127–8, 186, 188; on HV power lines, 148; on occupational exposure, 180; on Texas decision, 173; Smith contact, 86, 149; Smith investigation, 150–3, 164
Baker, R. D., 37, 139, 155, 163, 186
Baker, Robin R., 51
Ballarajan, Dr, 202
Banks, M. J. J., 150, 151
Barker, A. T., 61
Barlow, Philip, 202
Barnothy, Madeleine F., 239, 280
Barr, M. L., 45
Bassett, A., 86
Bawin, S. M., 182
Beadon, C. V., 242
Béchamp, Pierre Jacques Antoine, 289
Beck, M. T., 36
Beck, Robert, 227
Becker, Robert O.: Beischer encounter, 219; New York testimony, 134–5, 138, 171; on bone healing, 61, 75, 86, 135; on electrobiology, 127; on EMF levels, 177; on Greenham, 233; on muscle contractions, 11; on power lines, 168; on psychiatric illness, 41; on Schwan, 215–16; on synergistic effects, 140–1; on Woodpecker, 227–8
Becquerel, Henri, 68, 76
Behrens, Kaye, 102, 118, 122, 240
Beischer, Dietrich, 218–20
Bellamy, D., 203

Bell, B., 41–2
Bell, D. A., 63
Bentwich, Z., 284
Benveniste, Jacques, 100, 112, 271, 282, 283–4
Beral, V., 197
Berger, Hans, 73
Bernal, J. D., 14
Bertell, Rosalie, 233, 235
Besly, Kim, 235
Best, Simon T.: *Guardian* article, 187; Innsworth Inquiry, 137; military chapter, 7; on EMF allergy case, 200; on geopathic stress, 246, 288; Scottish transmitter, 221; Torness Inquiry, 142
Bigg, E. A., 41
Binks, Frank, 202
Birge, Robert, 236–7
Blackman, Carl, 182
Bloch, Felix, 29, 78
Bloembergen, N., 58
Boericke, W., 159
Boffey, P. M., 219
Bohlen, Charles, 214
Bohr, Niels, 28
Boltzmann, Ludwig, 21, 23, 25, 27
Bonnell, John, 138, 145, 147, 186, 187, 190
Bouchat, J., 177
Bowen, E., 37
Bowman, Joseph, 191
Box, W. R., 150
Bracken, Michael, 185
Bradley, D. A., 37
Braganza, L. F., 142, 204
Brahe, Tycho, 12
Braun, Werner von, 218
Brier, G. W., 37
Brillouin, L., 8
Britton, M., 288
Broadbent, D. E., 186, 187
Broadbent, M., 186, 187
Brodeur, Paul, 209, 210, 218–19, 229
Bronowski, J., 21
Brooker, Charles, 47, 241, 245, 255–6
Brown, Edgar, 102, 118, 122, 240
Brown, Frank A., Jr., 37
Brown, H., 206
Brown, P., 221
Brucato and Stephenson, 112
Brügemann Institute, 256

Buchner, Eduard, 54
Bullock, T. H., 65
Bunning, E., 41
Burr, Harold, 38, 264
Burrows, W., 225
Busch, Harvey, 145
Butrous, G. S., 186
Bydder, 78
Byrne, Valentine, 167
Byus, C. V., 172

Calderwood, J. H., 2
Calle, E. E., 180
Callinan, P., 112, 114
Cameron, J. R., 79
Cannon, W. B., 113
Carlson, S., 255
Carlton Lee, 87
Carmody, Paschal, 166
Carpenter, R. L., 177
Cartensen, E. L., 168
Cartwright, R. A., 189
Celan, Eugene, 116
Charpentier, L., 245
Chattopadhyay, S., 206
Chiabrera, A., 34
Chiang Huai, 205
Chinchon, Countess of, 111
Chizhevsky, Aleksandr, 39–40
Chomet, J., 236
Chow, C. S., 37
Choy, R., 200
Clarke, June, 204
Clausius, Rudolf, 21
Clayton, E. B., 79
Clegg, J. S., 68
Coggon, D., 188
Coghill, Roger, 119, 287
Coleman, M., 143, 187
Cole, Philip, 171
Colfox, Sir John and Lady, 202
Collier, R. J., 121
Colligan, 266
Collyer, John, 231
Cook-Mozaffari, P., 199
Cope, F. W., 52
Cox, Hugh, 117
Cox, Robin, 189–90
Cremer-Bartels, G., 49
Cremonese, G., 15
Cunningham, Joseph, 166
Cunningham, J. R., 77

Name index

Curie, Marie, 68, 77
Curie, Pierre, 68, 77
Currie, R., 41
Curry, P., 253
Czerski, Dr, 182

Damadian, Raymond, 228
Danielsson, Bengt, 234
Danilin, V. A., 134
Darras, Jean-Claude, 106
D'Auria, D., 199
Davenas, E., 112, 271, 284
Davis, C. C., 141
Dawe, T., 224
Day, L., 122
Dean, G., 253
Debye, P., 283
Defouw, R. J., 41–2
De La Warr, George, 122–4
Del Blanco, 263
Delgado, Jose, 138, 140
Del Giudice, E., 22, 26, 280–1, 282
Deutsch, S., 77
Dewey, Edward, 40
Dixey, R., 203
Dixon, B., 190
Donaldson, D. D., 177
Donarski, R. J., 121
Douglas, J. B., 177
Downer, J., 41
Dowson, David, 4, 190
Driori, J., 223
Drown, Ruth, 123
Dubrov, Aleksandr, 42, 46–7, 51
Dukes, 17
Dunne, B. J., 283
Dutta, S. K., 168

Edwards, G. S., 250
Egely, G., 106
Einstein, Albert, 27–8, 283
Eley, D. D., 58
Evans, M., 225
Eysenck, Hans, 254–5

Faraday, Michael, 56, 255
Farmer, C. B., 51
Farrow, Stephen, 233
Fidler, J. Havelock, 122, 243, 269
Field, J. W., 251
Fishman, S. N., 70
Fitzgerald, P., 224

Fleming, Alexander, 58
Florig, H. K., 168
Foulds, I. S., 61
Fowler, Norman, 195–6
Frank, 15
Franklin, Benjamin, 9, 12
Freeman, R., 222
Friedman, H., 41
Friedrich, W., 68
Fröhlich, Herbert: influence, 4, 53, 85, 172; on cell division, 58; on dielectrics, 55–6; on quantisation, 29, 273; on superconductivity, 2, 52; on synergistic interactions, 200; physicist's view, 53; predictions, 176; recommended reading, 168, 279
Fulton, J. P., 192

Gabor, D., 15
Galen, 10
Galilei, G., 9
Galvani, Luigi, 11
Gamow, R. I., 65
Gandhi, Om, 226
Ganong, W. F., 49
Gauquelin, Françoise, 252–3
Gauquelin, Michel, 41, 252–5
Geddes, L. A., 11
Geller, Uri, 239
Gendrin, R., 50
Genzel, L., 250
George III, 9
Gerratt, Malcolm, 1
Gilbert, William, 10
Gilling, Dick, 85–6
Goldberg, David, 156–8
Goldhaber, G., 196
Golding, Edward, 152
Goodman, Neville, 194
Gordon, R., 246
Gorter, 58
Goudau, G., 282
Graham Smith, F., 226
Grant, Edward, 236
Graves, H. B., 174
Graves, Tom, 241–3, 244
Green, J. H., 69
Grissett, James, 220
Grundler, W., 58
Gulyayev, Yuri, 39
Gurwitsch, Aleksandr Gavrilovich, 15

Gutfreund, H., 115
Guy, Bill, 76, 204

Hahnemann, Samuel, 6, 67, 111
Haldane, J., 115
Hamblin, T. J., 234
Hamilton, Archie, 221
Hanson, C., 231
Harris, J. F., 65
Hawkins, Leslie H., 4, 120, 136, 199, 204
Hayashi, Hidemitsu, 100
Heim, Burkhard, 283
Heisenberg, Werner, 26
Hell, Fr., SJ, 12, 238
Hertz, Heinrich Rudolf, 68
Hewitt, Roger, 152
Hiatt, R., 196
Hickey, Ted, 165–6
Hicks, N., 185
Hieronymus, T. G., 262
Hildyard, N., 148
Hill, D., 72
Hill, S., 35
Hippocrates, 119
His, Wilhelm, 70
Hochenegg, Leonhard, 284
Hodges, H., 105, 248
Hoff, H. E., 11
Hollows, F. C., 177
Hondors, D., 283
Hughes, C., 221
Humboldt, Friedrich Wilhelm von, 11
Hume, E. D., 289
Hyder, K., 224
Hyland, G. J., 2

Illingworth, Cynthia, 61

Jacobi, E., 49
Jacobson, Cecil, 212
Jaffary-Asl, A. H., 59, 154, 200
Jaffe, L. F., 62
Jahn, Robert, 283
Jhon, Mu Shik, 100
Johns, H. E., 77
Johnson, C. C., 185
Johnston, Russell, 221, 222
Jones, David, 220
Jones, D. S., 51
Jussal, R. L., 112–13
Justensen, Don, 204–5

Kauffman, G. B., 36
Kaune, Bill, 173
Keane, Frieda, 166
Keeton, W. T., 45
Kelly, I. W., 41
Kendall, 289
Kenyon, Julian, 39, 83, 105, 106–8, 124
Kepler, Johannes, 12, 251–2
Kervran, L. C., 94, 117, 279, 288
Kidd, P. M., 30, 200
Kirlian, Semyon D. and Valentina Kh., 118–19
Kirschrink, J. L., 51
Klinowska, M., 41
Knipping, P., 68
Kohler, Bodo, 285
Kollerstrom, N., 41, 252
König, H. L., 50
Koslov, Samuel, 166, 212, 215, 216
Kropp, Werner, 285
Krueger, Albert, 132

Lacoste, B., 225
Lakhovsky, Georges, 14–16, 75, 119, 241, 245
Landscheidt, T., 254
Larson, S. L., 81
Laue, Max von, 68
Lauterbur, Paul, 78
Lavoisier, Antoine-Laurent, 12
Laws, Cecil, 132
Lee, John, 221
Leeper, E., 143, 150, 163, 166, 170, 172–3, 179, 183, 185, 186, 192–3, 281
Le Lorrain, Fr., SJ, 238
Leonardo da Vinci, 209
Leopold, M., 224
Lester, J. R., 178–9, 237
Levine, S. A., 30, 200
Liboff, Abraham, 168
Lieber, A. L., 41
Li, K. H., 97
Lilienfeld, Abraham, 214
Lillie, Frank, 128
Lin, R. S., 192
Lippmann, Gabriel Jonas, 69
Lopez, Juan, 111
Loschmidt, Johann Joseph, 111
Louis XVI, 12
Lovell, B., 226
Lowther, W., 225

Name index

Ludwig, Wolfgang, 113, 116, 151, 282
Luette, J. P., 50
Lunt, M. J., 203
Lynes, B., 289

McAuliffe, K., 141, 203, 212
McClelland, David, 265–6
McDonald, F., 167
McDowell, M. E., 143, 186
McManus, T., 168
MacFadden, B. J., 51
McGillion, F., 254
Macmillan, Ian S., 168, 174
Maddock, Brian, 182
Maddox, J., 284
Mallard, John, 78
Malmivuo, J., 289
Mandel, P., 119
Mandino, O., 40
Manners, P. G., 124
Mansfield, Andrew, 78
Mansfield, P., 200
Marconi, Guglielmo, 81
Marino, Andrew A.: interview, 136; New York testimony, 134–5, 138; on Mount Wilson, 177; on muscle contraction, 11; on semiconduction, 127, 135; recommended reading, 168, 279–80; Szmigielski contribution, 217–18
Marriott, I. A., 196
Marsol, C., 177
Matteucci, Carlo, 11
Matthews, R., 231
Maxey, E. S., 281
Mayer-Gross, W., 81
Meda, E., 134
Meecham, W., 179
Melville, David, 4, 142, 204
Merritt, J. H., 179
Mesmer, Antoine, 4, 11–13, 119
Michaelangelo, 209
Michaelis-Menton, 115
Michelson, Albert, Abraham, 19
Michaelson, Solomon, 215
Middendorf, Dr von, 51
Milham, Samuel, 143, 175, 181, 191
Miller, George, 171
Miller, J. B., 87, 88, 112
Millikan, R., 28
Millis, R. M., 168
Mirakian, R., 202

Mishra, R. K., 112
Modan, Baruch, 197
Molyneux, D. H., 63
Monro, Jean: allergen dilutions, 87–8, 98, 274; allergy work, 6, 87, 202–3; Breakspear Hospital, 86; demonstration, 1; electromagnetic sensitivity work, 133, 144, 156, 187, 200; ESP in patients, 264, Rudd case, 201–2; Smith contact, 3; torch observation, 106; tubes, 87, 98
Montaigne, Michel de, 145
Moon, M. J., 100
Moore, D. F., 178–9, 237
Morley, Edward Williams, 19
Morris, Robert, 262
Mott, N. F., 19
Myers, A., 188, 189, 190, 192

Nadel, L., 265
Nagelschmidt, 75
Napoleon Bonaparte, 11
Napoleon III, 54
Narkevitch-Todko, Yakov, 118
Neumann, John von, 72
Nias, D. B., 254
Nordenström, Bjorn, 61–2, 75, 203
Norris, W. T., 187, 188
Northrop, Professor, 38
Norton-Taylor, R., 224
Nunraw, Abbot of, 142–3, 155

Obolensky, A. G., 18
O'Brien, P. J., 177
Oesterline, Fraulein, 12
O'Keefe, J., 265
Oldfield, H., 119
Olsen, R. G., 189
O'Neill, John J., 13
Ostrander, S., 121, 263
Overall, R., 62

Pappas, P. T., 18
Paracelsus, 40, 119
Park, 37
Parkinson, Cecil, 194
Parr, G., 72
Parry, G., 233, 235
Pasteur, Louis, 54, 289
Patrovsky, V., 242
Patterson, Margaret, 81, 86
Paz, Jacob, 191

Pearce, N. E., 175
Pearl, L., 186, 190
Perry, F. Stephen, 4, 138–9, 149, 155, 166, 172, 183, 186, 189, 190, 281, 287
Persinger, M. A., 89, 102
Peters, John, 185
Pethig, Ron, 128, 261, 275
Phillips, Jerry, 145, 171, 172, 174
Phillips, Richard, 138, 171
Piccardi, Giorgio, 36–7, 117
Pienaar, J., 194
Piper, S. E., 172
Pissarro, Camille, 130
Pissarro, Lucien, 130
Pius XI, Pope, 15
Planck, Max, 19, 21
Plante, Michel, 175
Plato, 10
Platts, Gabriel, 238
Playfair, Guy, L., 35, 239, 284
Pohl, G. F. von, 94, 245
Pohl, Herbert, 58–9, 68
Poitevin, B., 284
Polen, M., 196
Polk, C., 168
Polo, Marco, 10
Polson, P., 179
Popp, F.-A., 22, 26, 103, 116, 258, 268, 280
Postow, E., 168
Powell, J. W., 250
Prentice, T., 198
Preparata, G., 280–1
Pressler, Paul, 174
Preuss, J., 246–7, 251
Pringle, John, 9
Prohofsky, E., 250
Puharich, Andrija, 265
Purcell, Edward, 78

Rabi, Isidor, 78
Ravitz, Leonard, 38
Rawlins, D., 253
Ray, J., 138, 168
Rea, William J.: concept of allergy, 6; Dallas work, 86, 98, 156, 200; on EM sensitivity, 85; on environmental care costs, 277; pendulum demonstration, 240; Professorship, 202
Reichenbach, Karl Ludwig, 119
Reich, Wilhelm, 120–1

Reilly, D. T., 112, 284
Rein, G., 203
Reiter, R., 15
Renner, Fr. Frumentius, 242
Riazi, Abbas, 226
Riesch, Hubert, 242
Rife, R., 289
Rocard, Yves, 117, 239–40
Roman, Dr, 197
Romero-Sierra, 263
Röntgen, Wilhelm Conrad, 67–8, 76, 118
Rosen, D., 57
Rosenow, 289
Rose, Steven, 236
Ross, Stella, 140, 147, 186, 190
Roth, N., 17
Rothschild, Lord, 2
Rotton, J., 41
Rounds, H. D., 41
Royds, John, 4, 167
Rudd family, 201–2
Rutherford, E., 68, 77

Sacks, A. D., 113
Sadcikova, M. N., 177
Sagan, Leonard, 171
Sainsbury, Timoth, 222
Salzinger, Kurt, 170
Samoilenko, I. I., 163, 199–200, 227
Sances, A., Jr., 81
Savage, B., 127
Savitz, D. A.: New York testimony, 171; on cancer risk enhancement, 150, 163, 166, 167, 170, 172–3, 183, 185; on leukaemia, 179, 180, 281; on period of risk, 192; re-checked work, 193
Scheele, Carl Wilhelm, 13
Schiefelbein, S., 212, 215–16
Schmitt, O. H., 241
Schroeder, L., 121, 263
Schwan, Herman P., 79, 215–16
Scott, Elizabeth, 203
Searle, S., 242
Seba, D. B., 162
Selden, G., 11, 61, 75, 135, 168, 215, 216, 227–8
Selikoff, Irving, 197
Semm, P., 44
Seymour, Percy, 253–4
Shallis, Michael, 264, 284

Name index

Shaw, N., 179
Shaw, T. M., 57
Sheppard, A. R., 143
Sigler, A. T., 177
Skofronick, J. G., 79, 82
Slawinska, D., 113, 116, 249
Slawinski, J., 113, 116, 249, 268–9
Slesin, Louis, 4, 169, 181, 279
Smith, C. U. M., 54
Smith, Cyril W.: background, 85–6; Benveniste lab visit, 284; cataract study, 176; dowsing lesson, 242; enzyme work, 53; fan-mail, 156; Fishpond involvement, 132, 149, 186, 188; on allergic responses, 63, 88, 133, 200, 222, 248; on biological superconductivity, 52; on biosensors, 42, 65; on dental specimens, 153; on *E.coli*, 142; on effects of magnetic fields, 139, 155, 222, 240; on fabrics, 96; on neutralising frequencies, 98–9; on periodicity, 37; on pineal gland, 45; on proton NMR conditions, 59–60; on radiation emissions, 250–1, 272; on stimulation of endogenous opiates, 3, 144–5, 156; on sweeping magnetic field, 255; on water's 'remembering' structure, 112, 115, 239, 246, 269; safety recommendations, 163
Smith, David, 136–7, 150, 186
Smith, N., 165
Smoker, P., 97, 231
Snyder, W. Z., 177, 213
Soddy, Frederick, 68
Speers, M., 192
Spicer, Jim, 134
Spicer, Michael, 195
Spitz, M. R., 185
Stanway, A., 104, 109, 121, 122
Stark, F., 255
Startup, M., 255
Stead, G., 68
Stefant, R., 50
Stern, F. B., 180
Stevens, Richard G., 186, 193
Stewart, Alice, 129, 198–9
Stewart, Donald, 221
Stillings, D., 17
Stoessel, Walter, 141, 214
Stossel, Thomas, 213
Strong, P., 69, 82

Strumza, M. V., 132
Stuchly, M. A., 196
Sulman, Professor, 120
Sweeney, B. M., 41
Sweeney, J., 322
Swerdlow, A. J., 187
Swicord, Mays L., 141, 236
Sykes, J. M., 204
Symes, R. F., 150
Szent-Gyorgyi, Albert von, 127–8, 135
Szmigielski, Stanislaw, 217–18, 222

Taubes, G., 62, 75
Taylor, A. J. P., 16–17, 97, 241
Tell, R., 177
Tenforde, Tom, 181
Teresa, Mother, 265–6
Tesla, Nikola, 5, 13–14, 75
Thatcher, Margaret, 202–3
Theriault, Gilles, 175
Thompson, Llewellyn, 214
Thomson, G. M., 265
Tomenius, L., 143, 166, 172–3, 185, 187, 192
Tornquist, S., 180
Towne, Joe, 179
Trelles, M., 106
Trevithick, John, 176
Trincher, 51
Tromp, Solco, 40
Tucker, R. D., 241
Tumanyan, M. A., 163, 199, 227

Underwood, Guy, 241

Van Zandt, K., 250
Vernejoul, Professor Dr De, 106
Vesalius, 10
Vitiello, G., 280
Volta, Alessandro, 11
Vonier, Abbot A., 266–7

Wagner, Hildebert, 288
Waibel, R., 150
Wallace, D., 235
Waller, 68
Wallis, P., 235
Walsh, C., 166
Walter, 68
Wareham, Jean, 150, 151
Watkins, Alfred, 241
Watson, Bernard, 142, 203–4

Watterson, J. G., 115
Welkowitz, W., 77
Wellenstein, G., 133
Wertheimer, N., 143, 150, 163, 166, 170, 172–3, 179, 183, 185, 192–3, 281
Wever, Rutger, 47–50, 105, 142
White, David, 174
Whiteman, Winifred, 134
Whitmer, R. M., 283
Williams, I., 232
Wilson, B., 40
Williams, P., 235
Wilson, B. W., 185, 287
Wilson, Harold, 235

Wiseman, A., 39
Witherow, J., 224, 231
Wolkowski, Zbigniew William, 280
Woodbury, M. A., 37
Wright, Peter, 235
Wright, W. E., 143
Wrixon, A., 199

Young, I. R., 78
Young, Louise, 133, 144
Yousef, G., 201

Zaret, Milton, 129, 140, 176–7, 212–13, 237
Ziff, S., 94

Subject index

acupuncture: 105–8; electro-, 81; points, 71, 83, 265; popularity, 104; survival, 128
AIDS, 287
air-conditioning, 131
Alexandria, library of, 128
allergens, 102–3, 200
allergy: concept of, 6, 65, 86–8; electromagnetic, 63–5, 88–9, 200; in Fishpond, *see* Fishpond; in Mesmerism, 13; multiple, 63, 88, 200–1, 273; Tesla's case, 13–14; testing, 87–8, 89–95
Allergy and Environmental Medicine Hospital, 86, 200, 202
alternative medicine, 83–4, 104–5, 256–7
Alzheimer's disease, 78, 166
American National Standards Institute, (ANSI) 181–3, 216
animals: cataracts, 176; communication with, 263; lunar influence, 41; ELF effects, 134, 170, 228; *see also* bees, hens, pigeons
Antarctic, 50
Arctic, 51
astrology, 35, 251–5
astronauts, 47, 262
Australia, 173–5
Avogadro's Number, 99–100, 111

Bach remedies, 108, 110
bacteria, 142, 149, 151, 199, 203, 289
Base Installation Security System, 235
Bedlam Hospital, 40
bees, 45, 133, 139, 146–7
Bible, 7, 246–51, 268, 288
'Big Boy', Project, 213
biofeedback, 108, 110
biological tides, 41
blind people, 109, 265
Boltzmann's Constant, 21
bone fracture healing, 61, 75, 86, 203
bosons, 27
brain: calcium efflux, 182; immune control system, 287; rhythms, 73; structure, 72; theta frequencies, 265, 281; tumours, 180; Woodpecker effect, 227–8
Breakspear Hospital, 86, 200, 202
British Medical Association, 104
British Standards Institute, 82

Canada, 175–6
cancer: bacterium theory, 289; breast, 186; brain, 180; capacitance of tissue, 6; childhood, 170, 172–3, 179, 188, 194, 198–9; Colorado study, 192; EMR effects, 172; European Year of, 289; experiments, 234; eye, 187; Fishpond, 146–7; HV lines, 141, 143, 145, 167; Lakhovsky's plants, 15–16; leukaemia, *see* leukaemia; Moscow, 214–15, 223; Muroroa Atoll, 234; radar effects, 178–9, 217–18; radionics, 122; radiotherapy, 77; risk

cancer (contd)
    enhancement, 150, role of water, 16;
    steady current therapy, 75; tumours,
    see tumours
cardiovascular system, 134
cars, computer controlled, 232–3
cataracts: at Fishpond, 147; infra-red
    study, 198; microwave-induced, 129,
    140, 176–7, 212–13, 237; radar
    technicians, 179; risks denied, 195;
    Smith study, 176
cattle, 142, 144–5
CAT scan, 77
cell(s): array, 269; division, 58, 62, 77;
    membrane, 64–6, 176, 203–4, 206;
    nerve, 60, 62; resonances in, 64;
    shielded cultures, 46; tumour, 174,
    and see tumours; water in, 51–2, 68,
    77
Central Electricity Generating Board
    (CEGB): Fishpond, 132, 135–8,
    142–5, 148, 153; IIAC Report, 196;
    litigation hazards, 195, 206, 276;
    studies, 186–90, 193–4, 198
central heating, 131
Centre for Complementary Health
    Studies, 124–5
cerebral morphogenetic radiation
    (CMR), 287
CFCs, 50–1
Chartres Cathedral, 245
Chernobyl, 31, 227, 278
China, 105–6, 159, 205, 244
chiropractic, 104
circadian rhythms, 47–9, 102
coherence, 22, 25–7, 33, 52, 273, 281–2
colour therapy, 108–10
Committee on the Medical Aspects of
    Radiation in the Environment
    (COMARE), 198
communications, 25, 262
computer networks, 231
Consumer's Association, 104, 110
control systems, 32, 66, 115
cosmic ray activity, 41
cosmobiology, 35
cows, 144–5, 156
Creation, 268, 288
Crown Proceedings (Armed Forces) Act,
    223, 237
curare, 70
cyclic phenomena, 40

death, 268–9, 274
dental fillings, 94
depression, 81, 127, 138–9, 186, 190,
    215
diathermy, 75, 79–80
dielectrics, 55–6
dielectrophoresis, 58–9
dilutions, serial, 99–100, 112, 250,
    282–4
dioxin, 162
dissymmetry, 51
DNA, 26, 77, 141, 142, 236, 263
domestic appliance fields, 173, 185
Dove Project, 124
Down's Syndrome, 177
dowsing: 238–44; allergic responses,
    118; cancer zones, 16; geopathic
    stress, 94; history, 7; radiesthesia,
    122; survival, 128; Tromp's research,
    40
drug addiction, 81
Dudin's Resonator, 76

earthworms, 133
EEC, 125, 197, 199, 276
electrical safety, 81–3, 181–3, 205–8,
    275
electric blankets, 185, 193
electric currents in therapy:
    high-frequency, 75–6; micro, 75, 103;
    pulses, 74–5; steady, 73–4
electric field enhancement, 136–7, 144
electricity, animal, 11
Electric Power Research Institute
    (EPRI), 180, 185
electroacupuncture, 81
electro-anaesthesia, 81
electrocardiography (ECG), 68–70
electrocautery, 80
electro-convulsive therapy, 81
electroencephalography (EEC), 72–3
electrogastrography, 69
electrolysis, 73
electromagnetic: compatibility, 97,
    231–2; dosimeter, 176; emissions,
    100–2, 107, 274; frequencies, 26–7,
    95–6, 127, 181–2; interference
    (EMI), 231–3; pulse (EMP), 229–33;
    term, 8–9
electromyography (EMG), 69, 70–1
electronystagmography, 69
electrophoresis, 62, 73

Subject index

electrophysiology, 73
electro-sleep, 81
electrosurgery, 80
ELF (extremely-low-frequency): effects, 142–4, 148; Fishpond, 132–8; L-field, 38; pineal gland, 42; research, 169; risks, 167, 192–3, 209; Sanguine Project, 218, 220–2; screening, 102, 105; sensitivity, 101; shielding experiments, 46–9; widespread, 129; Woodpecker, 227–8
EMPRESS, 229–30
entropy, 258
enzymes, 53–5, 65, 114, 172
Environmental Medicine Foundation, 202–3
epilepsy, 140, 146, 147
Escherichia coli, 142, 149
extrasensory perception (ESP), 263–6
eyes, 80, 129, 140, 141, 176, 187, 197–8

fabrics, 96–7
feedback, 113–16
fertility, 134, 138, 140
fingertip regeneration, 61
fish, 62, 65, 273
Fishpond, Dorset, 4, 86, 130–48, 149–64, 186–8
fluorescent lighting, 93, 139, 145, 154, 197
fluoroscopy, 77
formaldehyde, 103, 116, 119, 163, 249
free radicals, 30–1, 34, 279
frequencies: effects of, 127; estimating, 101–2; neutralising, 95–6, 97, 99; range of, 26–7
frogs, 61, 62

galvanic skin response (GSR), 71–2
gamma-rays, 77, 78, 199
General Health Questionnaire, 156–9
geomagnetic field (GMF), 41, 42–7, 51, 101, 129
geopathic stress, 94, 242, 244–6, 288
geopathic zones, 16
gravitational force, 18, 41
Greenham Common, 225, 233, 235–6
Greenpeace, 235
growth rate, 134, 138
GWEN, 230–1

Hazards of Electromagnetic Radiation to Ordnance (HERO), 230–1
healing: Biblical, 251; bone fracture, 61, 75, 86, 203; electromedical apparatus, 83–4; electrophysiology, 73; laying on of hands, 110; magnetic, 10–11; Mesmerism, 12
heart, 68–70, 74–5, 145, 219–20
Heim's Theory, 283
Heisenberg Uncertainty Principle, 26
heliobiology, 39
Helmholtz Double-Layer, 107
hens, 138, 141
herbalism, 104, 110–11
high current configuration (HCC), 192
high-rise flats, 189–90, 191
homeostasis, 31–4, 56 113–14
homoeopathy, 6, 98–9, 104, 111–16, 256
hormones, 60
Houston, Texas, 145, 147–8, 162, 173–4, 184, 195, 276
hydropathy, 116–17
hypersensitivity, electromagnetic: demonstration, 1; dowsing, 240; frequencies, 95–6, 99; possibilities, 269; Tesla's case, 5, 13–14; testing, 88, 89–95, 274, 281; treating, 88

Industrial Injuries Advisory Council (IIAC), 195–6, 197
immune system, 218, 266, 287
information, 22, 258–62
infra-red, 39, 60, 109, 198, 226
Innsworth, Gloucestershire, 133, 135–40, 142, 148, 186, 188
insulating materials, 2
interference, electronic, 97
interferential therapy, 127
International Radiological Protection Association (IRPA), 175, 183
ionisation, 119, 131–2, 204, 136
ions, 119–20
Ireland, 165–8
irradiation, ionizing, 234–5

Japanese atrocities, suppression of, 235
jet-lag, 142
Josephson Effect, 52, 66, 273

kinesiology, 117–18
Kirlian photography, 118–19

lasers, 27, 29, 220–1
left/right-handed structures, 51, 285
legislation, 173–85, 205–8, 276–7
Leischmania, parasite, 63
leucocyte count, 134
leukaemia; CEGB study, 189; Moscow embassy, 141, 213–15; occupational, 143, 175, 180–1, 187, 188; risks studies, 193; Savitz study, 170, 172, 179
ley-lines, 141, 241–4
L-field, 38
Librium, 166
lie detectors, 71
light: quantum effects, 28–30; velocity of, 18–19
limb regeneration, 61
loadstone, 10
Loschmidt's Number, 99, 111
luminescence, 106
lunar cycles, *see* moon
Luxembourg Effect, 50, 262
lysozyme, 57, 58, 98

magnetic field: Earth's, *see* geomagnetic; sweeping, 255–6
magnetism, animal, 9, 11–13, 119
magnetite, 51
malaria, 111
Materia Medica, 98, 151, 159
melatonin, 49, 185–6, 287
membranes, biological, 2, 64–6
microscope, 9–10
microwaves: airport study, 179; bio-effects, 129, 236; Chinese birth control studies, 205; diathermy, 79–80; drug potentiation, 166; military uses, 226; Moscow embassy, 210–18; NMR carrier, 59; ocular effects, 176–7, *see also* cataracts; risks, 140–1; safety standards, 174, 275; yeast cell effects, 66
migrations, animal and bird, 20
Miller Technique, 88
Ministry of Defence (MoD), 196, 221–2, 231–4
miscarriages, 166, 185, 193, 197
mitosis, 58
modulation, 33–4, 64
moon, 35, 37, 38, 40–2, 262
Moscow, 76, 141, 210–18, 237
moths, 62

Mount Wilson, 177
multiple sclerosis (MS), 78, 204
Multiple Wave Oscillator, 75
multi-storey buildings, 189–90, 191
Muroroa Atoll, 234–5
muscle contraction, 11, 69, 70–1, 117–18
myalgic encephalomyelitis (ME), 201–2

National Academy of Sciences' National Research Council (NAS-NRC), 169
National Council on Radiation Protection, (NCRP) 182
National Radiological Protection Board, (NRPB), 136, 182–3, 196, 208
naturopathy, 119
navigation, 51
negative ion therapy, 119–20
nerve cells, 60, 62
nerve fibres, 60–1
NeuroElectric Therapy, 81
New York State Power Lines Project (NYSPLP), 3, 86, 156, 169–72, 188, 193, 196
New Zealand, 175, 276
Nightingale Hospital, 86
Non-Ionising Radiation Committee, 208; *see also* radiation
Norway, 50
nuclear magnetic resonance (NMR), 58–60, 78–9, 228
nuclear weapons, 230–1

occupational hazards, 143, 174–83, 185, 186, 191–2, 223
Official Secrets Act, 210, 278
opiates, stimulation of endogenous, 86, 145, 156
orgone therapy, 120–1
oscillations, 21–2, 33, 52, 58, 79
osteopathy, 104, 121
ozone layer, 50–1

pacemakers, 74–5, 186
pain relief, 109–10
Pandora, Project, 212–13
parapsychology, 262–3
pattern therapy, 121
pearl chains, 58–9
pendulum, 118, 122, 240, 243
peripheral nervous system, 134
pesticide, 161–2